THE SUPREME YOGA

Yoga Vāsiṣṭha

The Supreme Yoga

Yoga Vāsiṣṭha

Translated by

SWAMI VENKATESANANDA

Foreword by

SRI SWAMI RANGANATHANANDA

SWAMI MUKTANANDA PARAMAHAṀSA

RT. HON. SIR S. RAMGOOLAM, P.C.

MOTILAL BANARSIDASS PUBLISHERS
PRIVATE LIMITED • DELHI

Reprint: Delhi: 2005, 2006, 2010
Indian First Edition: Delhi, 2003

First Edition: South Africa 1976 in 2 Volumes
Second Edition: Australia 1981 in 1 Volume
Third Edition: Australia, 1984

ISBN: 978-93-90713-48-6 (Cloth)
ISBN: 978-93-90713-49-3 (Paper)

MOTILAL BANARSIDASS
41 U.A. Bungalow Road, Jawahar Nagar, Delhi 110 007
8 Mahalaxmi Chamber, 22 Bhulabhai Desai Road, Mumbai 400 026
203 Royapettah High Road, Mylapore, Chennai 600 004
236, 9th Main III Block, Jayanagar, Bangalore 560 011
Sanas Plaza, 1302 Baji Rao Road, Pune 411 002
8 Camac Street, Kolkata 700 017
Ashok Rajpath, Patna 800 004
Chowk, Varanasi 221 001

Printed in India

By Jainendra Prakash Jain at Shri Jainendra Press,
A-45 Naraina, Phase-I, New Delhi 110 028
and Published by Narendra Prakash Jain for
Motilal Banarsidass Publishers Private Limited,
Bungalow Road, Delhi 110 007

This publication is dedicated to my Gurudev Swami Sivananda. His life was a symphony whose constant refrain was: "In all conditions I am Knowledge-Bliss Absolute." Sage Vasiṣṭha incarnated as Swami Sivananda to embody the supreme yoga. In Gurudev Yoga Vāsiṣṭha was alive.

Venkatesa

ACKNOWLEDGEMENTS

Grateful thanks are offered to Sri Swami Ranganathananda, Swami Muktananda Paramahaṁsa, and the Right Honourable Sir Seewoosagur Ramgoolam for their gracious Foreword.

CONTENTS

CONTENTS

FOREWORD

The book, *The Supreme Yoga,* is a translation into English accompanied by brief expositions, by Swami Venkatesananda of the Divine Life Society, Rishikesh, India, of the well-known Vedanta treatise in Sanskrit, *The Yoga Vāsiṣṭha.*

The Swami has arranged the verses of the book in such a way as to convert them into a rosary of daily thoughts throughout the year, on the lines of his two other books published, namely *The Srimad Bhāgavataṁ* or *Book of God,* and *The Bhagavad Gītā* or *The Song of God.*

The *Yoga Vāsiṣṭha* has been a favourite book of spiritual seekers in India these several centuries. Its special appeal lies in its thoroughly rational approach, and in its presentation of Vedanta as a philosophy which dares, like the *Bhagavad Gītā,* to bridge the gulf between the secular and the sacred, action and contemplation, in human life, through a comprehensive and lofty spirituality. The reader will come across passages such as the verse entry for 31st January, highlighting the importance of reason:

'The remark of even a child is to be accepted, if it is in accordance with reason; but the remark of even Brahmā Himself, the creator of the world, is to be rejected like a piece of straw, if it does not accord with reason.'

It is this philosophy of a comprehensive spirituality, rational and practical, that man in the modern age needs to rescue himself from his stagnation of worldliness and put him on the high road of creative living and fulfilment.

Swami Venkatesananda, who has been working untiringly for decades to spread the life-giving message of Yoga and Vedanta in East and West, has done a great service to spiritual seekers far and wide by bringing out this translation of *The Yoga Vāsiṣṭha* in the wake of his translation of the other two great books.

The Chiltern Yoga Trust of Elgin, South Africa, deserves the silent thanks of readers for publishing these three books of the Swami and helping to broadcast far and wide the life-giving, purifying, and inspiring ideas of Eternal India, *Amar Bharat,* in her Vedanta.

20 December 1975 Swami Ranganathananda

President, Ramakrishna Math, Hyderabad, A.P., India.

BLESSINGS

The *Yoga Vāsiṣṭha* is a unique work of Indian philosophy. It is highly respected for its practical mysticism. The study of this great scripture alone can surely help one to attain to God-consciousness. For aspirants of the highest beatitude, the *Yoga Vāsiṣṭha* is like nectar. It is a storehouse of wisdom. Like the *Amritanubhava* of Śrī Jñāneshwar, the path shown in this work is for those who are highly spiritually evolved, almost to the state of a Siddha. It expounds the highest doctrine with many stories and illustrations. Not only philosophers, but even the modern psychologists and scientists will certainly find in it something related to their own discoveries.

Most of the scriptures were narrated by God to His devotees, but the *Yoga Vāsiṣṭha* was narrated to God Himself. It is the teaching of the sage Vasiṣṭha imparted to Lord Rāma. It contains true understanding about the creation of the world. The philosophy of the *Yoga Vāsiṣṭha* is very similar to that of *Kashmir Shaivism*. Its main teaching is that everything is Consciousness, including the material world, and that the world is as you see it. This is absolutely true. The world is nothing but the play of Consciousness.

Abhinavagupta, the tenth century scholar of *Kashmir Shaivism*, once said, "Shiva, the independent and pure Self that always vibrates in the mind, is the Parashakti that rises as joy in various sense experiences. Then the experience of this outer world appears as its Self. I do not know where this word 'saṁsāra' has come from." This is also the unparalleled philosophy of the *Yoga Vāsiṣṭha*.

In translating this monumental work, Swami Venkatesananda has worked hard to make its philosophy comprehensible to ordinary people. In doing so, he has done a great service to seekers of the Truth. Swamiji is a pure person, full of knowledge and therefore worthy of translating this work of supreme yoga.

Let this book bring true knowledge to its readers.

Swami Muktananda

PRIME MINISTER'S OFFICE
MAURITIUS

FOREWORD

It gives me great pleasure to write a foreword to Swami Venkatesananda's "the Supreme Yoga", a sequel to the first edition.

In this book Swami Venkatesananda has masterfully translated the Yoga Vasistha, the well known Vedanta treatise in Sanskrit so that it is understood not only by scholars but by laymen as well.

As a true diciple of Gurudev Sivananda, Swami Venkatesananda has been tirelessly spreading the life-giving message of the Vedanta and Yoga in both East and West, thus paving the way for a greater understanding of Indian Philosophy.

I am sure that Supreme Yoga spread far and wide the message of love and peace.

S. Ramgoolam

Sir Seewoosagur Ramgoolam.
Prime Minister

5th June, 1981

INTRODUCTION

Scholars speculate about the author of this monumental scripture and such other academic matters: may God bless them with success.

The Yoga Vāsiṣṭha is the greatest help to the spiritual awakening and the direct experience of the Truth. This is certain. If this is what you want, you are welcome to the Yoga Vāsiṣṭha.

The text abounds in repetitions which are, however, not repetitious. If you do not like (or need) repetition, then read just this one verse:

> "This world appearance is a confusion: even
> as the blueness of the sky is an optical
> illusion. I think it is better not to let
> the mind dwell on it, but to ignore it." (I-3/2)

This verse occurs several times in the scripture and it seems to be the very essence of the teaching.

If that is not quite clear to you now, read the scripture. The numerous ways in which this truth is revealed will open your mind.

It is wise to read just one page a day. The teaching is revolutionary.
The biased mind does not readily accept it. After the daily reading, meditate.
Let the message soak through.

II

An oft recurring expression in this scripture is 'kākatālīya' — a crow alights on the cocoanut palm tree and at that very moment a ripe cocoanut falls. The two unrelated events thus seem to be related in time and space, though there is no causal relationship.

Such is life. Such is 'creation'. But the mind caught up in its own trap of logic questions why, invents a 'why' and a 'wherefore' to satisfy itself, conveniently ignoring the inconvenient questions that still haunt an intelligent mind.

Vasiṣṭha demands direct observation of the mind, its motion, its notions, its reasoning, the assumed cause and the projected result, and even the observer, the observed and the observation — and the realisation of their indivisible unity as the infinite consciousness.

That is the uniqueness of this scripture which hence declares itself to be supreme:

"Except through this scripture, one cannot gain what is good, now or at any time. Therefore, for perfect realisation of the supreme truth, one should fervently investigate this scripture alone." (VI.2-103)

It is, however, the teaching that is supreme; not a book nor a sage. Hence, Vasiṣṭha is bold enough to say:

"If, however, one thinks it is not authoritative because it is of human origin, one can resort to the study of any other scripture dealing with self-knowledge and final liberation." (VI.2-175)

Whichever be the scripture taught by whomever, and whichever be the path you choose, stop not till the psychological conditioning ceases entirely. Hence, Vasiṣṭha exhorts the seeker:

"One should study at least a small part of this scripture daily. The beauty of this scripture is that its student is not abandoned to his despair; if something is not clear in the first instance, a further study of the scripture makes it clear." (VI.2-175)

III

A number of friends and publishers have asked for a one-volume version of this great classic. The co-operation of a number of friends, especially Mrs Priya Hart of Israel and Lakshmi of Australia, brought about an 'instant revision'.

In this edition, the extract from the Laghu Yoga Vāsiṣṭha has been omitted. In addition, the second part of the Nirvāṇa Prakaraṇaṁ has also been left out — almost, except for a couple of interesting stories which have been wedged into the first part of the Nirvāṇa Prakaraṇaṁ. The first part seems to conclude the dialogue with the great śakti-pāṭa episode and Rāma's self-absorption. Though the second part contains some gems, in some respects it seems an anti-climax and after-thought. The gems have been retained. In addition to the two stories mentioned above, some other brilliant declarations have been gathered and added to the end of the volume under the heading "Thus Spake Vasiṣṭha". Thus nothing of value has been left out and yet the two volumes of the previous edition have been combined into one!

May God bless you! Dust of Gurudev's Feet

Venkatesa

SCHEME OF TRANSLITERATION

VOWELS: a ā i ī u ū ṛ ṝ ḷ e ai o au ṁ ḥ

CONSONANTS:

gutturals	k kh g gh ṅ
palatals	c ch j jh ñ
cerebrals	ṭ ṭh ḍ ḍh ṇ
dentals	t th d dh n
labials	p ph b bh m
semi-vowels	y r l v
sibilants	s as in sun
	ś palatal sibilant
	ṣ cerebral sibilant — as in shun
aspirate	h

The above scheme does not facilitate the pronunciation of the syllable jña which occurs often in the Yoga Vāsiṣṭha as also in yoga literature (jñāna means knowledge). The j is not really pronounced as j but almost as a g. It is followed by the ñ which partakes of the character of the guttural and the palatal n. Added to all this there is also a suggestion of y before the appropriate vowel completes the syllable.

In this edition, the anglicization of plurals of sanskrit words and their adjectival forms has been abandoned. For plurals the last vowel has been 'elongated' irrespective of the correct grammatical form. We crave the indulgence of scholars.

On top of the page you have, for example:

I 1st JANUARY 1

Here I is the number of the section of the book (there are six such sections) and 1 is the number of the chapter in that section.

One verse from the relevant chapter is given in transliteration. This verse is 'freely' translated and printed in bold type in the body of the story on the same page.

On each page is given a faithful summary of the chapter selected for the day. Every effort has been made not to ignore any important teaching. Only non-essential repetition has been omitted.

OM TAT SAT

Om Namaḥ Śivānandāya
Om Namo Nārāyaṇāya
Om Namo Veṅkaṭeśāya

PRAYER BEFORE THE DAILY READING

yataḥ sarvāṇi bhūtāni pratibhānti sthitāni ca
yatrai 'vo 'paśamaṁ yānti tasmai satyātmane namaḥ (1)

jñātā jñānaṁ tatha jñeyaṁ draṣṭā darśana dṛśyabhūḥ
kartā hetuḥ kriyā yasmāt tasmai jñaptyātmane namaḥ(2)

sphuranti sīkarā yasmād ānandasyā 'ṁbare 'vanau
sarveṣāṁ jīvanaṁ tasmai brahmānandātmane namaḥ (3)

Salutations to that reality in which all the elements and all the animate and inanimate beings shine as if they have an independent existence, and in which they exist for a time and into which they merge.

Salutations to that consciousness which is the source of the apparently distinct threefold divisions of knower, knowledge and known; seer, sight and seen; doer, doing and deed.

Salutations to that bliss absolute (the ocean of bliss) which is the life of all beings whose happiness and unfoldment are derived from the shower of spray from that ocean of bliss.

The Supreme Yoga

ubhābhyām eva pakṣābhyāṁ yathā khe pakṣiṇaḥ gatiḥ
tathai 'va jñāna karmābhyāṁ jāyate paramaṁ padaṁ (7)

SUTĪKṢṆA, the sage, asked the sage Agastya:

O sage, kindly enlighten me on this problem of liberation — which one of the two is conducive to liberation, work or knowledge?

AGASTYA replied:

Verily, **birds are able to fly with their two wings: even so both work and knowledge together lead to the supreme goal of liberation.** Not indeed work alone nor indeed knowledge alone can lead to liberation: but, both of them together form the means to liberation. Listen: I shall narrate to you a legend in answer to your question. There once lived a holy man by name Kāruṇya who was the son of Agniveśya. Having mastered the holy scriptures and understood their purport, the young man became apathetic to life. Seeing this, Agniveśya demanded why Kāruṇya had abandoned the due performance of his daily duties. To which Kāruṇya replied: "Do not the scriptures declare on the one hand that one should fulfil scriptural injunctions till the end of one's life, and on the other that immortality can be realised only by the abandonment of all action? Caught between these two doctrines, what shall I do, O my guru and father?" Having said this, the young man remained silent.

AGNIVEŚYA said:

My son, listen: I shall narrate to you an ancient legend. Duly consider its moral and then do as you please. Once upon a time, a celestial nymph named Suruci was seated on a peak in the Himālayā, when she saw a messenger of Indra the king of gods fly past. Questioned by her, he informed her of his mission which was as follows: "A royal sage by name Ariṣṭanemi entrusted his kingdom to his son and was engaged in breath-taking austerities in Gandhāmadana hill. Seeing this, Indra asked me to approach him with a bevy of nymphs and escort the royal sage to heaven. The royal sage however wanted to know the merits and the demerits of heaven. I replied: In heaven, the best, the middling and the least among pious mortals receive appropriate rewards, and once the fruits of their respective merits have been exhausted they return to the world of mortals. The royal sage refused to accept Indra's invitation to heaven. Indra once again sent me to the royal sage with the request that he should seek the counsel of the sage Vālmiki before turning the offer down."

The royal sage was then introduced to the sage Vālmīki. He asked Vālmīki, "What is the best way to rid oneself of birth and death?" In reply, Vālmiki narrated to him the dialogue between Rāma and Vasiṣṭha.

ahaṁ baddho vimukttaḥ syām iti yasyā 'sti niścayah
nā 'tyantam ajño no taj jñaḥ so 'smiñ chāstre 'dhikāravān (2)

VĀLMĪKI said:

He is qualified to study this scripture (the dialogue between Rāma and Vasiṣṭha) who feels 'I am bound, I should be liberated', who is neither totally ignorant nor enlightened. He who deliberates on the means of liberation propounded in this scripture in the form of stories surely attains liberation from the repetitive history (of birth and death).

I had composed the story of Rāma earlier and I had imparted it to my beloved disciple Bharadvāja. Once when he went to the Mount Meru, Bharadvāja narrated it to Brahmā, the creator. Highly pleased with this, the latter granted a boon to Bharadvāja. Bharadvāja sought a boon that 'all human beings may be freed from unhappiness' and begged of Brahma to find the best way to achieve this.

Brahmā said to Bharadvāja: "Go to the sage Vālmīki and pray to him to continue to narrate the noble story of Rāma in such a way that the listener may be freed from the darkness of nescience." Not content with that, Brahmā accompanied by the sage Bharadvāja arrived at my hermitage.

After receiving due worship at my hands Brahmā said to me: "O sage, your story of Rāma should be the raft with which men will cross the ocean of samsāra (repetitive history). Hence, continue its narration and bring it to a successful completion." Having said this, the Creator instantly disappeared from the scene.

As if puzzled by the abrupt command of Brahmā, I requested the sage Bharadvāja to explain to me what Brahmā had just said. Bharadvāja repeated Brahmā's words: "Brahmā would like you to reveal the story of Rāma in such a manner that it would enable all to go beyond sorrow. I, too, pray to you, O sage: kindly tell me in detail, how Rāma, Lakṣmaṇa and the other brothers freed themselves from sorrow."

I then revealed to Bharadvāja the secret of the liberation of Rāma, Lakṣmaṇa and the other brothers, as also their parents and members of the royal court. And, I said to Bharadvāja: "My son, if you, too, live like them you will also be freed from sorrow here and now."

bhramasya jāgatasyā 'sya jātasyā 'kāśavarṇavat
apunaḥ smaraṇaṁ manye sādho vismaraṇaṁ varaṁ (2)

VĀLMĪKI continued:

This world-appearance is a confusion, even as the blueness of the sky is an optical illusion. I think it is better not to let the mind dwell on it, but to ignore it. Neither freedom from sorrow nor realisation of one's real nature is possible as long as the conviction does not arise in one that the world-appearance is unreal. And this conviction arises when one studies this scripture with diligence. It is then that one arrives at the firm conviction that the objective world is a confusion of the real with the unreal. If one does not thus study this scripture, true knowledge does not arise in him even in millions of years.

Mokṣa or liberation is the total abandonment of all vāsanā or mental conditioning, without the least reserve. Mental conditioning is of two types — the pure and the impure. The impure is the cause of birth; the pure liberates one from birth. The impure is of the nature of nescience and ego-sense; these are the seeds, as it were, for the tree of re-birth. On the other hand, when these seeds are abandoned, the mental conditioning that merely sustains the body, is of a pure nature. Such mental conditioning exists even in those who have been liberated while living: it does not lead to re-birth as it is sustained only by past momentum and not by present motivation.

I shall now narrate to you how Rāma lived an enlightened life of a liberated sage: knowing this you will be freed from all misunderstanding concerning old age and death.

Upon his return from the hermitage of his preceptor, Rāma dwelt in his father's palace sporting in various ways. Desirous of touring the whole country and visiting the holy places of pilgrimage, Rāma sought the presence of his father and asked to be permitted to undertake such a pilgrimage. The king chose an auspicious day for the commencement of this pilgrimage; and on that day, after receiving the affectionate blessings of the elders of the family, Rāma departed.

Rāma toured the whole country from the Himālāya downwards, along with his brothers. He then returned to the capital to the delight of the people of the country.

kopaṁ viṣāda kalanāṁ vitataṁ ca harṣaṁ
nā 'lpena kāraṇavaśena vahanti santaḥ
sargeṇa saṁhṛtijavena vinā jagatyāṁ
bhūtāni bhūpa na mahānti vikāravanti (5/15)

VĀLMĪKI continued:

Upon entering the palace Rāma devoutly bowed to his father, the sage Vasiṣṭha and other elders and holy men. The whole of the city of Ayodhya put on a festive appearance for eight days, to celebrate the return of Rāma from the piligrimage.

For some time Rāma lived in the palace duly performing his daily duties. However, very soon a profound change came over him. He grew thin and emaciated, pale and weak. The king Daśaratha was worried over this sudden and unaccountable change in his beloved son's appearance and behaviour. Whenever he questioned Rāma concerning his health, the latter replied that there was nothing wrong. When Daśaratha asked Rāma, "Beloved son, what is worrying you?" Rāma politely replied, "Nothing, father" and remained silent.

Inevitably Daśaratha turned to the sage Vasiṣṭha for the answers. The sage enigmatically answered: "Surely, there is some reason why Rāma behaves in this manner. **Even as in this world no great changes take place before the coming into being of their cause, viz., the cosmic elements; changes like anger, despondency and joy do not manifest in the behaviour of noble ones without proper cause."** Daśaratha did not wish to probe further.

Soon after this, there arrived at the palace the sage Viśvāmitra of world renown. When the king was informed of the holy visit, he rushed forward to greet him.

DAŚARATHA said:

Welcome, welcome, O holy sage! Your arrival at my humble abode makes me happy. It is as welcome to me as vision to a blind man, rain to parched earth, son to a barren woman, resurrection of a dead man, recovery of lost wealth. O sage, what may I do for you? Pray, whatever be the wish with which you have come to me, consider that wish already fulfilled. You are my worshipful deity. I shall do thy bidding.

kāle kāle pṛthag brahman bhūri vīrya vibhūtayaḥ
bhūteṣv abhyudayaṁ yānti pralīyante ca kālataḥ (8/29)

VĀLMĪKI continued:

Viśvāmitra was delighted to hear Daśaratha's words and proceeded to reveal his mission. He said to the king:

O king, I need your assistance in the fulfilment of a religious rite undertaken by me. Whenever I undertake a religious rite, the demons who are the followers of Khara and Dūṣana invade the holy place and desecrate it. Under the vows of the religious rite, I am unable to curse them.

You can help me. Your son Rāma can easily deal with these demons. And, in return for this help, I shall confer manifold blessings upon him which will bring you unexcelled glory. Do not let your attachment to your son overpower your devotion to duty. In this world the noble ones do not consider any gift beyond their means.

The moment you say yes, that very moment I consider that the demons are dead. For, I know who Rāma is; even so does the sage Vasiṣṭha and the other holy ones in this court. Let there be no procrastination, O king: send Rāma with me without delay.

Hearing this highly unwelcome request, the king remained stunned and silent for a while and then replied: "O sage, Rāma is not even sixteen years old and is, therefore, not qualified to wage a war. He has not even seen a combat, except what goes on in the inner apartment of the palace. Command me to accompany you; command my vast army to accompany you to exterminate the demons. But I cannot part with Rāma. Is it not natural for all living beings to love their young; do not even wise men engage themselves in extraordinary activities for the love of their children; and do not people abandon their happiness, their consorts and wealth rather than their children? No, I cannot part with Rāma.

I have heard of the might demon Rāvana. Is he the one that causes disturbance to your religious rite? In that case, nothing can be done to help you, for I know that even the gods are powerless against him. **Time and again, such powerful beings are born on this earth; and in time they leave the stage of this world.**"

Viśvāmitra was angry. Seeing this, the sage Vasiṣṭha intervened and persuaded the king not to back out on his promise, but to send Rāma with Viśvāmitra. "O king, it is unworthy of you to go back on your promise. A king should be an exemplar of righteous conduct. Rāma is safe in the care of Viśvāmitra, who is extremely powerful and who has numerous invincible missiles."

nirastā 'stho nirāśo 'sau nirīho 'sau nirā 'spadaḥ
na mūḍho na ca muktto 'sau tena tapyāmahe bhṛśaṁ (45)

VĀLMĪKI continued:

In obedience to the wishes of the preceptor Vasiṣṭha, the king Daśaratha ordered an attendant to fetch Rāma. This attendant returned and announced that Rāma would follow in a minute, and added "The prince seems to be dejected and he shuns company". Bewildered by this statement, Daśaratha turned to Rāma's chamberlain and wished to know the facts concerning Rāma's state of mind and health.

The CHAMBERLAIN was visibly distressed and he said:

Lord, since his return from the pilgrimage, a great change has come over the prince. He does not seem to be interested even in bathing and in the worship of the deity. He does not enjoy the company of the people in the inner apartments. He is not interested in jewels and precious stones. Even when offered charming and pleasing objects, he looks at them with sad eyes, uninterested. He spurns the palace dancers, regarding them as tormentors! He goes through the motions of eating, walking, resting, bathing and sitting, like an automaton, like one who is deaf and dumb. Often he mutters to himself "What is the use of wealth and prosperity, what is the use of adversity or of house? All this is unreal." He is silent most of the time and is not amused by entertainment. He relishes only solitude. He is all the time immersed in his own thought. We do not know what has come over our prince, what he contemplates in his mind, nor what he is after. Day by day he gets more and more emaciated.

Again and again, he sings to himself, "Alas, we are dissipating our life in various ways, instead of striving to reach the supreme! People wail aloud that they are suffering and they are destitute, but no one sincerely turns away from the sources of their suffering and destitution." Seeing all this and hearing all this, we, his humble servants, are extremely distressed. We do not know what to do. **He is bereft of hope, he is bereft of desire, he is attached to nothing and he depends on nothing, he is not deluded nor demented, and he is not enlightened either.** At times, however, it looks as if he is overwhelmed by suicidal thoughts spurred by the feelings of despondency: 'What is the use of wealth or of mothers and relations, what is the use of the kingdom, and what is the use of ambition in this world?' Lord, only you can find the appropriate remedy for this condition of the prince.

kiṁ nāme 'daṁ bata sukhaṁ yeyaṁ saṁsārasantatiḥ
jāyate mṛtaye loko mriyate jananāya ca (12/7)

VIŚVĀMITRA said:

If that be the case, may Rāma be requested to come here. His condition is not the result of delusion but is full of wisdom and dispassion, and it points to enlightenment. Bring him here and we shall dispel his despondency.

VĀLMĪKI said:

Thereupon the king urged the chamberlain to invite Rāma to the court. In the meantime Rāma himself got ready to meet his father. Even from a distance he saw and saluted his father and the sages; and they saw that though young, his face shone with the peace of maturity. He bowed to the feet of the king, who embraced him, lifted him up and said to him: "What makes you so sad, my son? Dejection is an open-invitation to a host of miseries." The sages Vasiṣṭha and Viśvāmitra concurred with the king.

RĀMA said:

Holy sir, I shall duly answer your question. I grew up happily in my father's abode; I was instructed by worthy teachers. Recently I went on a pilgrimage. During this period a trend of thought has taken hold of me, robbing me of all hope in this world. My heart begins to question: **what do people call happiness and can it be had in the ever-changing objects of this world? All beings in this world take birth but to die, and they die to be born!** I do not perceive any meaning in all these transient phenomena which are the roots of suffering and sin. Unrelated beings come together; and the mind conjures up a relationship between them. Everything in this world is dependent upon the mind, upon one's mental attitude. On examination, the mind itself appears to be unreal! But, we are bewitched by it. We seem to be running after a mirage in the desert to slake our thirst!

Sir, surely we are not bond slaves sold to a master; yet we live a life of slavery, without any freedom whatever. Ignorant of the truth, we have been aimlessly wandering in this dense forest called the world. What is this world? What comes into being, grows and dies? How does this suffering come to an end? My heart bleeds with sorrow, though I do not shed tears, in deference to the feelings of my friends.

bhāro 'vivekinaḥ śāstraṁ bhāro jñānaṁ ca rāgiṇaḥ
aśāntasya mano bhāro bhāro 'nātmavido vapuḥ (14/13)

RĀMA continued:

Equally useless, O sage, is wealth which deludes the ignorant. Unsteady and fleeting, this wealth gives birth to numerous worries and generates an insatiable craving for more. Wealth is no respecter of persons: both the good and the wicked can become wealthy. However, people are good, compassionate and friendly only till their hearts are hardened by the passionate pursuit of wealth. Wealth taints the heart even of the wise scholar, a hero, a man of gratitude and a dexterous and soft-spoken person. Wealth and happiness do not dwell together. Rare is that wealthy man who does not have rivals and enemies who scandalise him. To the lotus of right action, wealth is the night; to the white-lotus of sorrow, it is the moonlight; to the lamp of clear insight, it is the wind; to the wave of enmity, it is the flood; to the cloud of confusion, it is the favourable wind; to the poison of despondency, it is the aggravating agent. It is like the serpent of evil thoughts and it adds fear to one's distress; it is destructive snow-fall to the creeper of dispassion; it is the night-fall to the owl of evil desires; it is the eclipse of the moon of wisdom; in its presence a person's good nature shrivels. Indeed, wealth seeks him who has already been chosen by death.

Even so is the life-span, O sage. Its duration is like that of a water droplet on a leaf. The life-span is fruitful only to those who have self-knowledge. We may encompass the wind, we may break up space, we may string waves into a garland, but we cannot pin our faith on the life-span. Man vainly seeks to extend his life-span, and thereby he earns more sorrow and extends the period of suffering. Only he lives who strives to gain self-knowledge, which alone is worth gaining in this world, thereby putting an end to future births; others exist here like donkeys. **To the unwise, knowledge of scriptures is a burden; to one who is full of desires, even wisdom is a burden; to one who is restless, his own mind is a burden; and to one who has no self-knowledge, the body (the life-span) is a burden.**

The rat of time gnaws at the life-span without respite. The termite of disease eats (destroys) the very vitals of the living being. Just as a cat intent on catching a rat looks at it with great alertness and readiness, death is ever keeping a watch over this life-span.

cittaṁ kāraṇam arthānāṁ tasmin sati jagat trayaṁ
tasmin kṣīṇe jagat kṣīṇaṁ tac cikitsyaṁ prayatnataḥ (16/25)

RĀMA continued:

Holy sir, I am bewildered and scared when I contemplate the coming into being of the dreadful enemy of wisdom known as egotism. It comes into being in the darkness of ignorance, and flourishes in ignorance. It generates endless sinful tendencies and sinful actions. All suffering surely revolves around egotism (it is the 'I' who suffers); and egotism is the sole cause of mental distress. I feel that egotism is my worst disease! Spreading the net of worldly objects of pleasure, it is this egotism that traps living beings. Indeed, all the terrible calamities in this world are born of egotism. Egotism eclipses self-control, destroys virtue and dissipates equanimity. Giving up the egotistic notion that 'I am Rāma' and giving up all desires, I wish to rest in the self. I realise that whatever I have done with an egoistic notion is vain — non-egotism alone is truth. When I am under the influence of egotism, I am unhappy; when I am free from egotism I am happy. Egotism promotes cravings; without it they perish. It is this egotism alone, without rhyme or reason, that has spread the net of family and social relationships to catch the unwary soul. I think I am free from egotism; yet, I am miserable. Pray, enlighten me.

Bereft of the grace earned through the service of the holy ones, the impure mind-stuff remains restless as the wind. It is dissatisfied with whatever it gets and grows more and more restless by the day. The sieve can never be filled with water; nor can the mind ever reach the state of fulfilment however much of worldly objects one acquires. The mind flits in all directions all the time, but is unable to find happiness anywhere. Unmindful of the possibility of reaping great suffering in hell, the mind seeks pleasure here, but even that it does not get. Like the lion in a cage, the mind is ever restless, having lost its freedom yet not happy with its present state.

Alas, O holy one, I am bound by the knots of craving to the net that has been spread by the mind. Even as the rushing waters of a river uproot the trees on its bank, the restless mind has uprooted my whole being. I am being wafted like a dry leaf in the wind by the mind. It does not let me rest anywhere. **It is this mind alone which is the cause of all objects in the world; the three worlds exist because of the mind-stuff. When the mind vanishes the worlds vanish too.**

bhiṣayaty api dhīraṁ māṁ andhayaty api sekṣaṇaṁ
khedayaty api sānandaṁ tṛṣṇā kṛṣṇeva śarvarī (16)

RĀMA continued:

It is really when the mind-stuff is enveloped by craving that innumerable errors arise in the darkness of ignorance thus caused. This craving dries up the good and noble qualities of the mind and heart, like sweetness and gentleness of disposition, and makes me hard and cruel. In that darkness, craving in its different forms dances like a goblin.

Though I adopt various methods to restrain the craving, the latter overpowers me in a moment and helplessly drives me astray, even as a gale carries away a straw. Whatever hope I entertain of developing dispassion and such other qualities, craving cuts that hope away even as a rat snaps a thread. And I helplessly revolve, caught in the wheel of craving. Like birds caught in a net, we are unable, though we have the wings for it, to fly to our goal or abode of self-knowledge. Nor can this craving be ever appeased, even if I were to quaff nectar. The characteristic of this craving is that it has no direction: it drives me in one direction now and the very next moment it takes me away in another direction, like a mad horse. It spreads in front of us a very wide net of son, friend, wife and other relations.

Though I am a hero, this craving makes me a frightened coward; though I have eyes to see, it makes me blind; though I am full of joy, it makes me miserable; it is like a dreadful goblin. It is this dreadful goblin craving that is responsible for bondage and misfortune; it breaks the heart of man and creates delusion in him. Caught by this Goblin, man is unable to enjoy even the pleasures that are within his reach. Though it appears as if the craving is for happiness, this craving leads neither to happiness nor to fruitfulness in this life; on the contrary, it involves vain effort and leads to every kind of inauspiciousness. Even when it occupies the stage called life on which several happy and unhappy situations play, this craving, like an aged actress, is incapable of performing anything good and noble and suffers defeat and discomfiture at every turn. Yet it does not give up dancing on the stage!

Craving now ascends to the skies, now dives into the depths of the nether world; it is ever restless. For it is based on the emptiness of the mind. In the mind the light of wisdom momentarily shines, but there is delusion the next moment. It is a wonder that sages are able to cut this with the sword of self-knowledge.

baddhāsthā ye śarīreṣu baddhāsthā ye jagatsthitau
tān moha madironmattān dhigdhig astu punaḥ punaḥ (52)

RĀMA continued:

This pitiable body composed of veins, arteries and nerves is also a source of pain. Inert, it appears to be intelligent: one does not know if it is sentient or insentient, and it engenders only delusion. Delighted with a little gratification and distressed by the least adversity, this body is indeed highly despicable.

I can only compare a tree to the body: with branches for arms, trunk for the torso, holes for eyes, fruits for head, leaves for numerous illnesses — it is a resting place for living beings. Who can say that it is one's own? Hope or despair in relation to it is futile. It is but a boat given to one for crossing this ocean of birth-and-death; but one should not regard it as one's self.

This tree which is the body is born in the forest known as saṁsāra (repetitive existence), the restless monkey (mind) plays on it, it is the abode of crickets (worries), it is constantly eaten by the insects (of endless suffering), it shelters the venomous serpent (of craving), and the wild crow (of anger) dwells on it. On it are the flowers (of laughter), its fruits are good and evil, it appears to be animated by the wind (of life-force), it supports the birds (of senses), it is resorted to by the traveller (lust or desire) for it provides the shade of pleasure, the formidable vulture (egotism) is seated on it and it is hollow and empty. It is certainly not meant to promote happiness. Whether it lives for long or falls in a short time, it is still useless. It is composed of flesh and blood; it is subject to old age and death. I am not enamoured of it. It is completely filled with impure substances and afflicted with ignorance. How can it fulfil my hopes?

This body is the home of illness, the field for mental distress and changing emotions and mental states. I am not enamoured of it. What is wealth, what is kingdom, what is the body? All these are mercilessly cut down by time (death). At death this ungrateful body abandons the soul that dwelt in it and protected it — what hope shall I repose in it? Shamelessly it indulges again and again in the same actions! Its only certain purpose seems to be to burn in the end. Unmindful of old age and death that are common to the rich and the poor, it seeks wealth and power. **Shame, shame upon those who are bound to this body, deluded by the wine of ignorance! Shame on those who are bound to this world!**

aśakttir āpadas tṛṣṇā mūkatā mūḍhabuddhitā
gṛdhnutā lolatā dainyaṁ sarvaṁ bālye pravartate (2)

RĀMA said:

Even childhood, the part of life which people ignorantly regard as enjoyable and happy, is full of sorrow, O sage. **Helplessness, mishaps, cravings, inability to express oneself, utter foolishness, playfulness, instability, weakness — all these characterise childhood.** The child is easily offended, easily roused to anger, easily bursts into tears. In fact, one may say boldly that the child's anguish is more terrible than that of a dying person, an aged man, a sick man or any other adult. For in childhood one's state is comparable truly to that of an animal living at the mercy of others.

The child is exposed to the countless happenings around it; they puzzle the child, confuse the child, and arouse in it various phantasies and fears. The child is impressionable and is easily influenced by the wicked: in consequence, the child is subjected to control and punishment by its parents. Childhood seems to be a period of subjection and nothing else!

Though the child may appear to be innocent, the truth is that all sorts of defects, sinful tendencies, and neurotic behaviour lie hidden and dormant in it, even as an owl lies hidden in a dark hole during the day-time. O sage, I pity those people who foolishly imagine that childhood is a happy period.

What can be worse suffering than a restless mind? And, the child's mind is extremely restless. Unless the child gets something new every day, it is unhappy. Crying and weeping seem to be the child's foremost activity. When the child does not get what it wants, it looks as if its heart is broken.

When the child goes to school, it receives punishment in the hands of its teachers; and all this adds to its unhappiness.

When the child cries, its parents, in order to pacify it, promise to give it the world; and from then on the child begins to value the world, to desire the worldly objects. The parents say, "I shall give you the moon for a toy," and the child, believing their words, thinks that it can hold the moon in its hands. Thus are the seeds of delusion sown in the little heart.

Though the child feels heat and cold, it is unable to avoid it — how is it better than a tree, then? Like the animals and birds the child vainly reaches out to get what it wants; and it is fearful of every elder in the house.

udbodhayati doṣālim nikṛntati guṇāvalim
narāṇām yauvanollāso vilāso duṣkṛtaśriyām (29)

RĀMA continued:

Leaving this period of childhood behind, the human being goes on to the stage of youth, but he is unable to leave the unhappiness behind! There he is subjected to numerous mental modifications and he progresses from misery to greater misery, for he abandons wisdom and embraces the terrible goblin known as lust that resides in his heart. His life is full of desire and anxiety. They who have not been robbed of their wisdom in their youth can withstand any onslaught.

I am not enamoured of this transient youth in which shortlived pleasure is quickly followed by long-lasting suffering, and deluded by which man regards the changing to be changeless. What is worse still, it is during youth that one indulges in such actions that bring unhappiness to many others.

Even as a tree is consumed by a forest fire, the youth's heart is consumed by the fire of lust when his beloved leaves him. However much he may strive to develop purity of heart, the youth's heart is stained with impurity. Even when his beloved is not present near him, he is distracted by the thoughts of her beauty. Such a person who is full of cravings is naturally not held in high esteem by good men.

Youth is the abode of diseases and mental distress. It can be compared to a bird whose wings are good and evil acts. Youth is like a sandstorm that disperses and dissipates one's good qualities. **Youth aroses all sorts of evils in the heart and suppresses the good qualities that may exist there; it is thus the promoter of evil.** It gives rise to delusion and attachment. Though youthfulness appears to be very desirable to the body, it is destructive to the mind. In youth, the man is tempted by the mirage of happiness and in its pursuit he falls into the well of sorrow. Hence I am not enamoured of youth.

Alas, even when youth is about to leave the body, the passions that had been aroused by youth burn the more fiercely and bring about one's quick destruction. He who delights in this youth is surely not a man, but an animal in human garb.

They are adorable, they are great souls and they alone are men who are not overcome by the evils of youth and who survive that stage of life without succumbing to its temptations. For, it is easy to cross a great ocean; but to reach the other shore of youth without being overcome bv its likes and dislikes is indeed difficult.

na jitāḥ śatrubhiḥ saṁkhye praviṣṭā ye 'drikotare
te jarā jirṇa rākṣasyā paśyā "śu vijitā mune (22/31)

RĀMA continued:

In his youth, man is a slave of sexual attraction. In the body which is no more than the aggregate of flesh, blood, bone, hair and skin, he perceives beauty and charm. Even if this 'beauty' is permanent, there is some justification to the imagination; but, alas, it does not last very long. On the contrary, very soon the very flesh that contributed to the attractiveness, the charm and the beauty of the beloved is transformed first into the shrivelled ugliness of old age, and later consumed by fire, or by worms, or by vultures. Yet, while it lasts this sexual attraction consumes the heart and the wisdom of the man. By this is the creation maintained; when this attraction ceases, this saṁsāra (birth-death cycle) also ceases.

When the child is dissatisfied with its childhood, youth takes over; when youth is plagued by dissatisfaction and frustration, old age overpowers it — how cruel is life. Even as wind tosses a dew-drop from a leaf, old age destroys the body. Even as a drop of poison when it enters the system soon pervades it, senility soon pervades the entire body and breaks it down and makes it the laughing stock of other people.

Though the old man is unable to satisfy his desires physically, the desires themselves flourish and grow. He begins to ask himself, "Who am I? What should I do?" etc., when it is too late for him to change his life's course, alter his life-style, or make his life more meaningful. With the onset of senility all the distressing symptoms of a physical break-down, like cough, white hairs, hard breathing, dyspepsia and emaciation, manifest themselves.

Perhaps, the deity presiding over death sees the white-roofed head of the old man as salted melon and rushes to take it. As a flood cuts away the roots of trees standing on the river-bank, senility vigorously cuts the root of life. Death follows and carries it away. Senility is like the royal attendant who precedes the king, death.

Ah, how mysterious and how astounding it is! **They who have not been overcome by enemies and who have taken their abode in inaccessible mountain-peaks — even they have been afflicted by the demoness known as senility and degeneracy.**

yuga vatsara kalpākhyaiḥ kiñcit prakaṭatāṁ gataḥ
rūpair alakṣya rūpātmā sarvam ākramya tiṣṭhati (23/7)

RĀMA continued:

All enjoyments in this world are delusion, like the lunatic's enjoyment of the taste of fruits reflected in a mirror. All the hopes of man in this world are consistently destroyed by Time. Time alone, O sage, wears everything out in this world; there is nothing in creation which is beyond its reach. Time alone creates innumerable universes, and in a very short time Time destroys everything.

Time allows a glimpse of itself through its partial manifestation as the year, the age, and the epoch; but its essential nature is hidden. This Time overpowers everything. Time is merciless, inexorable, cruel, greedy and insatiable. Time is the greatest magician, full of deceptive tricks. This Time cannot be analysed; for however much it is divided it still survives indestructible. It has an insatiable appetite for everything — it consumes the smallest insects, the biggest mountains, and even the king of heaven! Even as a young boy plays with a ball for his pastime, Time uses the two balls known as the sun and the moon for its pastime. It is indeed Time alone that appears as the destroyer of the universe (Rudra), the creator of the world (Brahmā), the king of heaven (Indra), the lord of wealth (Kubera), and the nothingness of cosmic dissolution. It is indeed this Time that successively creates and dissolves the universe again and again. Just as even the great and mighty mountain is rooted on earth, this mighty Time is also established in the absolute being (Brahman).

Even though Time creates endless universes, it is not wearied, nor does it rejoice; it does not come, nor does it go; it does not rise, nor does it set.

Time, the gourmet, sees that the objects of this world have been ripened by the fire of the sun, and when he finds them fully ripe he consumes them! Each epoch of time is decked, as it were, by the lovely jewels of colourful beings for the pleasure of Time that wipes them all out playfully.

To the lotus of youthfulness, Time is the nightfall; to the elephant of life-span, Time is the lion. In this world there is nothing, high or low, that Time does not destroy. Even when all these are destroyed, Time is not destroyed. Just as a man after a day's activity rests in sleep, as if in ignorance, even so Time after the cosmic dissolution sleeps or rests with the creation-potential hidden in it. No one really knows what this Time is.

dānavā api dīryante dhruvā 'py adhruva jīvitāḥ
amarā api māryante kaivā ''sthā mādṛśe jane (26/26)

RĀMA continued:

Besides the Time I have just described, there is another Time which is responsible for birth and death; people refer to it as the deity presiding over death.

Yet again there is another aspect of this Time, known as kṛtānta — the end of action, its inevitable result or fruition. This kṛtānta is like a dancer with niyati (the law of nature) for his wife: the two together bestow on all beings the inevitable fruit of their actions. During the course of the existence of the universe, they are indefatigable in their labour, unwinking in their vigilance and unflagging in their zeal.

When Time thus dances in this universe, creating and destroying everything, what hope can we entertain? Kṛtānta holds sway even over those whose faith is firm, and makes them restless. On account of this kṛtānta everything in this world is constantly undergoing change; there is no permanency here.

All beings in this world are tainted with evil; all relationships are bondage; all enjoyments are great diseases; and desire for happiness is only a mirage. One's own senses are one's enemies; the reality has become unreal (unknown); one's own mind has become one's worst enemy. Egotism is the foremost cause for evil; wisdom is weak; all actions lead to unpleasantness; and pleasure is sexually oriented. One's intelligence is governed by egotism, instead of being the other way round. Hence there is no peace nor happiness in one's mind. Youth is fading. Company of holy ones is rare. There is no way out of this suffering. The realisation of truth is not to be seen in anyone. No one is happy at the prosperity and happiness of others, nor is compassion to be found in anyone's heart. People are getting baser and baser by the day. Weakness has overcome strength, cowardice has overpowered courage. Evil company is easily had, good company is hard to come by. I wonder whither Time is driving humanity.

Holy one, this mysterious power that governs this creation **destroys even powerful demons, robs whatever has been considered to be eternal of its permanency, kills even the immortals — is there then any hope for simple folk like me?** This mysterious being seems to dwell in all, and its individualised aspect is regarded as egotism, and there is nothing that is not destroyed by it. The entire universe is under its control; its will alone prevails here.

taranti mātaṅga ghaṭā taraṅgaṁ raṇāmbudhiṁ ye mayi te na śūrāḥ
śūrāsta eve manasastaraṅgaṁ dehe 'ndriyāmbodhim imaṁ taranti (9)

RĀMA continued:

O sage, thus neither in childhood nor in youth nor in old age does one enjoy any happiness. None of the objects in this world is meant to give happiness to anyone. The mind vainly seeks to find such happiness in the objects of this world. Only he is happy who is free from egotism and who is not swayed by craving for sense-pleasure: but such a person is extremely rare in this world. Indeed, **I do not regard him as a hero who is able to battle successfully against a mighty army; only him I consider a hero who is able to cross the ocean known as the mind and the senses.**

I do not regard that as a 'gain' which is soon lost: only that is a gain which is not lost — and there is no such gain available to man in this world, however hard he may struggle. On the other hand, both fleeting gains and temporary adversities come to a man even without his seeking. I am puzzled, holy sir, that a man roams here and there seemingly busy throughout the day and is all the time engaged in selfish activity, and though he does not do one good turn during the day, he is still able to sleep at night!

Yet, even though the busy man overcomes all his earthly enemies and surrounds himself with wealth and luxury, and even when he boasts that he is happy, death creeps in upon him. How it finds him, only God knows.

In ignorance, man binds himself to wife, son and friends; he knows not that this world is like a large pilgrim centre where countless people come together fortuitously — and they whom he calls his wife, son and friends are among them.

This world is like a potter's wheel: the wheel looks as if it stands still though it revolves at a terrific speed — even so to the deluded person this world appears to be stable even though in fact it is constantly changing. This world is like a poison tree: one who comes into contact with it is knocked unconscious and stupified. All points of view in this world are tainted; all countries in the world are territories of evil; all the people of the world are subject to death; all actions are deceitful.

Many aeons have come and gone; they are but moments in time — for there is essentially no difference between an epoch and a moment, both being measures of time. From the viewpoint of the gods even an epoch is but a moment. Even so the whole earth is but a modification of the earth-element! How futile to pin our faith and our hope on it!

iti me doṣadāvāgni dagdhe mahati cetasi
prasphuranti na bhogāśā mṛgatṛṣṇā sarahsv iva (29/1)

RĀMA continued:

O holy one! Whatever appears to be permanent or transient in this world — it is all like a dream. What is a crater today was a mountain before, what is a mountain today becomes a hole in the earth in a short while, what is a dense forest today is soon transformed into a big city, what is fertile soil now becomes arid desert. Similar is the change in one's body and in one's life-style and fortune.

This life-and-death cycle appears to be a skilful dancer whose skirt is made up of living souls, and her dancing gestures consist of lifting the souls up to heaven, hurling them down in hell, or bringing them back to this earth. All the mighty deeds, even the great religious rites that people perform here, are soon consigned to one's memory. Human beings are born as animals and vice versa; gods lose their divinity — what is unchanging here? I see even the creator Brahmā, the protector Viṣṇu, the redeemer Rudra and others inexorably going towards destruction. In this world sense-objects appear to be pleasant to one only till he remembers his inevitable destruction. Just as a child playing with earth makes different designs with a clod, the ordainer of the universe keeps creating new things and destroying them soon.

This perception of the defects of the world has destroyed the undesirable tendencies in my mind; and therefore desire for sense-pleasure does not arise in my mind, even as a mirage does not appear on the surface of water. This world and its delights appear bitter to me. I am not fond of wandering in the pleasure-gardens. I do not relish the company of girls, I do not value the acquisition of wealth. I wish to remain at peace within myself. I am constantly enquiring: "How can I wean my heart completely away from even thinking of this ever-changing phantasm called the world?" I do not long for death, nor do I long to live; I remain as I am, free from the fever of lust. What shall I do with the kingdom, pleasure or wealth, all of which are the playthings of egotism which is absent in me?

If I do not get established in wisdom now, when shall another opportunity arise? For, indulgence in sense-pleasure poisons the mind in such a way that its effects last several life-times. Only the man of self-knowledge is free from this. Therefore, O sage, I pray to thee: instruct me in such a way that I may forever be free from anguish, fear and distress. With the light of your instruction destroy the darkness of ignorance in my heart.

apahastita sarvārtham anavasthitir āsthitā
gṛhītvotsṛjya cā "tmānaṁ bhavasthitir avasthitā (30/8)

RĀMA continued:

By reflecting on the pitiable fate of living beings thus fallen into the dreadful pit of sorrow, I am filled with grief. My mind is confused, I shudder, and at every step I am afraid. **I have given up everything but I have not established myself in wisdom; hence I am partly caught and partly freed.** I am like a tree that has been cut but not severed from its root. I wish to restrain my mind but do not have the wisdom to do so.

Hence, pray tell me: what is that condition or state in which one does not experience any grief? How can one who is involved in the world and its activities, as I am, reach the supreme state of peace and bliss? What is that attitude that enables one not to be influenced by various kinds of activities and experiences? Pray tell me: how do you people who are enlightened live in this world? How can the mind be freed from lust and made to view the world both as one's own self and also as no more valuable than a blade of grass? The biography of which great one shall we study in order to learn the path of wisdom? How should one live in this world? Holy sir, instruct me in that wisdom which will enable my otherwise restless mind to be steady like a mountain. You are an enlightened being; instruct me so that I may never again be sunk in grief.

Obviously this world is full of pain and death; how does it become a source of joy, without befuddling one's heart? The mind is obviously full of impurities; how can it be cleansed and with what cleanser prescribed by what great sage? How should one live here so as not to fall a victim to the twin currents of love-and-hate? Obviously there is a secret that enables one to remain unaffected by the grief and suffering in this world even as mercury is not affected when it is thrown into the fire. What is that secret? What is the secret that counteracts the habit of the mind that is spread out in the form of this universe?

Who are those heroes who have freed themselves from delusion? And what methods did they adopt to free themselves. If you consider that I am neither fit nor capable of understanding this, I shall fast unto death.

VĀLMĪKI said:

Having said so, Rāma remained silent.

**sakala loka camatkṛti kāriṇo 'py abhimataṁ yadi rāghavacetasaḥ
phalati no tad ime vayam eva hi sphuṭataraṁ munayo hatabuddhayaḥ (33/46)**

VĀLMĪKI said:

All those who had assembled in the court were highly inspired by the flaming words of Rāma's wisdom which is capable of dispelling the delusion of the mind. They felt as if they themselves had been rid of all their doubts and deluded misunderstanding. They drank the nectarine words of Rāma with great delight. As they sat in the court listening to Rāma's words, it appeared as though they were no longer living beings but painted figures — they were so still with rapt attention.

Who listened to Rāma's discourse? Sages like Vasiṣṭha and Viśvāmitra, the ministers, members of the royal family including king Daśaratha, citizens, holy ones, servants, caged birds, animal pets, the horses of the royal stable, and the celestials including the perfected sages and heavenly musicians. Surely, even the king of heaven and the chiefs of the nether world listened to Rāma.

Thrilled to hear Rāma's speech, all of them acclaimed "Bravo, bravo" with one voice and this joyous sound filled the air. To felicitate Rāma, there was a shower of flowers from heaven. Everyone assembled in the court cheered him. Surely, no one but Rāma who was full of dispassion could have uttered the words that he gave expression to — not even the preceptor of the gods. We were indeed extremely fortunate to have been able to listen to him. While we listened to him, it seemed as though we were filled with the feeling that there is no happiness even in heaven.

THE PERFECTED SAGES in the assembly said:

Surely, the answers that the holy ones are about to give to the weighty and wise questions of Rāma are worthy of being heard by all beings in the universe. O sages, come, come, let us all gather in the court of king Daśaratha to listen to the answer of the supreme sage Vasiṣṭha.

VĀLMĪKI said:

Hearing this, all the sages of the world hastened to the court, where they were duly received, honoured and seated in the court. Surely, **if in our heart the lofty wisdom of Rāma is not reflected, we shall indeed be the losers; whatever be our abilities and faculties, we shall thereby prove that we have lost our intelligence!**

yaśaḥ prabhṛtinā yasmai hetunai 'va vinā punaḥ
bhuvi bhogā na rocante sa jīvanmuktta ucyate (2/8)

VIŚVĀMITRA said:

O Rāma, you are indeed the foremost among the wise, and there is really nothing further for you to know. However, your knowledge needs confirmation, even as the self-knowledge of Śuka needed confirmation from Janaka before Śuka could find the peace that passeth understanding.

Just like you, Śuka also arrived at the truth concerning existence after deep contemplation of the evanescence of this world. Yet because it was self-acquired knowledge, he could not positively affirm to himself 'This is the truth'. He had of course arrived at the state of extreme and supreme dispassion.

One day, this Śuka approached his father Vedavyāsa and asked him: "Sir, how did this diversity of world-creation come into being; and how will it come to an end?" Vedavyāsa gave a detailed answer to this question: but Śuka thought 'All this I knew already; what is new in this?' and was not impressed. Vedavyāsa also sensed this, and hence he said to Śuka: "My son, I do not know anything more than this; but there is the royal sage Janaka on earth who knows more than this. Kindly approach him.

Śuka thereupon came to Janaka's palace. Informed by the palace guards of the young Śuka's arrival, Janaka ignored him for a week while Śuka patiently waited outside. The next week Janaka had Śuka brought into the palace and waited upon by dancers and musicians. Śuka was unmoved by this, too. After this, Śuka was ushered into the royal presence, and Janaka said: "You know the truth; what else shall I tell you now. This diversity arises on account of mental modifications and it will cease when they cease." Thus when his self-knowledge had been confirmed. Śuka attained peace and remained in nirvikalpa samādhi.

Like Śuka, Rāma too has gained the highest wisdom. The surest sign of a man of the highest wisdom is that he is unattracted by the pleasures of the world, for in him even the subtle tendencies have ceased. When these tendencies are strong, there is bondage; when they have ceased, there is liberation. **He is truly a liberated sage who by nature is not swayed by sense-pleasure, without the motivation of fame or other incentives. And I pray that the sage Vasistha should so instruct Rāma that he will be confirmed in his wisdom and we, too, may be inspired.**

VASIṢṬHA said:

I shall surely accede to your request. And, O Rāma, I shall now impart to you the wisdom which was revealed to me by the divine creator Brahmā, himself. O Rāma, countless have been the universes that have come into being and that have been dissolved. In fact, even the countless universes that exist at this moment are impossible to conceive of. All this can immediately be realised in one's own heart, for these universes are the creations of the desires that arise in the heart, like castles built in the air. Neither the world of matter nor the modes of creation are truly real; yet the living and the dead think and feel they are real. Ignorance of this truth keeps up the appearance.

paraṁ pauruṣam āśritya dantair dantān vicūrṇayan
śubhenā 'śubham udyukttaṁ prākttanaṁ pauruṣaṁ jayet (5/9)

VASIṢṬHA continued:

O Rāma, even as water remains water whether there are waves or no waves, whatever be the external appearance of the liberated sage his wisdom remains unchanged. The difference is only in the eyes of the ignorant spectator. Therefore, O Rāma, listen to what I am about to say; this instruction is sure to remove the darkness of ignorance.

In this world whatever is gained is gained only by self-effort; where failure is encountered it is seen that there has been slackness in the effort. This is obvious, but what is called fate is fictitious, and is not seen. Self-effort, Rāma, is that mental, verbal and physical action which is in accordance with the instructions of a holy person well versed in the scriptures. It is only by such effort that Indra became king of heaven, that Brahmā became the creator, and the other deities earned their places.

Self-effort is of two categories: that of past births and that of this birth. The latter effectively counteracts the former. Fate is none other than self-effort of a past incarnation. There is constant conflict between these two in this incarnation; and that which is more powerful triumphs.

Self-effort which is not in accord with the scriptures is motivated by delusion. When there is obstruction in the fruition of self-effort one should examine it to see if there is such deluded action, and if there is it should be immediately corrected. There is no power greater than right action in the present. Hence, **one should take recourse to self-effort, grinding one's teeth, and one should overcome evil by good and fate by present effort.**

The lazy man is worse than a donkey. One should never yield to laziness but strive to attain liberation, seeing that life is ebbing away every moment. One should not revel in the filth known as sense-pleasures as a worm revels in pus.

One who says: "Fate is directing me to do this" is brainless, and the goddess of fortune abandons him. Hence, by self-effort acquire wisdom and then realise that this self-effort is not without its own end, in the direct realisation of the truth. If this dreadful source of evil named laziness is not found on earth, who will ever be illiterate and poor? It is because laziness if found on earth that people live the life of animals, miserable and poverty-stricken.

VĀLMĪKI said: At this stage, it was time for evening prayers and the assembly broke up for the day.

śāstraiḥ sadācara vijṛmbhita deśadharmair
yatkalpitaṁ phalam atīva cira prarūḍhaṁ
tasmin hṛdi sphurati copanam eti cittam
aṅgāvali tad anu pauruṣam etad āhuḥ (6/40)

VASIṢṬHA began the second day's discourse:

As is the effort so is the fruit, O Rāma: this is the meaning of self-effort, and it is also known as fate (divine). When afflicted by suffering people cry 'Alas what tragedy' or 'Alas, look at my fate', both of which mean the same thing. What is called fate or divine will is nothing other than the action or self-effort of the past. The present is infinitely more potent than the past. They indeed are fools who are satisfied with the fruits of their past effort (which they regard as divine will) and do not engage themselves in self-effort now.

Sometimes it happens that without effort someone makes a great gain: for example, the state elephant chooses (in accordance with an ancient practice) a mendicant as the ruler of a country whose king suddenly died without leaving an heir; this is certainly neither an accident nor some kind of divine act, but the fruit of the mendicant's self-effort in the past birth.

Sometimes it happens that a farmer's efforts are made fruitless by a hailstorm; surely, the hailstorm's own power was greater than the farmer's effort and the farmer should put forth greater effort now. He should not grieve over the inevitable loss. If such grief is justified, why should he not weep daily over the inevitability of death? The wise man should of course know what is capable of attainment by self-effort and what is not. It is ignorance however to attribute all this to an outside agency and to say that God sends me to heaven or to hell or that an outside agency makes me do this or that — such an ignorant person should be shunned.

One should free oneself from likes and dislikes and engage oneself in righteous self-effort and reach the supreme truth, knowing that self-effort alone is another name for divine will. We only ridicule the fatalist. **That alone is self-effort which springs from right understanding that manifests in one's heart which has been exposed to the teachings of the scriptures and the conduct of holy ones.**

O Rāma, one should, with a body free from illness and mind free from distress, pursue self-knowledge so that he is not born again here. Such self-effort has a threefold root and therefore threefold fruit: an inner awakening in the intelligence, a decision in the mind and the physical action.

aśubheṣu samāviṣṭaṁ śubheṣv evā 'vatārayet
prayatnāc cittam ity eṣa sarva śāstrā 'rtha saṁgrahaḥ (7/12)

VASIṢṬHA continued:

Self-effort is based on these three: knowledge of scriptures, instructions of the preceptor and one's own effort. Fate (or divine dispensation) does not enter here. Hence, he who desires salvation **should divert the impure mind to pure endeavour by persistent effort — this is the very essence of all scriptures.**

Rāma, the tendencies brought forward from past incarnations are of two kinds — pure and impure. The pure ones lead you towards liberation, and the impure ones invite trouble. You are indeed consciousness itself, not inert physical matter. You are not impelled to action by anything other than yourself. Hence you are free to strengthen the pure latent tendencies in preference to the impure ones. The holy ones emphasise: persistently tread the path that leads to the eternal good. And the wise seeker knows: the fruit of my endeavours will be commensurate with the intensity of my self-effort and neither fate nor a god can ordain it otherwise. Indeed, such self-effort alone is responsible for whatever man gets here; when he is sunk in unhappiness, to console him people suggest that it is his fate. This is obvious: one goes abroad and one appeases one's hunger, by undertaking a journey and by eating food — not on account of a fate. No one has seen such a fate or a god, but everyone has experienced how an action (good or evil) leads to a result (good or evil). Hence, right from one's childhood one should endeavour to promote one's true good (salvation) by a keen intelligent study of the scriptures, by having the company of the holy ones and by right self effort.

Fate or divine dispensation is merely a convention which has come to be regarded as truth by being repeatedly declared to be true. If this god or fate is truly the ordainer of everything in this world, of what meaning is any action (even like bathing, speaking or giving), and whom should one teach at all? No. In this world, except a corpse, everything is active and such activity yields its appropriate result. No one has ever realised the existence of a fate or divine dispensation. People use such expressions as 'I am impelled by fate or divine dispensation to do this' for self-satisfaction, but this is not true. For example, if an astrologer predicts that a young man would become a great scholar, does that young man become a scholar without study? No. Then, why do we believe in divine dispensation? Rāma, this sage Viśvāmitra became a Brahmā-Ṛṣi by self-effort; all of us have attained self-knowledge by self-effort alone. Hence, renounce fatalism and apply yourself to self-effort.

Note: The word used in the text for fate is 'daivaṁ' which also means 'god'.

imām mokṣa kathām śrutvā saha sarvair vivekibhiḥ
param yāsyasi nirduḥkham nāśo yatra na vidyate (8)

VASIṢṬHA continued:

The cosmic order that people refer to as fate, daivam or niyati and which ensures that every effort is blessed with appropriate fruition, is based on omnipresent and omnipotent omniscience (known as Brahman). By self-effort therefore restrain the senses and the mind, and with a mind that is one-pointed calmly listen to what I am going to say.

This narrative deals with liberation; listening to it with other wise seekers who are assembled here, you will realise that supreme being where there is no sorrow nor destruction. This was revealed to me by the creator Brahmā himself in a previous age.

O Rāma, the omnipresent omniscience (the cosmic being) shines eternally in all beings. When a vibration arises in that cosmic being, lord Viṣṇu is born, even as a wave arises when the surface of the ocean is agitated. From that Viṣṇu, Brahmā the creator was born. Brahmā began to create the countless varieties of animate and inanimate, sentient and insentient beings in the universe. And the universe was as it was before the cosmic dissolution.

The Creator saw that all living beings in the universe were subject to disease and death, to pain and suffering. In his heart there arose compassion, and he sought to lay down a path that might lead living beings away from all this. He thereupon instituted centres of pilgrimage and noble virtues like austerity, charity, truthfulness and righteous conduct. But these were inadequate; they could bestow only temporary relief from suffering, and not final liberation from sorrow.

Reflecting thus, the Creator brought me into being. He drew me to himself and drew the veil of ignorance over my heart. Instantly I forgot my identity and my self-nature. I was miserable. I begged of Brahmā the creator, my own father, to show me the way out of this misery. Sunk in my misery I was unable and unwilling to do anything, and I remained lazy and inactive.

In response to my prayer, my father revealed to me the true knowledge which instantly dispelled the veil of ignorance that he himself had spread over me. The Creator then said to me: "My son, I veiled the knowledge and revealed it to you so that you may experience its glory; for only then will you be able to understand the travail of ignorant beings and to help them." Rāma, equipped with this knowledge, I am here and I will continue to be here till the end of creation.

mokṣadvāre dvārapālāś catvāraḥ parikīrtitāḥ
śamo vicāraḥ santoṣaś caturthaḥ sādhusaṅgamaḥ (59)

VASIṢṬHA continued:

Even so, in every age the Creator wills into being several sages and myself for the spiritual enlightenment of all. And, in order to ensure the due performance of the secular duties by all, Brahmā also creates kings who rule justly and wisely over parts of the earth. These kings, however, are soon corrupted by lust for power and pleasure: conflict of interests leads to wars among them which in turn give rise to remorse. To remove their ignorance, the sages used to impart spiritual wisdom to them. In days of yore, O Rāma, kings used to receive this wisdom and cherish it; hence it was known as Rāja-Vidyā (Kingly Science).

The highest form of dispassion born of pure discrimination has arisen in your heart, O Rāma, and it is superior to dispassion born of a circumstantial cause or an utter disgust. Such dispassion is surely due to the grace of God. This grace meets the maturity of discrimination at the exact moment when dispassion is generated in the heart.

As long as the highest wisdom does not dawn in the heart, the person revolves in this wheel of birth and death. Pray, listen to my exposition of this wisdom with a concentrated mind.

This wisdom destroys the forest of ignorance. Roaming in this forest one undergoes confusion and seemingly interminable suffering. One should therefore approach an enlightened teacher and by asking the right question with the right attitude, elicit the teaching. It then becomes an integral part of one's being. The fool asks irrelevant questions irreverently; and the greater fool is he who spurns the sage's wisdom. He is surely not a sage who responds to the vain questions of a foolish questioner.

O Rāma, you are indeed the best among all seekers, for you have duly reflected over the truth and you are inspired by the best form of dispassion. And I am sure that what I am going to say to you will find a firm seat in your heart. Indeed, one should positively strive to enthrone wisdom in one's heart, for the mind is unsteady like a monkey. And, one should then avoid unwise company.

Rāma, **there are four gate-keepers at the entrance to the Realm of Freedom (Mokṣa). They are self-control, spirit of enquiry, contentment and good company.** The wise seeker should diligently cultivate the friendship of these, or at least one of them.

prasanne cittatve hṛdi śamabhave valgati pare
śamā bhogī bhūtāsv akhila kalanā dṛṣṭiṣu puraḥ
samaṁ yāti svāntaḥkaraṇa ghaṭanāsvādita rasaṁ
dhiyā dṛṣṭe tattve ramaṇamaṭanaṁ jāgatam idaṁ (12/21)

VASIṢTHA continued:

With a pure heart and a receptive mind, and without the veil of doubt and the restlessness of the mind, listen to the exposition of the nature and the means of liberation, O Rāma. For, not until the supreme being is realised will the dreadful miseries of birth and death come to an end. If this deadly serpent known as ignorant life is not overcome here and now, it gives rise to interminable suffering not only in this but in countless lifetimes to come. One cannot ignore this suffering, but one should overcome it by means of the wisdom that I shall impart to you.

O Rāma, if you thus overcome this sorrow of repetitive history (saṁsāra), you will live here on earth itself like a god, like Brahmā or Viṣṇu! For when delusion is gone and the truth is realised by means of enquiry into self-nature, when the mind is at peace and the heart leaps to the supreme truth, when all the disturbing thought-waves in the mind-stuff have subsided and there is unbroken flow of peace and the heart is filled with the bliss of the absolute, when thus the truth has been seen in the heart, then this very world becomes an abode of bliss.

Such a person has nothing to acquire, nor anything to shun. He is untainted by the defects of life, untouched by its sorrow. He does not come into being nor go out, though he appears to come and go in the eyes of the beholder. Even religious duties are found to be unnecessary. He is not affected by the past tendencies which have lost their momentum: his mind has given up its restlessness, and he rests in the bliss that is his essential nature. Such bliss is possible only by self-knowledge, not by any other means. Hence, one should apply oneself constantly to self-knowledge — this alone is one's duty.

He who disregards holy scriptures and holy men does not attain self-knowledge. Such foolishness is more harmful than all the illnesses that one is subject to in this world. Hence, one should devoutly listen to this scripture which leads one to self-knowledge. He who obtains this scripture does not again fall into the blind well of ignorance. O Rāma, if you want to free yourself from the sorrow of saṁsāra (repetitive history) receive the wholesome instructions of sages like me and be free.

sthito 'pi na sthita iva na hṛṣyati na kupyati
yaḥ suṣuptasamaḥ svasthaḥ sa śānta iti kathyate (76)

VASIṢṬHA continued:

In order to cross this formidable ocean of saṁsāra (repetitive history), one should resort to that which is eternal and unchanging. He alone is the best among men, O Rāma, whose mind rests in the eternal and is, therefore, fully self-controlled and at peace. He sees that pleasure and pain chase and cancel each other, and in that wisdom there is self-control and peace. He who does not see this sleeps in a burning house.

He who gains the wisdom of the eternal here is freed from saṁsāra and he is not born again in ignorance. One may doubt that such unchanging truth may not exist! If it does not, one comes to no harm by enquiring into the nature of life; seeking the eternal will soften the pain caused by the changes in life. But, if it exists, then by knowing it one is freed.

The eternal is not attained by rites and rituals, by pilgrimages nor by wealth; it is to be attained only by the conquest of one's mind, by the cultivation of wisdom. Hence everyone — gods, demons, demi-gods or men should constantly seek (whether one is walking, falling or sitting) the conquest of the mind and self-control which are the fruits of wisdom.

When the mind is at peace, pure, tranquil, free from delusion or hallucination, untangled and free from cravings, it does not long for anything nor does it reject anything. This is self-control or conquest of mind — one of the four gatekeepers to liberation which I mentioned earlier.

.... that is good and auspicious flows from self-control. All evil is dispelled by self-control. No gain, no pleasure in this world or in heaven is comparable to the delight of self-control. The delight one experiences in the presence of the self-controlled is incomparable. Everyone spontaneously trusts him. None (not even demons and goblins) hates him.

Self-control, O Rāma, is the best remedy for all physical and mental ills. When there is self-control, even the food you eat tastes better, else it tastes bitter. He who wears the armour of self-control is not harmed by sorrow.

He who even while hearing, touching, seeing, smelling and tasting what is regarded as pleasant and unpleasant, is neither elated nor depressed — he is self-controlled. He who looks upon all beings with equal vision, having brought under control the sensations of pleasure and pain, is self-controlled. **He who, though living amongst all is unaffected by them, neither feels elated nor hates, is self-controlled.**

vicārāj jñāyate tattvaṁ tattvād viśrāntir ātmani
ato manasi śāntatvaṁ sarva duḥkha parikṣayaḥ (53)

VASIṢṬHA continued:

Enquiry (the second gate-keeper to liberation) should be undertaken by an intelligence that has been purified by a close study of the scripture, and this enquiry should be unbroken. By such enquiry the intelligence becomes keen and is able to realise the supreme; hence enquiry alone is the best remedy for the long-lasting illness known as saṁsāra.

The wise man regards strength, intellect, efficiency and timely action as the fruits of enquiry. Indeed kingdom, prosperity and enjoyment, as well as final liberation, are all the fruits of enquiry. The spirit of enquiry protects one from the calamities that befall the unthinking fool. When the mind has been rendered dull by the absence of enquiry, even the cool rays of the moon turn into deadly weapons, and the childish imagination throws up a goblin in every dark spot. Hence, the non-enquiring fool is really a store-house of sorrow. It is the absence of enquiry that gives rise to actions that are harmful to oneself and to others, and to numerous psychosomatic illnesses. Therefore, one should avoid the company of such unthinking people.

They in whom the spirit of enquiry is ever awake illumine the world, enlighten all who come in contact with them, dispel the ghosts created by an ignorant mind, and realise the falsity of sense-pleasures and their objects. O Rāma, in the light of enquiry there is realisation of the eternal and unchanging reality; this is the supreme. With it one does not long for any other gain nor does one spurn anything. He is free from delusion, attachment; he is not inactive nor does he get drowned in action; he lives and functions in this world and at the end of a natural life-span he reaches the blissful state of total freedom.

The eye of spiritual enquiry does not lose its sight even in the midst of all activities; he who does not have this eye is indeed to be pitied. It is better to be born as a frog in the mud, a worm in dung, a snake in a hole, but not be one without this eye. What is enquiry? To enquire thus: 'Who am I? How has this evil of saṁsāra (repetitive history) come into being?' is true enquiry. **Knowledge of truth arises from such enquiry; from such knowledge there follows tranquillity in oneself; and then arises the supreme peace that passeth understanding, and the ending of all sorrow.**

(Vicāra or enquiry is not reasoning nor analysis; it is directly looking into oneself.)

santoṣaḥ paramo lābhaḥ satsaṅgaḥ paramā gatiḥ
vicāraḥ paramaṁ jñānaṁ śamo hi paramaṁ sukhaṁ (16/19)

VASIṢṬHA continued:

Contentment is another gate-keeper to liberation. He who has quaffed the nectar of contentment does not relish craving for sense-pleasures; no delight in this world is as sweet at contentment which destroys all sins.

What is contentment? To renounce all craving for what is not obtained unsought and to be satisfied with what comes unsought, without being elated or depressed even by them — this is contentment. As long as one is not satisfied in the self, he will be subjected to sorrow. With the rise of contentment the purity of one's heart blooms. The contented man who possesses nothing owns the world.

Satsaṅga (company of wise, holy and enlightened persons) is yet another gate-keeper to liberation. Satsaṅga enlarges one's intelligence, destroys one's ignorance and one's psychological distress. Whatever be the cost, however difficult it may be, whatever obstacles may stand in its way, satsaṅga should never be neglected. For, satsaṅga alone is one's light on the path of life. Satsaṅga is indeed superior to all other forms of religious practices like charity, austerity, pilgrimage and the performance of religious rites.

One should by every means in one's power adore and serve the holy men who have realised the truth and in whose heart the darkness of ignorance has been dispelled. They, on the other hand, who treat such holy men disrespectfully, surely invite great suffering.

These four — contentment, satsaṅga (company of wise men), the spirit of enquiry, and self-control, are the four surest means by which they who are drowning in this ocean of saṁsāra (repetitive history) can be saved. **Contentment is the supreme gain. Satsaṅga is the best companion to the destination. The spirit of enquiry itself is the greatest wisdom. And, self-control is supreme happiness.** If you are unable to resort to all these four, then practise one: by diligent practice of one of these, the others will also be found in you. The highest wisdom will seek you of its own accord. Until you tame the wild elephant of your mind with the help of these noble qualities, you cannot have progress towards the supreme, even if you become a god, demi-god or a tree. Therefore, O Rāma, strive by all means to cultivate these noble qualities. He who is endowed with the qualities that I have enumerated thus far is qualified to listen to what I am about to reveal. You are indeed such a qualified person, O Rāma.

yukttí yukttam upādeyaṁ vacanaṁ bālakād api
anyat tṛṇam iva tyājyam apy ukttaṁ padmajanmanā (18/3)

VASIṢṬHA continued:

One who sows the seed of the knowledge of this scripture soon obtains the fruit of the realisation of truth. Though human in origin, an exposition of truth is to be accepted; otherwise even what is regarded as divine revelation is to be rejected. **Even a young boy's words are to be accepted if they are words of wisdom; else, reject it like straw even if uttered by Brahmā the creator.**

He who listens to and reflects upon the exposition of this scripture enjoys unfathomable wisdom, firm conviction and unperturbable coolness of spirit. Soon he becomes a liberated sage whose glory is indescribable.

One who studies this scripture and comprehends its teaching is no longer deluded by world-appearance. When one sees that the yonder deadly snake is a life-like painting, one is no longer afraid of it. When the world-appearance is seen as an appearance it does not produce either elation or sorrow. It is indeed a great pity that even when such a scripture exists, people seek sense-pleasures which lead to great sorrow.

O Rāma, when a truth that has not been personally experienced is expounded, one does not grasp it except with the help of an illustration. Such illustrations have been used in this scripture with a definite purpose and a limited intention. They are not to be taken literally, nor is their significance to be stretched beyond the intention. When the scripture is thus studied, the world appears to be a dream-vision. These indeed are the purpose and the purport of the illustrations. Let no one of perverted intellect misinterpret the illustrations given in this scripture.

Again, study of this scripture should continue till the truth is realised; one should not stop short of complete enlightenment. A little knowledge of the scripture results in confusion worse confounded. Non-recognition of the existence of supreme peace in the heart and the assumption of the reality of imaginary factors, are both born of imperfect knowledge and the consequent perverted logic.

Even as the ocean is the substratum of all the waves, direct experience alone is the basis for all proofs — the direct experience of truth as it is. That substratum is the experiencing intelligence which itself becomes the experiencer, the act of experiencing, and the experience.

Even as movement is inherent in air, manifestation (as the subtle perceiving mind and as the gross objects it perceives) is inherent in this experiencing intelligence. And the perceiving mind, on account of ignorance, thinks 'I am such and such an object' and thence becomes that. The object is experienced only in the subject, not elsewhere!

yathā rasaḥ padārtheṣu yathā tailaṁ tilādiṣu
kusumeṣu yathā "modas tathā draṣṭari dṛśyadhīḥ (43)

VASIṢṬHA continued:

I shall now declare to you the creation and its secret. For, it is only as long as one invests the perceived object with reality that bondage lasts; once that notion goes, with it goes bondage. Here in this creation only that which is created grows, decays and then goes either to heaven or to hell, and it gets liberated.

During the cosmic dissolution the entire objective creation is resolved into the infinite being which is variously designated as Ātmā, Brahman, Truth, etc., by the wise, to facilitate communication and dialogue. This same infinite self conceives within itself the duality of oneself and the other. Thence, mind arises, as a wave arises when the surface of the calm ocean is disturbed. But, please bear in mind that just as a bracelet of gold is but gold (and though gold exists without being a bracelet, bracelet does not exist without gold or other metal), the qualities and the nature of the created and the potentiality of creation are inherent in the Creator. The mind is non-different from (has no existence independent of) the infinite self.

Even as the mirage appears to be a very real river of water, this creation appears to be entirely real. And, as long as one clings to the notion of the reality of 'you' and 'I', there is no liberation. Not by merely and verbally denying such a notion of existence is it obliterated; on the contrary, such denial itself becomes a further distraction.

Rāma, if the creation is in fact real then there is no possibility of its cessation: for it is an immutable law that the unreal has no real existence and the real does not cease to be. Austerity, meditation and such other practices can therefore not cause its cessation nor enlightenment. As long as the notion of creation lasts, even the contemplation (samādhi) in which there is no movement of thought (nirvikalpa) is not possible. Even if it were possible, the moment one returns from such contemplation, the creation with its sorrow arises in the mind. Movement of thought creates the notion of created objects.

Even as the essence exists in all things, as oil exists in sesame seeds, as aroma exists in flowers, the faculty of objective perception exists in the perceiver. Even as the dream-objects are experienced only by the dreamer, the objects of perception are experienced by the perceiver. Just as from a seed the sprout arises in due time, this potentiality becomes manifest as the notion of creation.

ātivāhikam evā 'ntar vismṛtyā dṛḍharūpayā
ādhibhautikabodhena mudhā bhāti piśācavat (3/22)

VASIṢṬHA continued:

In the Creator there is neither a seer nor an object of perception. Yet, he is known as self-created. He shines in cosmic consciousness as a painting in the mind of an artist.

In the Creator there is no memory of the past since he had no previous karma. He does not even have a physical body; the unborn is of spiritual substance. Mortal beings have two bodies, as it were, one physical and the other spiritual, but the unborn Creator has only the spiritual, since the cause that gives rise to the physical does not exist in him.

He was not created, but he is the Creator of all beings. Surely, the created (like a bracelet) is of the same substance as that of which it was created (gold). The Creator's thought being the cause of this manifold creation and the Creator himself having no physical body, the creation, too, is truly of the nature of thought, without materiality.

A throbbing arose in the Creator whose thought had spread out as the universe. This throb brought into being the subtle body (made of intelligence) of all beings. Made only of thought, all these beings only appeared to be, though they felt that that appearence was real. However, this appearence, thus imagined to be real, produced realistic results or consequences, even as sexual enjoyment in a dream does. Similarly, even the Creator (the holy man of the story) though he has no body, appears to have a body.

The Creator is also of a dual nature: consciousness and thought. Consciousness is pure, thought is subject to confusion. Hence, he appears to come into being (arise), though he does not so arise. He is the intelligence that supports the entire universe, and every thought that arises in that intelligence gives rise to a form. **Though all these forms are of the nature of pure intelligence, on account of self-forgetfulness of this, and of the thought of physical forms, they freeze into the physical forms, even as goblins though formless are seen to have forms on account of the perceiver's delusion.**

The Creator, however, is not subject to such delusion. Hence, he is always of a spiritual nature, not materialistic. The Creator is spiritual; and even so, his creation, too, is in reality spiritual in essence. This creation is causeless. Hence, it is essentially spiritual even as the supreme being, Brahman is. The materiality of the creation is like the castle in the air, an illusory projection of one's own mind — imaginary.

The Creator is the mind; mind or pure intelligence is his body. Thought is inherent in the mind. The object of perception is inherent in the perceiver. Who has ever discovered a distinction between the two?

na dṛśyam asti sadrūpaṁ na draṣṭā na ca darśanaṁ
na śūnyaṁ na jaḍaṁ no cic chāntam evedam ātataṁ (70)

VĀLMĪKI said:

At this stage the sun sped towards the western hills as if eager to meditate upon the sage's words and to illumine other parts of the earth. The assembly dispersed for prayers. The next morning all the members of the court reassembled as before.

RĀMA asked:

O Holy sage! Pray, tell me what the mind really is.

VASIṢṬHA replied:

Even as empty, inert nothingness is known as space, mind is empty nothingness. Whether the mind is real or unreal, it is that which is apprehended in objects of perception. Rāma, thought is mind; there is no distinction between the two. The self that is clothed in the spiritual body is known as mind; it is that which brings the material or physical body into existence. Ignorance, saṁsāra (repetitive history), mind-stuff, bondage, impurity, darkness and inertia are all synonyms. Experience alone is the mind; it is none other than the perceived.

This entire universe is forever non-different from the consciousness that dwells in every atom, even as an ornament is non-different from gold. Just as an ornament potentially exists in gold, the object exists in the subject. But when this notion of the object is firmly rejected and removed from the subject, then consciousness alone exists without even an apparent or potential objectivity. When this is realised, evils like attraction and repulsion, love and hate, cease in one's heart, as also the false notions of the world, you, I, etc. Even the tendency to objectify ceases; this is freedom.

RĀMA asked:

Holy sir, if the object of perception is real, then it shall not cease to be. If it is unreal, then we do not see it as unreal; so how can we overcome this?

VASIṢṬHA said:

Yet, O Rāma, we see that there are holy ones who have overcome this! External objects like space, etc. and psychological factors like 'I' etc. exist only in name. **In reality neither the objective universe, nor the perceiving self, nor perception as such, nor void, nor inertness exists; only one is — cosmic consciousness (cit).** In this it is the mind that conjures up the diversity, diverse actions and experiences, the notion of bondage and the desire for liberation.

yasmād viṣṇvādayo devāḥ sūryādiva maricayah
yasmāj jaganty anantāni budbudā jaladher iva (5/9)

RĀMA asked:

O holy sage! What is the source of this mind and how did it arise? Kindly enlighten me on these.

VASIṢṬHA replied:

After the cosmic dissolution and before the next epoch dawned, the entire objective universe was in a state of perfect equilibrium. There then existed the supreme Lord, the eternal, unborn, self-effulgent, who is the all and who is omnipotent. He is beyond conception and description; though he is known by various names like Ātmā etc., these are viewpoints and not the truth. He is, yet he is not realised by the world; he is within the body, too, yet he is far. **From him emerge countless divinities like lord Viṣṇu, even as countless rays emerge from the sun; from him emerge infinite worlds as ripples arise from the surface of the ocean.**

He is the cosmic intelligence into which countless objects of perception enter. He is the light in which the self and the world shine. He ordains the characteristic nature of every created thing. In him the worlds appear and disappear, even as a mirage appears and disappears repeatedly. His form (the world) vanishes, but his self is unchanging. He dwells in all. He is hidden and he overflows. By his mere presence this apparently inert material world and its inhabitants are ever active. Because of his omnipresent omnipotent omniscience, his very thoughts materialise.

This supreme self cannot be realised, O Rāma, by means other than wisdom — not indeed by exerting oneself in religious practices. This self is neither far nor near; it is not inaccessible nor is it in distant places: it is what in oneself appears to be the experience of bliss, and is therefore realised in oneself.

Austerity and penance, charity and the observances of religious vows do not lead to the realisation of the Lord; only the company of holy men and the study of true scriptures are helpful, as they dispel ignorance and delusion. Even when one is convinced that this self alone is real, one goes beyond sorrow, on the path of liberation.

Austerity or penance is self-inflicted pain. Of what value is charity performed with wealth earned by deceiving others — only they derive the fruits of such charity! Religious observances add to one's vanity. There is only one remedy for ignorance of the Lord: the firm and decisive renunciation of craving for sense-pleasure.

draṣṭṛ dṛśya kramo yatra sthito 'py astamayaṅgataḥ
yad anākāśam ākāśaṁ tad rūpaṁ paramātmanaḥ (21)

RĀMA asked:

Where does this Lord dwell, and how can I reach him?

VASIṢṬHA replied:

He who has been described as the Lord is not very far: He is the intelligence dwelling in the body. He is the universe, though the universe is not He. He is pure intelligence.

RĀMA remarked:

Even a little boy says that the Lord is intelligence; what need is there for special instruction concerning this?

VASIṢṬHA replied:

Ah, one who knows that pure intelligence is the objective universe knows nothing. Sentient is the universe, and sentient is the soul (jiva). The sentient creates the knowable and gets involved in sorrow. When there is cessation of the knowable, and the flow of attention is towards that which is not knowable (pure intelligence), then there is fulfilment and one goes beyond sorrow.

Without the cessation of the knowable, one's attention cannot be finally turned away from the knowable. Mere awareness of the involvement of the jīva in this saṁsāra is of no use. But, if the supreme Lord is known, this sorrow comes to an end.

RĀMA asked: Holy sir, please describe the Lord.

VASIṢṬHA replied:

The cosmic intelligence in which the universe, as it were, ceases to be, is the Lord. **In him the subject-object relationship appears to have ceased, as such. He is the void in which the universe appears to exist.** In him even cosmic consciousness stands still like a mountain.

RĀMA asked again:

How can we realise the Lord, and realise the unreality of the universe that we have come to regard as real?

VASIṢṬHA answered: The Lord can be realised only if one is firmly established in the unreality of the universe even as the blueness of the sky is unreal. Dualism presupposes unity, and non-dualism suggests dualism. Only when the creation is known to be utterly non-existent the Lord is realised.

yo jāgarti suṣuptastho yasya jāgran na vidyate
yasya nirvāsano bodhaḥ sa jivanmukttaḥ ucyate (9/7)

RĀMA asked:

Holy sir, by what method is this known, and what should I know by which the knowable comes to an end?

VASIṢṬHA replied:

The wrong notion that this world is real has become deep rooted on account of persistent wrong thinking. However, it can be removed that very day on which you resort to the company of holy men and to the study of the holy scripture. Of all scriptures this Mahārāmāyanaṁ is best. What is found here is found elsewhere; what is not found here is not found anywhere else. However, if one does not wish to study this, one is welcome to study any other scripture — there is no objection to this.

When the wrong notion is dispelled and the truth realised, that realisation so thoroughly saturates one, that one thinks of it, speaks of it, rejoices in it and teaches it to others. Such people are sometimes called Jīvanmuktā and also Videhamuktā.

RĀMA asked:

Lord, what are the characteristics of Jīvanmuktā (liberated while living) and Videhamuktā (liberated ones who have no body)?

VASIṢṬHA replied:

He who, while living an apparently normal life, experiences the whole world as an emptiness, is a Jivanmukta. He is awake but enjoys the calmness of deep sleep; he is unaffected in the least by pleasure and pain. **He is awake in deep sleep; but he is never awake to this world. His wisdom is unclouded by latent tendencies.** He appears to be subject to likes, dislikes and fear; but in fact he is as free as the space. He is free from egotism and volition; and his intelligence is unattached whether in action or in inaction. None is afraid of him; he is afraid of none. He becomes a Videhamukta when, in due time, the body is dropped.

The Videhamukta is, yet is not, is not 'I' nor the 'other'. He is the sun that shines, Viṣṇu that protects all, Rudra that destroys all, Brahmā that creates; he is space, the earth, water and fire. He is in fact cosmic consciousness — that which is the very essence in all beings. All that which is in the past, present and future — all indeed is he and he alone.

draṣṭṛ darśana dṛśyānāṁ madhye yad darśanaṁ sthitaṁ
sādho tad avadhānena svātmānam avabuddhyase (75)

RĀMA asked again:

Lord, my perception is distorted: how can I attain to that state you have indicated?

VASIṢṬHA replied:

What is known as liberation, O Rāma, is indeed the absolute itself, which alone is. That which is perceived here as 'I', 'you' etc., only seems to be, for it has never been created. How can we say that that Brahman has become all these worlds?

O Rāma, in ornaments I see only gold, in waves I see only water, in air I see only movement, in space I see only emptiness, in mirage I see only heat, and naught else; similarly, I see only Brahman the absolute, not the worlds.

The perception of 'the worlds' is beginningless ignorance. Yet it will vanish with the help of enquiry into truth. Only that ceases to be which has come into being. This world has never really come into being, yet it appears to be — the exposition of this truth is contained in this chapter on creation.

When the previous cosmic dissolution took place, all that appeared to be before disappeared. Then the infinite alone remained; it was neither emptiness nor a form, neither sight nor the seen, and one could not say that it was, nor that it was not. It has no ears, no eyes, no tongue, and yet it hears, sees and eats. It is uncaused and uncreated; and it is the cause of everything as water is the cause of waves. This infinite and eternal light is the heart of all; and in its light the three worlds shine, as a mirage.

When the infinite vibrates, the worlds appear to emerge; when it does not vibrate, the worlds appear to submerge: even as when a firebrand is whirled fast a fiery circle appears, and when it is held steady, the circle vanishes. Vibrating or not vibrating, it is the same everywhere at all times. Not realising it, one is subject to delusion; when it is realised all cravings and anxieties vanish.

From it is time; from it is perception of the perceivable object. Action, form, taste, smell, sound, touch and thinking — all that you know is it alone; and it is that by which you know all this! **It is in the seer, sight and seen as the very seeing; when you know it, you realise your self.**

pūrṇāt pūrṇaṁ prasarati saṁsthitaṁ pūrṇam eva tat
ato viśvam anutpannaṁ yac cotpannaṁ tad eva tat (29)

RĀMA said:

Holy sir, how can it be said to be not empty, not to be illuminated and not dark? By such contradictory expressions you confuse me!

VASIṢṬHA replied:

Rāma, you are asking immature questions. Yet, I shall elucidate the correct meaning.

Even as the uncarved image is forever present in a block, the world whether you regard it as real or unreal is inherent in the absolute, which is therefore not void. Just as one cannot say that there are no waves present in a calm ocean, the absolute is not empty of the world. Of course, these illustrations have limited application and should not be exceeded.

In truth, however, this world does not arise from the absolute nor does it merge in it. The absolute alone exists now and for ever. When one thinks of it as a void, it is because of the feeling one has that it is not void; when one thinks of it as not-void, it is because there is a feeling that it is void.

The absolute is immaterial and so material sources of light like the sun, do not illumine it. But it is self-luminous, and therefore it is not inert or dark. This absolute cannot be realised or experienced by another; only the absolute can realise itself.

The infinite (space of) consciousness is even purer than infinite space; and the world is even as that infinite is. But, one who has not tasted capsicum does not know its taste; even so, one does not experience consciousness in the infinite in the absence of objectivity. Hence, even this consciousness appears to be inert or insentient, and the world is experienced as such too. Even as in tangible ocean tangible waves are seen, in the formless Brahman the world also exists without form. **From the infinite the infinite emerges and exists in it as the infinite; hence the world has never really been created — it is the same as that from which it emerges.**

When the notion of self is destroyed by the withdrawal of the fuel of ideas from the mind, that which is, is the infinite. That which is not sleep nor inert, is the infinite. It is on account of the infinite that knowledge, knower and known exist as one, in the absence of the intellect.

ādāv eva hi yan nā 'sti kāraṇāsaṁbhavāt svayaṁ
vartamāne 'pi tan nā 'sti nāśaḥ syāt tatra kīdṛśaḥ (13)

RĀMA said:

Lord, during the cosmic dissolution, this world which is clearly seen now -- where does it go?

VASIṢṬHA said:

From where does the son of a barren woman come, and where does he go? A barren woman's son has no existence, ever. Even so, this world as such has no existence, ever. This analogy baffles you only because you have taken the existence of the world for granted.

Consider this: Is there a bracelet-ness in the golden bracelet, is it not just gold? Is there a thing called sky independent of the emptiness? Even so, there is no 'thing' called the world independent of Brahman the absolute. Just as coldness is inseparable from ice, what is called the world is inseparable from Brahman.

Water in the mirage does not come into being and go out of existence; even so this world does not come out of the absolute nor does it go anywhere. **The creation of the world has no cause, and therefore it has had no beginning. It does not exist even now; how can it reach destruction?**

If you concede that the world has not been created out of Brahman but assert that it is an appearance based on the reality of Brahman, then indeed it does not exist and Brahman alone exists. It is like a dream: in a state of ignorance the intelligence within oneself appears as numerous dream-objects, all of which are nothing other than that intelligence. Even so, in what is known as the beginning of creation, such an appearance happened; but it is not independent of Brahman, it does not exist apart from Brahman, hence it does not exist.

RĀMA said:

Holy sir, if that is so, how is it that this world has acquired such a sense of reality? As long as the perceiver is, the perceived exists, and vice versa, and only when both these come to an end is there liberation. If there is a clean mirror, it reflects something or other all the time: even so in the seer this creation will again and again arise. However, if the non-existence of creation is realised then the seer ceases to be. But, such a realisation is hard to get!

VASIṢṬHA said:

Rāma, I shall presently dispel your doubts with the help of a parable. You will then realise the non-existence of creation and lead an enlightened life in this world.

jagataḥ pañcakaṁ bījaṁ pañcakasya cid avyayā
yad bījaṁ tat phalaṁ viddhi tasmād brahmamayaṁ jagat (13/9)

VASIṢṬHA said:

O Rāma, I shall narrate to you how this creation appears to have emerged from the one pure undivided cosmic being, even as dreams appear in the consciousness of the sleeping person.

This universe is in fact the eternal effulgent infinite consciousness which generates within itself the knowable (which would be known as that which is to be) with an idea concerning its form (which is space), and with an enquiry concerning itself. Thus is space brought into being. When, after a considerable time the consciousness of creation becomes strong in the infinite being, the future jīva (living cosmic soul — also known as Hiraṇyagarbha) arises within it: and the infinite abandons, as it were, its supreme state, to limit itself as the jīva. However, even then Brahman remains the infinite, and there is no real transformation into any of these.

In space, the faculty of sound manifests itself. Then comes into being egotism which is vital to further creation of the universe, and, at the same time, the factor known as time. All this happens merely by the creative-thought inherent in the cosmic being, not as real transformations of the infinite.

By the similar exercise of the creative-thought, air is created. Consciousness which is surrounded by all these is called the jīva which gives rise to all the different elements in this world.

There are fourteen planes of existence, each with its own type of inhabitants. And all these are the manifestations of the creative-thought of consciousness. Even so, when this consciousness thought: 'I am light', sources of light like the sun, etc., were instantly created. Similarly water and earth were created.

All these fundamental elements continued to act upon one another — as experiencer and experience — and the entire creation comes into being like ripples on the surface of the ocean. And, they are interwoven and mixed up so effectively that they cannot be extricated from one another till the cosmic dissolution. These material appearances are ever changing and the reality exists unchanged; since these are all linked with consciousness, they instantly become gross physical substance, though all these are the infinite consciousness alone, which has undergone no change whatsoever.

The five elements are the seed of which the world is the tree; and the eternal consciousness is the seed for the elements. As is the seed, so is the fruit (tree). Therefore, the world is nothing but Brahman the absolute.

asatyām satyasaṁkāśām brahmā "ste jīvaśabdavat
ittham sa jīvaśabdārthaḥ kalanākulatām gataḥ (13/33)

VASIṢṬHA continued:

Rāma, I shall now tell you how the jiva (living soul) came to dwell in this body.

The jīva thought "I am atomic in nature and stature" and so it became atomic in nature. Yet, it only apparently became so, on account of its imagination which was false. Even as one may dream that he is dead and that he has another body, this jīva which in truth had an extremely subtle body of pure consciousness, now begins to identify itself with grossness and so becomes gross. Even as a mountain is reflected in a mirror and is seen as if it were in the mirror, the jīva reflects the external objects and activities, and soon begins to think that they are all within itself and that he is the doer of the actions and the experiencer of experiences.

When the jīva wishes to see, eyes are formed in the gross body. Even so the skin (tactile sense), ears, tongue, nose and the organs of action are formed as a result of the appropriate desire arising in the jīva. Thus in the body abides the jiva, which has the extremely subtle body of consciousness, imagining various external physical experiences and various internal psychological experiences. Thus resting in the unreal which however appears to be real, Brahman, now appearing to be jiva, becomes confused.

This same Brahman which has come to regard itself as a finite jīva and endowed with a physical body, apprehends the external world which on account of the veil of ignorance appears to be composed of matter. Someone thinks he is Brahma, someone else thinks he is something else — in this manner the jīva imagines it is this or that, and so binds itself to the illusion of world-appearance.

Rāma; there is neither one jīva nor many nor a conglomerate of jīvā. Jiva is only a name! What exists is only Brahman. Because he is omnipotent, his thought-forms materialise. One alone appears as diverse on account of ignorance; we do not experience this ignorance which disappears on enquiry even as darkness vanishes when light is brought in to look at it. Brahman alone is the cosmic (Mahajīva) soul and the millions of jīvā. There is naught else.

But all this is mere imagination or thought. Even now nothing has ever been created; the pure infinite space alone exists. Brahmā the creator could not create the world as it was before the cosmic dissolution, for Brahmā attained final liberation then. Cosmic consciousness alone exists now and ever; in it are no worlds, no created beings. That consciousness reflected in itself appears to be creation. Even as an unreal nightmare produces real results, this world seems to give rise to a sense of reality in a state of ignorance. When true wisdom arises, this unreality vanishes.

cetya saṁvedanāt jīvo bhavatyāyāti saṁsṛtiṁ
tad asaṁvedanād rūpaṁ samāyāti samaṁ punaḥ (36)

VASIṢṬHA continued:

By the apprehension of the perceived or the knowable, consciousness becomes jīva (the living soul) and is apparently involved in repetitive history (saṁsāra). When the false notion of a knowable apart from the knower (consciousness) ceases, it regains its equilibrium.

The mysterious power of consciousness which in an inexplicable and miraculous way produces this infinite diversity of names and forms (body) is known as egotism. When egotism has come into being, that egotism (which is non-different from consciousness) entertains notions of the various elements that constitute this universe, and they arise. In unity diversity arises. Rāma, give up all these false notions of 'I' and 'you', by renouncing even the notions of a jīva and its own cause. When all these have gone, you will realise the truth which is in the middle between the real and the unreal.

This consciousness is not knowable: when it wishes to become the knowable it is known as the universe. Mind, intellect, egotism, the five great elements, and the world — all these innumerable names and forms are all consciousness alone. A man and his life and works are indistinguishable, the static and the kinetic manifestations of the same factor. Jīva and the mind etc. are all vibrations in consciousness. This is the truth. People like to argue and confuse others; they are indeed confused. But, O Rāma, we are beyond confusion. Changes in the unchanging are imagined by ignorant and deluded people; but in the vision of sages who have self-knowledge no change whatsoever has taken place in consciousness.

When the notion of an external knowable has been removed, self-knowledge arises; and when in it there is the notion of inertia or ignorance, the state of deep sleep has come to it. Hence, since consciousness alone exists at all times, it may be said that space exists and does not exist, the world exists and does not exist.

Even as heat is to fire, whiteness is to a conch-shell, firmness is to a mountain, liquidity is to water, butter is to milk, coolness is to ice, brightness is to illumination, oil is to mustard seed, flow is to a river, sweetness is to honey, ornament is to gold, aroma is to a flower — the universe is to consciousness. The world exists because consciousness is: and the world is the body of consciousness. There is no division, no difference, no distinction. Hence the universe can be said to be both real and unreal; real because of the reality of consciousness which is its own reality, and unreal because the universe does not exist as universe, independent of consciousness.

But, because of the unreality of the universe, etc., it cannot be said that its own cause, namely, the consciousness, is also unreal: such a statement would only be a set of words with no meaning — for it runs counter to our experience, and the existence of consciousness cannot be denied.

(At this stage, the third evening set in: and the assembly dispersed.)

varjayitvā 'jñavijñānaṁ jagac chabdārtha bhājanaṁ
jagad brahma sva śabdānāmarthe nā 'styeva bhinnatā (10)

VASIṢṬHA continued:

O Rāma, even as from the waking state experience, there is no materiality in the objects seen in a dream (though while dreaming the objects appear to be solid) this world appears to be material yet in reality it is pure consciousness. There is not even a temporary or subtle river in the mirage: even so there is in no sense a real world, but only pure consciousness. **Only knowledge based on ignorance clings to the notion of a world; in reality, there is no difference in the meaning of the words 'world', 'Brahman or the infinite' and 'self'.** The world is as true in relation to Brahman as the dream-city is true in relation to the experience of the waking consciousness. Hence, 'world' and 'cosmic consciousness' are synonyms.

To make all this crystal clear, O Rāma, I shall now narrate to you the story of Maṇḍapa: pray, listen attentively.

Once upon a time, O Rāma, there was a king on earth called Padma. He was perfect in every respect; and by his own nature and conduct he enhanced the glory of his dynasty. He honoured religious traditions even as the ocean respects the authority of the shore. He subdued his enemies even as the sun routs darkness. Even as fire reduces hay to ashes, he destroyed evil in society. Holy men resorted to him even as gods resort to heaven. He was the abode of virtue. He made his enemies tremble on the battlefield even as a gale ruffles a creeper. He was highly learned and a master of arts. To him there was nothing impossible of achievement, even as to lord Nārāyaṇa there was no impossibility.

This king had a wife by name Līlā. She was highly accomplished as a woman and was very beautiful. It appeared as if she was goddess Lakshmī (consort of Nārāyaṇa) incarnate on earth. She was soft-spoken, her gait was slow and graceful and her smile radiated the cool delight of moonlight. She was fair. She was sweet as honey. Her arms were soft and delicate. Her body was as pure and clear as the waters of the holy river Gaṅgā; and even as a touch of the waters of the Gaṅgā gives rise to bliss, to touch her was to experience bliss. She was highly devoted to her husband Padma and knew how to serve him and to please him.

She was one with the king, and shared his joy and sorrow. She was in fact the alter ego of Padma — except that when the king became angry, she merely reflected fear.

cittākāśaṁ cidākāśaṁ ākāsaṁ ca tṛtīyakaṁ
dvābhyāṁ śūnyataraṁ viddhi cidākāśaṁ varānane (17/10)

VASIṢṬHA continued:

King Padma and queen Līlā lived an ideal life. They enjoyed their life in every possible and righteous way. They were young and youthful like the gods, and their love for each other was pure and intense, without any hypocrisy or artificiality. One day, the queen Līlā thought: "The most handsome king who is my husband is dearer to me than even my own life. What should I do in order that he and I may live forever enjoying the pleasures of life? I shall immediately undertake such austerities as the holy ones would suggest in order that I may fulfil my ambition." She sought the counsel of the holy ones, who said to her: "O queen, austerities or penance, repetition of mantrā and a disciplined life will surely bestow upon you all that it is possible for one to attain in this world; but physical immortality is not possible of attainment in this world!"

Līlā began to propitiate the goddess Sarasvatī immediately, without even discussing this project with her husband. The goddess Sarasvatī appeared before her and granted her the boons of her choice. Līlā prayed: "O Divine Mother, grant me two boons: (1) when my husband departs from his body, let his jīva remain in the palace, and (2) whenever I pray to you, let me see you." Sarasvatī granted these two boons and disappeared. Time inexorably passed. King Padma, who was mortally wounded on the battlefield, died in the palace. Queen Līlā was inconsolable with grief. When she was thus sunk in grief the ethereal voice of Sarasvatī said: "My child, cover the king's dead body with flowers; then it will not decay. He will not leave the palace.

(Līlā asked her: "Pray, tell me where my husband is".)

"O Līlā, there are three types of space — the psychological space, the physical space and the infinite space of consciousness. Of these the most subtle is the infinite space of consciousness. By intense meditation on this infinite space of consciousness you can see and experience the presence of one (like your husband) whose body is that infinite space, even though you do not see him here. That is the infinite space which exists in the middle when the finite intelligence travels from one place to another; for it is infinite. If you give up all thoughts you will here and now attain to the realisation of oneness with all. Normally only he who has realised the utter non-existence of the universe can experience this; but you will do so by my grace."

VASISTHA continued:

Līlā began to meditate. Immediately she entered the highest state of consciousness free from all distractions (nirvikalpa). She was in the infinite space of consciousness. There she saw the king once again, on a throne, surrounded by many kings who adored him — but they did not see her. She wondered: are they all dead, too! Again, by the grace of goddess Sarasvatī, she came back to her palace, and saw her attendants asleep. She woke them and asked them to request the members of the royal court to assemble at once.

ādarśe 'ntarbahiścaiva yathā śailo 'nubhūyate
bahirantaś cid ādarśe tathā sargo 'nubhūyate (18/5)

VASIṢṬHA continued:

Seeing all the members of the royal court, Līlā was puzzled: she thought, "This is strange, for these people seem to exist in two places at the same time — in that region which I saw in my meditation and here in front of me. **Just as a mountain is seen both inside the mirror and outside it, this creation is seen both within consciousness and outside it.** But; which of these is real and which the reflection? I must find out from Sarasvatī." She adored Sarasvatī and saw her seated in front of her.

LĪLĀ asked: Be gracious, O Goddess, and tell me this. That on which this world is reflected is extremely pure and undivided, and it is not the object of knowledge. This world exists both within it as its reflection and outside as solid matter: which is real and which the reflection?

SARASVATĪ asked: Tell me first: what do you consider real and what unreal?

LĪLĀ answered: That I am here and you are in front of me — this I consider real. That region in which my husband is now — that I consider unreal.

SARASVATĪ said: How can the unreal be the effect of the real? The effect is the cause, there is no essential difference. Even in the case of a pot which is able to hold water whereas its cause (clay) cannot, this difference is due to the co-operative causes. What was the material cause of your husband's birth? For only material effects are produced by material causes. Hence when you find no immediate cause for an effect, then surely the cause existed in the past — memory. Memory is like space, empty. All creation here is the effect of that emptiness — and hence the creation is empty, too. Even as the birth of your husband is an illusory product of memory, I see all this as the illusory and unreal effect of imagination.

I shall narrate to you a story which illustrates the dream-like nature of this creation. In pure consciousness, in a corner of the mind of the Creator, there was a dilapidated shrine covered with a blue dome. It had the fourteen worlds for rooms. The three divisions of space were holes in it. The sun was the light. In it there were little ant hills (the cities), little piles of earth (mountains) and little pools of water (the oceans). This is creation, the universe. In a very small corner of it there lived a holy man with his wife and children. He was healthy and free from fear. He performed his religious and social duties well.

That holy man was known as Vasiṣṭha and his wife was Arundhatī. One day he saw a colourful procession with a king riding a stately elephant, followed by an army and other royal paraphernalia. Looking at this a wish arose in his heart: "When will I ride a royal elephant like that and be followed by an army like this?"

yathaitat pratibhāmātraṁ jagat sargāvabhāsanaṁ
tathaitat pratibhāmātraṁ kṣaṇakalpāvabhāsanaṁ (20/29)

SARASVATĪ continued:

Some time after this the holy man grew old and then death overtook him. His wife, who was highly devoted to him, prayed to me and asked for the same boon that you had asked for: that her husband's spirit should not leave her house. I granted her that boon. Though that holy man was an ethereal being, on account of the power of his constant wish during the previous life-span he became a mighty king and ruled over a great empire which resembled heaven on earth. Arundhatī had also given up her body and attained reunion with her husband. It is eight days since this happened.

Līlā, it is the same holy man who is now your husband, the king; and you are the same Arundhatī who was his wife. On account of ignorance and delusion it seems that all this takes place in the infinite consciousness, though in reality nothing happens. I do not utter falsehood, but am telling the truth. It sounds incredible but this kingdom appears to be only in the hut of the holy man on account of his desire for a kingdom. The memory of the past is hidden, and you two have risen again. Death is but waking from a dream. Birth which arises from a wish is no more real than the wish, like waves in a mirage! Even after the 'creation' of all this in the holy man's house, it remained as it was before. Indeed, in every atom there are worlds within worlds.

LĪLĀ asked:

O Goddess, you said that it was only eight days ago that the holy man had died; and yet my husband and I have lived for a long time. How can you reconcile this discrepancy?

SARASVATĪ said:

O Līlā, just as space does not have a fixed span, time does not have a fixed span either. **Just as the world and its creation are mere appearances, a moment and an epoch are also imaginary,** not real. In the twinkling of an eye the jīva undergoes the illusion of the death-experience, forgets what happened before that, and in the infinite consciousness thinks 'I am this' etc., and 'I am his son, I am so many years old', etc.

Even as in a dream there is birth, death and relationship all in a very short time, and even as a lover feels that a single night without his beloved is an epoch, the jīva thinks of experienced and non-experienced objects in the twinkling of an eye. And, immediately thereafter, he imagines those things (the world) to be real. Even those things, which he had not experienced nor seen, present themselves before him as in a dream.

This world and this creation is nothing but memory, dream: distance and measures of time (like a moment and an age) are all hallucinations. This is one kind of knowledge — memory. There is another which is not based on memory of past experiences. This is the fortuitous meeting of atoms in consciousness which are then able to produce their own effects.

mahācidrūpam eva tvaṁ smaraṇaṁ viddhi vedanaṁ
kāryakāraṇatā tena sa śabdo na ca vāstavaḥ (23)

SARASVATĪ continued:

Liberation is the realisation of the total non-existence of the universe as such. This is different from a mere denial of the existence of the ego and the universe! The latter is only half-knowledge. Liberation is to realise that all this is pure consciousness.

Indeed, the prior hallucination of the creation of the holy man and his wife was due to the thought-form of Brahmā, the creator. He himself had no hidden thought-forms (memory), for before creation there was dissolution and at that time the Creator had attained liberation. At the beginning of this epoch, someone assumes the role of creator and thinks "I am the new Creator" — this is pure coincidence, even as one sees a crow alighting on a palm tree and the cocoanut falling, though these two are independent of each other. Of course, do not forget that even though all this seems to happen, there is no creation! **The one infinite consciousness alone is thought-form or experience: there is no cause and effect relationship. These ('cause' and 'effect') are only words, not facts.** The infinite consciousness is forever in infinite consciousness.

LĪLĀ said:

O Goddess, your words are truly enlightening. However, since I have never been exposed to them before, the wisdom is not well grounded. I wish to see the original house of the holy Vasiṣṭha.

SARASVATĪ said:

O Lilā, give up this form of yours and attain the pure spiritual insight. For only Brahman can really see or realise Brahman. My body is made of pure light, pure consciousness. Your body is not. With this body of yours you cannot even visit the places of your own imagination, then how can you enter the field of another's imagination? But if you attain the body of light, you will immediately see the holy man's house. Affirm to yourself, "I shall leave my body here and take a body of light. With that body, like the scent of incense I shall go to the house of the holy man." Even as water mixes with water, you will become one with the field of consciousness.

By the persistent practice of such meditation, even your body will become one of pure consciousness and subtle. For, I see even my body as consciousness. You do not, for you see the world of matter. Such ignorance arises of its own accord, but is dispelled by wisdom and enquiry. In fact such ignorance does not even exist! There is neither unwisdom, nor ignorance; neither bondage, nor liberation. There is but one pure consciousness.

taccintanaṁ tatkathanaṁ anyonyaṁ tat prabodhanaṁ
etad eka paratvaṁ ca tad abhyāsaṁ vidur budhāḥ (22/24)

SARASVATĪ said:

Dear Līlā, in dream, the dream-body appears to be real; but when there is an awakening to the fact of dream, the reality of that body vanishes. Even so, the physical body which is sustained by memory and latent tendencies is seen to be unreal when they are seen to be unreal. At the end of the dream, you become aware of the physical body; at the end of these tendencies, you become aware of the etheral body. When the dream ends, deep sleep ensues; when the seeds of thought perish, you are liberated. In liberation the seeds of thought do not exist: if the liberated sage appears to live and to think, he only appears to do so, like a burnt cloth lying on the floor. This is, however, not like deep sleep or unconsciousness, in both of which the seeds of thought lie hidden.

By persistent practice (abhyāsa) egotism is quietened. Then you will naturally rest in your consciousness; and the perceived universe heads towards the vanishing point. What is called practice?

Thinking of that alone, speaking of that, conversing of that with one another, utter dedication to that one alone — this is called abhyāsa or practice by the wise. When one's intellect is filled with beauty and bliss, when one's vision is broad, when passion for sensual enjoyment is absent in one – that is practice. When one is firmly established in the conviction that this universe has never even been created, and therefore it does not exist as such, and when thoughts like 'This is world, this I am' do not arise at all in one — this is abhyāsa or practice. It is then that attraction and repulsion do not arise; the overcoming of attraction and repulsion by the use of willforce is austerity, not wisdom.

(At this stage, evening set in; and the court dispersed. Early next morning the court assembled, and Vasiṣṭha continued his discourse.)

VASIṢṬHA continued:

O Rāma, Sarasvatī and queen Līlā immediately sat in deep meditation or nirvikalpa samādhi. They had risen above body-consciousness. Because they had given up all notions of the world, it had completely vanished in their consciousness. They roamed freely in their wisdom-bodies. Though it seemed that they had travelled millions of miles in space, they were still in the same 'room' but on another plane of consciousness. They saw all that was already in the mind of Sarasvatī and which Sarasvatī wanted to show to queen Līlā.

Having seen the oceans, mountains, the protectors of the universe, the kingdom of the gods, the sky and the very bowels of the earth, Līlā saw her own house.

paramāṇau paramāṇau sargavargā nirargalaṁ
mahāciteḥ sphuranty arkarucīva trasareṇavaḥ (27/29)

VASIṢṬHA continued:

O Rāma, the two ladies then entered into the holy man's house. The whole family was in mourning. On account of their grief the house itself had a depressing atmosphere. By the practice of the yoga of pure wisdom Līlā had acquired that faculty by which her thoughts instantly materialised. She wished, "These, my relations, should see me and Sarasvatī as if we were ordinary womenfolk." They appeared so to the mourning family. But the two ladies were of supernatural radiance which dispelled the gloom that pervaded the house. They asked the eldest son of the departed holy couple: "Tell us the cause of the sorrow which seems to afflict all these people here."

The son of the holy couple replied: "O ladies, in this very house there lived a pious man and his devoted wife, who were both devoted to a righteous life. Recently, they abandoned their children and grandchildren, their house and their cattle, and ascended to heaven. Therefore, to us the whole world appears to be empty." Hearing this, Līlā laid her hand on the young man's head: instantly he was relieved of his sorrow.

LĪLĀ asked Sarasvatī:

How was it that we were seen by this family of mine here, and we were not seen by my husband who was ruling a kingdom when we visited him?

SARASVATĪ answered:

Then you were still clinging to your notion 'I am Līlā'; now you have overcome that body-consciousness. Till the consciousness of duality is completely dispelled, you cannot act in the infinite consciousness; you cannot even understand it, even as one standing in the sun does not know the coolness of the shade of a tree. But now if you go to your husband you will be able to deal with him as before. Līlā, you and your husband have been through many incarnations, three of which you now know. In this incarnation the king has slipped deep into the snare of worldliness and he thinks "I am the lord, I am strong, I am happy, etc." Though from the spiritual standpoint the whole universe is experienced here, from the physical point of view millions of miles separate the planes. **In the infinite consciousness, in every atom of it, universes come and go like particles of dust in a beam of sunlight that shines through a hole in the roof.** These come and go like ripples on the ocean.

LĪLĀ reminisced: O Divinity! Since emerging as a reflection in the infinite consciousness I have had 800 births. Today I see this. I have been a nymph, a vicious human woman, a serpent, a forest tribal woman, and on account of evil deeds I became a creeper, and by the proximity of sages I became a sage's daughter; I became a king, and on account of evil deeds done then I became a mosquito, a bee, a deer, a bird, a fish; and again I became a celestial, after which I became a tortoise, and a swan, and I became a mosquito again. I have also been a celestial nymph when other celestials (males) used to fall at my feet. Just as the scales of balance seesaw constantly, I have also been caught up in the seesaw of this repetitive existence (saṁsāra).

ihaivā 'ṅguṣṭamātrānte tad vyomny eva padaṁ sthitaṁ
mad bhartṛ rājya samavagataṁ yojanakoṭibhāk (29/36)

RĀMA asked:

Holy sir, how was it possible for the two ladies to travel to distant galaxies in the universe, and how did they overcome the numerous barriers on the way?

VASIṢṬHA replied:

O Rāma, where is universe, where are galaxies, where are barriers? The two ladies remained in the queen's inner apartment. It was there that the holy man Vasiṣṭha was ruling as king Vidūratha; it was he who was king Padma before. All this happened in pure space: there is no universe, no distance, no barriers.

Conversing with each other, the two ladies emerged from the room and proceeded towards a village on top of a mountain.

On account of the intensity of her practice of the yoga of wisdom, Līlā had acquired full knowledge of the past, present and future. She recollected the past and said to Sarasvatī: "O Divinity, some time ago my husband and I lived an ordinary unenlightened life. We did not practise self-inquiry." After saying this, Līlā showed to Sarasvatī her previous dwelling, and continued: "See, this is my favourite calf. On account of my separation, it has been constantly weeping for the past eight days. In this place, my husband ruled the world. Because he was determined to be a great king soon, he had indeed become an emperor within the short span of eight days, though it looked like a long, long time. In this house my husband lives, unseen. **Here, in the space of the size of a thumb, we imagined the kingdom of my husband to be a million square miles.** O Divinity, surely both my husband and I are of pure consciousness; yet, on account of the mysterious illusory power, Māyā, my husband's kingdom appears to encompass hundreds of mountains. This is truly marvellous. I wish to enter into the capital city where my husband rules. Come let us go there: for what is impossible of achievement to the industrious?"

Sarasvatī and Līlā rose into space and saw the whole creation; and beyond that was pure consciousness. Because of the essential nature of this infinite consciousness, universes, jivā and forms keep arising and again arising, and by their own thought-force, return to a state of tranquillity; all this is like the spontaneous play of a child.

Of those countless universes, O Rāma, in some there are only plants; some have Brahmā, Viṣṇu, Rudra and others as the presiding deities, and some have none at all; in some there are only animals and birds; in some there is only an ocean; some are solid rocks, some are inhabited only by worms; some are pervaded by dense darkness; in some angels dwell; some are forever illumined. Some seem to be heading towards dissolution; some seem to be falling in space towards destruction. Since consciousness exists everywhere for ever, creation of these universes and their dissolution also goes on everywhere for ever. All these are held together by a mysterious omnipresent power. Rāma, everything exists in the one infinite consciousness; everything arises from it; it alone is everything.

yathā saṁvit tathā cittaṁ sā tathā 'vasthitiṁ gatā
parameṇa prayatnena nīyate 'nyadaśāṁ punaḥ (40/13)

VASIṢṬHA continued:

Having seen all this, Līlā saw the inner apartment of the palace where the corpse of the king lay buried under a heap of flowers. There arose in her an intense wish to behold her husband's other life. Instantly, she broke through the summit of the universe and entered into the realm where her husband now ruled.

At the same time, a mighty king who ruled over the Sindhu region was laying siege to her husband's kingdom. As the two ladies were coursing the space above the battlefield they encountered countless celestials who had assembled there to witness the battle and the exploits of the great heroes.

O Rāma, still standing in the sky, Līlā saw the two great armies closing in on each other, ready to engage themselves in battle.

As evening set in, Līlā's husband held council with his ministers concerning the events of the morning; and then he went to sleep.

The two ladies left the place where they stood watching the fierce battle, and travelling like a breath of air, entered unobstructed into the closed apartment where the king was asleep.

O Rāma, it is impossible for one who is rooted in the idea that he is a physical body to pass through a subtle hole. It is the innermost conviction 'I am the body which is obstructed thus in its movement' that in fact manifests as such obstruction: when the former is absent, the latter is absent, too. For the same infinite consciousness is also the individual consciousness (mind) and the cosmic space (material). Therefore the ethereal body can enter anything anywhere, and it goes where the wish of its heart leads.

Just as water ever remains water and flows down, and fire does not abandon its nature of rising up, consciousness remains for ever consciousness. But, he who has not understood this does not experience its subtlety or true nature. **As is his understanding so is his mind, for it is the understanding that is the mind; yet, its direction can be changed by great effort.** Normally, one's actions are in accordance with one's mind, (i.e., one's understanding).

O Rāma, everyone's consciousness is of this nature and power. In everyone's consciousness there is a different idea of the world. Death and other such experiences are like cosmic dissolution, the night of cosmic consciousness. When that comes to an end everyone wakes up to one's own mental creation, which is the materialisation of one's ideas, notions and delusions. Even as the cosmic being creates the universe after the cosmic dissolution, the individual creates his own world after his death.

dirgha svapnam idaṁ visvaṁ viddhy ahantādi saṁyutaṁ
atrā'nye svapna puruṣā yathā satyās tathā śṛṇu (42/8)

VASIṢṬHA continued:

The two ladies entered the apartment of the king like two divinities, resplendent like two moons. When Sarasvatī asked the king who he was, the minister informed the ladies that he was Vidūratha. Sarasvatī then blessed Vidūratha by laying her hand on his head, and inspired him to recollect the facts of his previous lives. Instantly, the king remembered everything and asked Sarasvatī: "How is it that though it is hardly one day since I died, it seems that I have lived in this body a full seventy years?"

SARASVATĪ replied:

O king, at the very moment of your death and in the very place of your death, all this that you are seeing here manifested. All this is where the holy man Vasiṣṭha lived, in the village on the hill. That is his world, and in that world is the world of king Padma, and in that world of king Padma is the world that you are in. Living in it you think: "These are my relations, these are my subjects, these are my ministers, these are my enemies"; you think that you are ruling, you are engaged in religious rites; you think that you have been fighting with your enemies and you were defeated by them; you think you are seeing us, worshipping us, and that you are receiving enlightenment from us. All this took no time to happen, even as in no time during a dream a whole life's drama is enacted. In reality, you are unborn and you do not die. To the enlightened person there is only one infinite consciousness, and there is no notion of 'I am' or 'these are'. (While Vasiṣṭha said this, another day came to an end.)

To an immature and childish person who is confirmed in his conviction that this world is real, it continues to be real. He who sees the glory of palaces, elephants and cities does not see the infinite consciousness which alone is true. **This universe is but a long dream. The ego-sense and also the fancy that there are others, are as real as dream-objects.** The sole reality is the infinite consciousness which is omnipresent, pure, tranquil, omnipotent, and whose very body and being is absolute consciousness (therefore not an object, not knowable): wherever this consciousness manifests in whatever manner, it is that. Because the substratum (the infinite consciousness) is real, all that is based on it acquires reality, though the reality is of the substratum alone. This universe and all beings in it are but a long dream. To me you are real, and to you I am real; even so the others are real to you or to me. And, this relative reality is like the reality of the dream-objects.

O king, you shall die in this war and then you will regain your previous kingdom. After your death in this body, you will come over to the previous city with your daughter and your ministers. We two shall go now as we came; and all of you will of course follow us in due course: for the nature of the motion of a horse, an elephant and a camel is different!

mṛtir janmany asadrūpā mṛtyāṁ janmā 'py asanmayaṁ
viśared viśarārutvād anubhūteś ca rāghava (44/26)

VASIṢṬHA continued:

Even as Sarasvatī was saying this to the king, a royal messenger rushed in to announce that the enemy forces had entered the capital and were destroying it.

In the meantime, the queen arrived there. The lady-in-waiting announced her to the king. She said: "Your Majesty, all the other ladies of the harem have been violently dragged away by the enemy. From this indescribable calamity that has befallen us, only Your Majesty can redeem us."

The king bowed to Sarasvatī and excused himself, "I shall myself go to the battle-front, O Goddess, to deal with the enemy; and this, my wife, will wait upon you during that time."

The enlightened Līlā was amazed to see that the Queen was a complete replica of herself. She asked Sarasvatī: "O Divinity, how is it that she is exactly what I am? Whatever I was in my own youth, she is now. What is the secret of this? Also: all these ministers, etc., who are here, are the same that were there, in our palace. If they are but a reflection or the objects of our fancy, are they sentient and are they also endowed with consciousness?"

SARASVATĪ replied:

O Līlā, whatever vision arises within oneself, that is immediately experienced. Consciousness (as subject) itself becomes, as it were, the object of knowledge. When in consciousness the image of the world arises, at that very instant it becomes so. Time, space, duration and objectivity do not arise from matter; for then they would be material. What is reflected in one's consciousness shines outside also.

What is regarded as the real objective world experienced in the waking state is no more real than that experienced during sleep (dream). During sleep, the world does not exist; and during the waking state, the dream does not exist! **Even so, death contradicts life: while living, death is non-existent, and in death, life is non-existent. Because, that which holds together either experience is absent in the other.**

One cannot say that either is real, or unreal, but one can only say that their substratum alone is real. The universe exists in Brahman only as a word, an idea. It is neither real nor unreal: just as a snake-in-a-rope is neither real nor unreal. Even so is the existence of the jīva. This jīva experiences its own wishes. It fancies that it experiences what it had experienced before; and some others are new experiences. They are similar at times and dissimilar at times. All these experiences, though essentially unreal, appear to be real. Such is the nature of these ministers and others. Even so this Līlā exists as the product of the reflection in consciousness. Even so are you, me and all others. Know this and rest in peace.

tapo vā devatā vā 'pi bhūtvā svaiva cid anyathā
phalaṁ dadāty atha svairaṁ nabhaḥ phala nipātavat (45/19)

THE SECOND LĪLĀ said to Sarasvatī:

O Divinity, I used to worship Sarasvatī and she used to appear to me in my dreams. You look exactly like her: I presume that you are Sarasvatī. I humbly beg of you to grant me a boon — when my husband dies on the battlefield, may I accompany him to whichever realm he goes, in this very body of mine.

SARASVATĪ replied:

O dear lady, you have worshipped me for a long time with intense devotion: therefore, I grant you the boon sought by you.

THE FIRST LĪLĀ thereupon said to Sarasvatī:

Truly, your words never fail, your wish always comes true. Pray, tell me why you did not allow me to travel from one plane of consciousness to another with the same body.

SARASVATĪ replied:

My dear Līlā, I do not really do anything to anyone. Every jīva earns its own state by its own deeds. I am merely the deity presiding over the intelligence of every being; I am the power of its consciousness and its life-force. Whatever form the energy of the living being takes within itself, that alone comes to fruition in course of time. You longed for liberation, and you obtained it. **You may consider it the fruit of your austerity or worship of the deity; but it is consciousness alone that bestows the fruit upon you — even as the fruit that seems to fall from the sky really falls from the tree.**

VASIṢṬHA continued:

As they were talking among themselves like this, the king Vidūratha ascended his resplendent chariot and proceeded to the battlefront. Unfortunately, he had not assessed the relative strength of his and the enemy's forces right up to the moment he actually entered into the enemy ranks.

The two Līlā, Sarasvatī, as also the princess who had received the blessings of Sarasvatī, were watching the terrible war from their apartment in the palace.

The sky was crowded with the missiles from both the armies. The battle cries of the warriors were heard everywhere. There was a pall of smoke and dust over the entire city.

Even as the king Vidūratha entered the ranks of the enemy, there was an intense tut-tut sound of intense crossfire. As the missiles collided, there were sounds like khut-khut, tuk-tuk, jhun-jhun.

yo yathā prerayati māṁ tasya tiṣṭhāmi tat phalā
na svabhāvo 'nyatāṁ dhatte vahner auṣṇyamivaiṣa me (47/5)

VASIṢTHA continued:

THE SECOND LĪLĀ asked Sarasvatī: O Goddess, please tell me why it is that though we are blessed by you, my husband cannot win the battle?

SARASVATĪ replied: No doubt, I was adored by king Vidūratha for a considerable time, but he did not pray for victory in battle. Being the consciousness that dwells in the understanding of every person, I bestow upon that person that which he seeks. **Whatever it be that a person asks of me, I bestow upon him that fruit: it is but natural that fires gives you heat.** He had asked for liberation; and he shall attain liberation. On the other hand, the king of Sindhu worshipped me and prayed for victory in battle. Hence, the king Vidūratha will be slain in battle, and he will rejoin you both and in course of time will attain liberation. This king of Sindhu will win the war and will rule the country as the victorious monarch.

At one stage both the kings lost their vehicles. As Vidūratha was about to ascend a new one he was cut down by the king of Sindhu. Seeing Vidūratha fall, the second Līlā fell unconscious. The first Līlā said to Sarasvatī: "O Goddess, see, this my husband is about to give up the ghost."

SARASVATĪ said: Dear one, all this terrible war, this destruction and death, are as real as a dream; for there is neither a kingdom nor the earth. All this took place in the house of the holy man Vasiṣṭha on top of the hill. This palace and this battlefield and all the rest of it is nowhere but the inner apartments of your own palace. In fact, the entire universe is there. For, within the house of the holy man is the world of the king Padma; and within the palace of that king in that world is all that you have seen here. All this is mere fancy, hallucination. What is, is the sole reality — which is neither created nor destroyed. It is that infinite consciousness that is perceived by the ignorant as the universe. Just as a whole city exists within the dreamer, the three worlds exist in a small atom; surely, there are atoms in those worlds, and each one of those atoms also contains the three worlds. The other Līlā who fell down unconscious has already reached that world in which your husband Padma's body is lying.

LĪLĀ asked: O Goddess, tell me: how did she go there already, and what are the people there telling her?

SARASVATĪ replied: Just as both of you are the fancied objects of the king, even so the king himself and I are dream-objects. One who knows this gives up looking for 'objects of perception'. In the infinite consciousness we have created each other in our fancy. The other youthful Līlā was indeed yourself. She worshipped me and prayed that she would never be widowed; hence, before the king Vidūratha died she left this place. Dear one, you are all individualised cosmic consciousness, but I am the cosmic consciousness: and I make all these things happen.

tasmin prathamataḥ sarge yā yathā yatra saṁvidaḥ
kacitās tās tathā tatra sthitā adyā 'pi niścalāḥ (54/13)

VASIṢṬHA continued:

O Rāma, the second Līlā who had obtained a boon from Sarasvatī rose into the sky and there met her daughter. The girl introduced herself to Līlā. And, Līlā requested her to guide her to where her husband the king was. The girl thereupon flew away with her mother.

Passing beyond even this universe, Līlā crossed over the oceans and other elements that envelop this universe, and entered into the infinite consciousness. In that infinite consciousness there are countless universes which do not know of one another's existence. Līlā entered one of those universes in which the body of king Padma lay covered with a heap of flowers. She thought, "By the grace of Sarasvatī I have physically reached this place. I am the most blessed among persons." She began to fan the king's body.

SARASVATĪ said to the first Līlā: The king, the servants of the royal household and all the rest of them, are only infinite consciousness. However, since the substratum is the reflection of the infinite consciousness which is real, and since there is a conviction in the order of fanciful creation, they recognise one another. She could not go in her own physical body to the new realm, because light cannot co-exist with darkness. When the wisdom concerning one's ethereal body arises, the physical body ceases to be recognised as true. This is the fruit of the boon that I granted her. The recipient of the boon thinks, "Just as you have made me think by your boon, so I am." Therefore, she thinks she has reached her husband's abode in her physical body. Only one who has arrived at wisdom can ascend to the ethereal realms, O Līlā, not others. This Līlā does not possess such wisdom; hence, she only fancied that she had reached the city where her husband dwelt.

THE ENLIGHTENED LĪLĀ said: Please tell me: how did the objects acquire their characteristics — like heat in fire, coolness in ice, solidity in earth?

SARASVATĪ said: Dear one, during the cosmic dissolution, the entire universe having disappeared, only the infinite Brahman remains in peace. It fancies the existence of a creation.

Whatever, wherever and however was conceived or fancied by the infinite consciousness during that first creation, all that has remained there and in that manner and with those characteristics even now. In fact, this order is inherent in infinite consciousness. All these objects and their characteristics were potentially present in it even during the cosmic dissolution: into what else could they dissolve? Moreover, how can something become nothing? Gold that appears as bracelet cannot become formless entirely.

Such is the order (niyati) in the universe, that nothing until now has been able to alter it.

jiva ity ucyate tasya nāmā 'ṇor vāsanāvataḥ
tatraivā "ste sa ca śavāgāre gaganake tathā (55/6)

SARASVATĪ continued:
According to the order that existed in the first creation, human beings were endowed with a life-span of one, two, three or four hundred years. The shortening or the lengthening of the life-span is dependent upon the purity or impurity of the following factors — country, time, activity, and the materials used and consumed. He who adheres to the injunctions of the scriptures enjoys the life-span guaranteed by those scriptures. Thus, the person lives a long or short life and reaches its end.

THE ENLIGHTENED LĪLĀ said:

O Goddess, kindly enlighten me concerning death: is it pleasant or unpleasant, and what happens after death?

SARASVATĪ said:

There are three types of human beings, my dear: the fool, one who is practising concentration and meditation, and the yogi (or intelligent one). The two latter types of human beings abandon the body by the practice of the yoga of concentration and meditation and depart at their sweet will and pleasure. But, the fool who has not practised concentration or meditation, being at the mercy of forces outside himself, experiences great anguish at the approach of death.

Such is the order established in the beginning of creation by the infinite consciousness. When life-breath does not flow freely, the person ceases to live. But all this is imaginary. How can infinite consciousness cease to be? The person is nothing but infinite consciousness. Who dies and when; to whom does this infinite consciousness belong and how? Even when millions of bodies die, this consciousness exists undiminished.

When there is cessation of the flow of the life-breath, the consciousness of the individual becomes utterly passive. Please remember, O Līlā, that consciousness is pure, eternal and infinite: it does not arise nor cease to be. It is ever there in the moving and unmoving creatures, in the sky, on the mountain and in fire and air. When life-breath ceases, the body is said to be 'dead' or 'inert'. The life-breath returns to its source — air — and consciousness freed from memory and tendencies remains as the self.

That atomic ethereal particle which is possessed of these memories and tendencies is known as jīva: and it remains there itself, in the space where the dead body is. And they refer to it as 'preta' (departed soul). That jīva now abandons its ideas and what it had been seeing till then, and perceives other things as in dreaming or day-dreaming.

After a momentary lapse of consciousness, the jīva begins to fancy that it sees another body, another world and another life-span.

na tu jāḍyaṁ pṛthak kiñcid asti nā 'pi ca cetanaṁ
nā 'tra bhedo 'sti sargādau sattā sāmānyake na ca (57)

SARASVATĪ continued:

Whatever the jīva sees, it experiences. For in this empty space of infinite consciousness there is nothing known as time, action, etc. Then the jīva fancies, 'the god of death has sent me to heaven (or hell)' and 'I enjoyed (or suffered) the pleasures (or tortures) of heaven (or hell)' and 'I am born as an animal, etc., as ordained by the god of death'. This goes on again and again till the jīva is enlightened by self-knowledge.

The mountains, the forests, the earth and the sky — all these are but infinite consciousness. That alone is the very being of all, the reality in all; and hence in the very beginning that pure infinite consciousness appeared to become whatever form it took whenever it manifested itself. Till now it continues to be so. When the life-breath enters into the bodies and begins to vibrate the various parts of the bodies, it is said that those bodies are living. Such living bodies existed right in the beginning of creation. When those bodies into which the life-breath had entered did not vibrate, they were known as trees and plants. It is indeed a small part of the infinite consciousness that becomes the intelligence in these bodies. This intelligence, entering into the bodies, brings into being the different organs like the eyes.

When that intelligence, which is part of the infinite consciousness, fancied itself to be a tree, it became a tree; or a rock, it became a rock; or grass, it became grass. **There is no distinction between the sentient and the insentient, between the intelligent and the inert: there is no difference at all in the essence of substances,** for the infinite consciousness is present everywhere equally. The differences are only due to the intelligence identifying itself as different substances.

The same infinite consciousness is known by different names in these different substances. In the same way, it is the same infinite consciousness that the intelligence identifies as the worms, ants and birds. In it there is no comparison, nor a sense of difference: just as the people living in the north pole do not know (and therefore do not contrast themselves with) the people of the south pole. Each independent substance identified as such by this intelligence exists by itself, without distinction from the other substances. Ascribing distinctions to them as 'sentient' and 'insentient' is like a frog born in a rock and a frog born outside it considering themselves different, one insentient and the other sentient!

O Līlā, I think that now the king Vidūratha wishes to enter into the heart of the body of the king Padma. He is proceeding towards it. Tuning himself to the ego-principle in the heart of Padma, Vidūratha fancies that he is proceeding to another world. Let us proceed along our own paths: one cannot tread the path of another!

dehād dehāntara prāptiḥ pūrva dehaṁ vinā sadā
ātivāhika dehe 'smin svapneṣv iva vinaśvari (57/22)

VASIṢṬHA continued:

In the meantime the life-breath left the body of the king Vidūratha. His intelligence rose into space, in an ethereal form. Līlā and Sarasvatī saw this and followed it. In a few moments that ethereal form became conscious, when the period of post-mortem unconsciousness came to an end. Līlā and Sarasvatī re-entered that beautiful palace and the room in which the embalmed body of Padma had been kept. All the royal attendants were fast asleep. There, seated near the body of king Padma, they saw the second Līlā who was devoutly fanning the king, but she did not see them.

RĀMA asked:

It was said that the first Līlā had temporarily left her body near the king and travelled with Sarasvatī in an ethereal body: but now the first Līlā's body is not mentioned at all.

VASIṢṬHA replied:

When the first Līlā became enlightened, the egoistic fancy of her ethereal real being abandoned its link with the gross physical form, and it melted away like snow. In fact, it was Līlā's ignorant fancy that made it appear as if she had a physical body. In the mind of the deluded the unreal manifests itself; and when the delusion has been dispelled there is no longer an ignorant fancy. This fanciful conviction that the unreal is real is deep rooted by repeated imagination.

Even without destroying it, one can move from one ethereal body to another, just as in dream one can take one form after another without abandoning the previous one. The yogi's body is truly invisible, ethereal, even though it appears to be visible in the eyes of the ignorant beholder. And it is such a beholder who, on account of his own ignorance, thinks and says "This yogi is dead". For, where is the body, what exists and what dies? That which is — is; only delusion vanished!

RĀMA asked:

Does a yogi's physical body become an ethereal body?

VASIṢṬHA replied:

How many times have I told you, O Rāma: yet you do not grasp it! The ethereal body alone is: by persistent fancy, it appears to be linked to a physical body. Just as an ignorant man, (who thinks he is the physical body) when he dies and the body is cremated, has a subtle body, even so the yogi on being enlightened while living, has an ethereal body.

sad vāsanasya rudhayam ativahika samvidi
deho vismrtim ayati garbhasamstheva yauvane (58/16)

VASIṢṬHA continued:

In the meantime, Sarasvatī restrained Vidūratha's jiva from entering into the body of king Padma.

THE ENLIGHTENED LĪLĀ asked Sarasvatī: O Goddess, from the time I sat here in contemplation till now, how much time has elapsed?

SARASVATĪ replied:

Dear one, it is a month since you entered into contemplation. During the first fifteen days your body, on account of the great heat generated by prāṇāyāma, became vaporised. Then it became like a dry leaf and fell down. Then it became rigid and cold. The ministers then thought that you had died of your own accord and cremated that body. Now, on account of your own wish you appear here in your ethereal body. In you there are no memories of past life nor latent tendencies brought forward from previous incarnation. **For when the intelligence is established in the conviction of its ethereal nature the body is forgotten, even as in youth one forgets life as a foetus.** Today is the thirty-first day and you are here. Come, let us reveal ourselves to this other Līlā.

When the second Līlā saw them before her, she fell at their feet and worshipped them. Sarasvatī asked her: "Tell us how you came here".

THE SECOND LĪLĀ replied: When I fainted in the palace of Vidūratha, I did not know anything for some time. I then saw that my subtle body rose to the sky and was seated in an aerial vehicle which brought me here. And, I saw that Vidūratha was lying here asleep in a garden of flowers. I thought he was fatigued from battle and without disturbing him, I fan him.

Sarasvatī immediately let Vidūratha's jīva enter the body. The king at once awoke as if from a slumber. The two Līlā bowed to him. The king asked the enlightened Līlā, "Who are you, who is she, and from where has she come?" The enlightened Līlā replied: "Lord, I am your wife in your previous incarnation and your constant companion, even as a word and its meaning are. This Līlā is your other wife; she is my own reflection, created by me for your pleasure. And, she who is seated on yonder golden throne is the goddess Sarasvatī herself. She is present here on account of our great good fortune." Hearing this, the king sat up and saluted Sarasvatī. Sarasvatī blessed him with long life, wealth and so on, and enlightenment.

Thus is the story of Līlā, O Rāma, which I have narrated in detail to you: contemplation of this story will remove from your mind the least faith in the reality of what is perceived.

duḥkhitasya niśā kalpaḥ sukhitasyaiva ca kṣaṇaḥ
kṣaṇaḥ svapne bhavet kalpaḥ kalpaś ca bhavati kṣaṇaḥ (60/22)

RĀMA said:

Pray, explain to me the mystery of time: in the story of Līlā sometimes a whole lifetime was spent in eight days, sometimes in one month. I am puzzled. Are there different time scales in different universes?

VASIṢṬHA replied:

O Rāma, whatever one thinks within oneself in his own intelligence, that alone is experienced by him. **To a suffering person a night is an epoch; and a night of revelry passes like a moment. In a dream a moment is non-different from an epoch.** But to the sage whose consciousness has overcome limitations, there is neither day nor night.

RĀMA asked:

How does the delusion of the notions of 'I' and 'the world' arise in the first place, without any cause?

VASIṢṬHA replied:

As all things are equally indwelt by intelligence, so at all times in every way the uncreated is all, the self of all. We use the expression 'all things': it is only a figure of speech, for only the infinite consciousness or Brahman exists. Just as there is no division between a bracelet and gold, there is no division between the universe and the infinite consciousness. The latter alone is the universe: the universe as such is not the infinite consciousness, just as the bracelet is made of gold but gold is not made of bracelet.

In that infinite consciousness there is an inherent non-recognition of its infinite nature: That appears to manifest as 'I' and 'the world'. Just as there is an image in a marble slab even if it has not been carved, even so this notion of 'I' and 'the world' exists in the infinite consciousness. That is known as its creation. The word 'creation' has no other connotation. No creation takes place in the supreme being or the infinite consciousness; and the infinite consciousness is not involved in the creation. They do not stand in a divided relationship to each other.

The infinite consciousness regards its own intelligence in its own heart, as it were, though it is non-different from it, even as wind is non-different from its own movement. At that very moment, when there is unreal division, there arises in that consciousness the notion of space, which, on account of the power of the consciousness, appears as the element known as space. That itself later believes itself to be air and then fire. From this notion there arises the appearance of fire and light. That itself further entertains the notion of water with its inherent faculty of taste; and that itself believes itself to be the earth with its inherent faculty of smell and also its characteristic of solidity. Thus do the water and the earth elements appear to have manifested themselves.

nā 'stameti na codeti kvacit kiñcit kadācana
sarvaṁ śāntam ajaṁ brahma cidghanaṁ suśilāghanaṁ (31)

VASIṢṬHA continued:

At the same time, the same infinite consciousness held in itself the notion of a unit of time equal to one-millionth of the twinkling of an eye: and from this evolved the time-scale right up to an epoch consisting of several revolutions of the four ages, which is the life-span of one cosmic creation. The infinite consciousness itself is uninvolved in these: for it is devoid of rising and setting (which are essential to all time-scales), and it is devoid of a beginning, middle and end.

The infinite consciousness alone is the reality, ever awake and enlightened: and with creation also it is the same. That infinite consciousness alone is the unenlightened appearance of this creation: and even after this creation it is the same always. It is ever the same. When one realises in the self by the self that consciousness is the absolute Brahman, then he experiences it as all — even as the one energy dwelling in all his limbs.

One can say that this world-appearance is real only so far as it is the manifestation of consciousness and because of direct experience; and it is unreal when it is grasped with the mind and the sense-organs. Wind is perceived as real in its motion, and it appears to be non-existent when there is no motion: even so this world-appearance can be regarded as both real and unreal. The mirage-like appearance of the three worlds exists as non-different from the absolute Brahman.

The creation exists in Brahman just as the sprout exists in the seed, liquidity in water, sweetness in milk and pungency in capsicum; but in ignorance it appears to be different from and independent of Brahman. There is no cause for the world's existence as a pure reflection in the absolute Brahman. When there is a notion of creation, the creation seems to be; and when through self-effort there is an understanding of non-creation, there is no world.

Nothing has ever been created anywhere at any time; and nothing comes to an end either. The absolute Brahman is all, the supreme peace, unborn, pure consciousness and permanent. Worlds within worlds appear in every atom. What can be the cause and how do these arise?!

As and when one turns away from the notions of 'I' and the 'world', one is liberated: the notion of 'I am this' is the sole bondage here. They who know the infinite consciousness as the nameless, formless substratum of the universe, gain victory over saṁsāra (repetitive history).

astīha niyatir brāhmī cic chakttiḥ spandarūpiṇī
avaśya bhavitavyaika sattā sakala kalpagā (62/8)

RĀMA asked:

It is evident that Brahman alone exists, O holy sage! But, then why do even these sages and men of wisdom exist in this world, as if so ordained by god — and what is god?

VASIṢṬHA replied:

There does exist, O Rāma, the power or energy of the infinite consciousness, which is in motion all the time; that alone is the reality of all inevitable futuristic events, for it penetrates all the epochs in time. It is by that power that the nature of every object in the universe is ordained. That power (cit śakti) is also known as Mahasāttā (the great existence), Mahāciti (the great intelligence), Mahāśakti (the great power), Mahādṛṣṭi (the great vision), Mahākriyā (the great doer or doing), Mahodbhavā (the great becoming), Mahāspandā (the great vibration). It is this power that endows everything with its characteristic quality. But this power is not different from or independent of the absolute Brahman: it is as real as a pie in the sky. Sages make a verbal distinction between Brahman and the power, and declare that creation is the work of that power.

The distinction is verbal, even as one speaks of the body (as a whole) and its parts. The infinite consciousness becomes aware of its inherent power, even as one becomes aware of the limbs of his body: such awareness is known as niyati (the power of the absolute that determines nature). It is also known as daiva or divine dispensation.

That you should ask me these questions is ordained by niyati; and that you should act upon my teaching is also ordained by niyati. If one says, 'The divine will feed me' and remains idle, that also is the work of niyati. This niyati cannot be set aside even by gods like Rudra. But, wise men should not give up self-effort because of this, for niyati functions only as and through self-effort. This niyati has two aspects, human and super-human: the former is seen where self-effort bears fruit and the latter where it does not.

If one remains idle, depending upon niyati to do everything for him, he soon discovers that his life departs — for life is action. He can, by entering into the highest superconscious state, stop the breath and attain liberation: but then that is indeed the greatest self-effort!

The infinite consciousness alone appears as one thing in one place and another in another place. There is no division between that consciousness and its power, as there is no division between wave and water, limbs and the body. Such division is experienced only by the ignorant.

brahmaṇaḥ sphuraṇaṁ kiñcid yad avātāmbudher iva
dīpasyevā 'py avātasya taṁ jīvaṁ viddhi rāghava (64/8)

RĀMA asked:

When the only reality is the infinite consciousness and its own inherent kinetic power, how does the jīva acquire an apparent reality in the secondless unity?

VASIṢṬHA replied:

This terrible goblin known as jīva arises as a reflected reality or appearance in the mind of the ignorant alone. No one, not even the men of wisdom or sages, can definitely say what it is; because it is devoid of any indications of its nature.

In the mirror of infinite consciousness are seen countless reflections which constitute the appearance of the world. These are the jīvā. **Jīva is like unto just a little agitation on the surface of the ocean of Brahman; or just a little movement of the flame of a candle in a windless room.** When in that slight agitation the infinitude of the infinite consciousness is veiled, limitation of consciousness appears to arise. This too is inherent in that infinite consciousness. And that limitation of consciousness is known as the jīva.

Just as when a spark from a flame comes into contact with flammable substance it bursts into an independent flame, even so this limitation of consciousness, when it is fed by latent tendencies and memories, condenses into egotism — 'I'-ness. This I-ness is not a solid reality: but the jīva sees it as real, like the blueness of the sky. When the egotism begins to entertain its own notions it gives rise to the mind-stuff, the concept of an independent and separate jīva, mind, Māyā or cosmic illusion, cosmic nature, etc.

The intelligence which entertains these notions conjures up the natural elements (earth, water, fire, air and space). Associated with these, the same intelligence becomes a spark of light, though it is the cosmic light in truth. It then condenses into countless forms — somewhere it becomes a tree, somewhere a bird, somewhere it becomes a goblin, somewhere it becomes demi-gods, etc. The first of such modifications becomes the creator Brahmā and creates others, by thought and will. Thus the vibration in consciousness alone is the jīva, karma, god; and all the rest follows.

Creation (of the mind) is but agitation in consciousness; and the world exists in the mind! It seems to exist because of imperfect vision, imperfect understanding. It is really not more than a long dream. If this is understood then all duality will come to an end, and Brahman, jīva, mind, Māyā, doer, action and the world, will all be seen as synonymous with the one non-dual infinite consciousness.

cidghanenaikatām etya yadā tiṣṭhati niścalaḥ
śāmyan vyavaharan vā 'pi tadā saṁśānta ucyate (66/12)

VASIṢṬHA continued:

The one never became many, O Rāma. When many candles are kindled from another it is the same flame that burns in all candles; even so, the one Brahman appears to be many. When one contemplates the unreality of this diversity he is freed from sorrow.

Jiva is nothing more than the limitation of consciousness; when the limitation goes, there is peace — even as for one who wears shoes the whole world is paved with leather. What is this world? Nothing but an appearance, even as a plantain stem is nothing but leaves. Even as liquor is able to make one see all sorts of phantasms in the empty sky, mind is able to make one see diversity in unity. Even as a drunkard sees a tree moving, the ignorant one sees movement in this world.

When the mind perceives duality then there is both duality and its counterpart, which is unity. When the mind drops the perception of duality there is neither duality nor unity. **When one is firmly established in the oneness of the infinite consciousness, whether he is quiet or actively engaged in work, then he is considered to be at peace with himself.** When one is thus established in the supreme state, that is also known as the state of non-self, or the state of knowledge of the void or emptiness.

On account of the agitation of the mind, consciousness appears to become the object of knowledge! Then there arise in the mind all sorts of false notions like 'I am born' etc. Such knowledge is not different from the mind. Hence it is known as ignorance or delusion.

To rid oneself of the disease of this saṁsāra or world-appearance, there is no remedy other than wisdom or self-knowledge. Knowledge alone is the cure for the wrong perception of a snake in the rope. When there is such knowledge, then there is no craving in the mind for sense-pleasure which aggravates the ignorance. Hence, if there is craving, do not fulfil it: what difficulty is there in this?

When the mind entertains notions of objects, there is agitation or movement in the mind; and when there are no objects or ideas, then there is no movement of thought in the mind. When there is movement, the world appears to be; when there is no movement, there is cessation of world-appearance. The movement of thought itself is called jīva, cause and action; that is the seed for world-appearance. Then follows the creation of the body.

yathā saṁpadyate brahmā kīṭaḥ saṁpadyate tathā
kīṭastu rūḍhabhūtaugha valanāt tucchakarmakaḥ (69)

VASIṢṬHA continued:

On account of various causes, there is this movement of thought; someone is freed from this in one lifetime, and someone else is freed in a thousand births. When there is movement of thought one does not see the truth; and then there is the feeling of 'I am', 'This is mine' etc.

The world-appearance is the waking state of consciousness; egotism is the dreaming state; the mind-stuff is the deep sleep state; and pure consciousness is the fourth state or uncontradicted truth. Beyond even this fourth state there is absolute purity of consciousness. One who is established in it goes beyond sorrow.

The world-appearance is said to have the absolute Brahman as its cause, in just the same way as the sky (space) is the cause of the growth of a tree (since the sky does not obstruct its growth, it promotes or causes it). In fact, Brahman is not an active causative factor; and this is revealed by enquiry. Even as one digging the solid earth finds empty space as he continues to dig, when the enquiry is continued you will find the truth that all this is none other than the infinite consciousness.

RĀMA asked: Pray, tell me how this creation becomes so extensive.

VASIṢṬHA continued:

The vibration in the infinite consciousness is not different from that consciousness itself. From that vibration, just as the jīva becomes manifest, even so from the jīva the mind becomes manifest because the jīva thinks. The mind itself entertains the notions of the five elements and it transforms itself into those elements. Whatever the mind thinks of, that alone it sees. After this, one by one the jīva acquires the sense-organs — the tongue, the eyes, the nose, the sense of touch, etc. In this there is no causal connection between the mind and the senses, but there is the coincidence of the thought and of the manifestation of the sense-organs — just as a crow sits on a palm tree, the fruit accidentally drops from it, and it appears that the crow dislodged it! Thus the first cosmic jīva came into being.

RĀMA asked: Holy sir, if ignorance is non-existent in truth, then why should one even bother about liberation or about enquiry?

VASIṢṬHA replied:

Rāma, that thought should arise in its own time, not now! Flowers bloom and fruits ripen in their due time.

The cosmic jīva utters OṀ and by pure will creates the various objects. **Just as the creator Brahmā was willed into being, even so is a worm brought into being: because the latter is caught up in impurity, its action is trivial.** The distinction is illusory. In truth, there is no creation and hence no division at all.

svārtha kriyogra sāmarthyād yāti bhāvanāya 'nyatām
padārtho 'bhimatāṁśāḍhyo niḥśvāseneva darpaṇaḥ (70/19)

VASIṢṬHA continued:

In connection with this, O Rāma, there is an ancient legend which I shall now narrate to you.

There once lived to the north of the Himālaya mountain a terrible demoness known as Karkaṭī. She was huge, black and dreadful to look at. This demoness could not get enough to eat, and she was ever hungry. She thought, "If only I can eat all the people living in Jambudvīpa continent in one meal, then my hunger will disappear. Let me engage myself in penance, for through penance is attained that which would otherwise be extremely difficult to attain."

Karkaṭī then went up one of the snow-peaks and commenced her penance. In course of time she had grown so thin that it looked as if she was a skeleton clad in transparent skin.

After a thousand years had passed, the creator Brahmā appeared before her, pleased with her penance. She bowed to him mentally. She thought, "I shall request that I should become a living steel pin (Sūcikā), an embodiment of disease. With this boon I shall simultaneously enter the hearts of all beings and fulfil my desire and appease my hunger." When Brahmā said to her, "I am pleased with your penance; ask a boon of your choice," she expressed her wish. Brahmā said: "So be it; you shall also be Viṣūcikā. Remaining a subtle thing, you will inflict pain on those who eat the wrong food and indulge in wrong living, by entering their heart.

Immediately, O Rāma, the demoness with a mountainous body began to shrink gradually to the size of a pin. She became so subtle that her existence could only be imagined. She was constantly followed by her other form known as Viṣūcikā (cholera). Though she was extremely subtle and unseen, her demoniacal mentality underwent no change at all. Viṣūcikā was radiant, and was as subtle as the aroma of flowers. Dependent upon the life-force of others, she was devoted to her own work. She had gained the boon of her choice; but she could not fulfil her desire to devour all beings! That is because she was of the size of a needle!! How strange: the deluded ones do not have foresight. **The selfish person's violent efforts to gain his selfish ends often lead to other results, even as a person is unable to see his face when he runs to the mirror puffing and panting — his own breath mists the mirror.**

Sūcikā entered into the physical bodies of people who, on account of previous illness, had been greatly debilitated or had become obese, and transformed herself into Viṣūcikā (cholera). Sūcikā entered into the heart of even a healthy and intelligent person, and perverted his intellect. In some cases, however, she left that person when the latter underwent a healing treatment either with the aid of the mantra or with drugs.

āpatadd hi mano moham pūrvamāpat prayacchati
paścād anartha vistāra rūpeṇa parijṛmbhate (71/72)

VASIṢṬHA continued:

Sūcikā had her numerous hiding places. Among them were: dust and dirt on the ground, (unclean) fingers, threads in a cloth, within one's body in the muscles, dirty skin covered with dust, unclean furrows on the palms and on other parts of the body (due to senility), places where flies abound, in a lustreless body, in places full of decaying leaves, in places devoid of healthy trees, in people of filthy dress, people of unhealthy habits, in tree-stumps caused by deforestation in which flies breed, in puddles of stagnant water, in polluted water, in open sewers running in the middle of roads, in rest houses used by travellers, and in those cities where there are many animals like elephants, horses, etc.

Unharmed and unprovoked by others, Sūcikā works for the destruction and death of others. Known also as Jiva-sūcikā, she moves in all beings as the life-force with the help of prāṇa and apāna, subjecting the jīva to sorrow by causing terribly sharp pain (of gout, rheumatism) which makes one lose his mind. She enters into the feet (like a needle) and drinks blood. Like all wicked people, she rejoices in other's sorrow.

(As Vasiṣṭha was saying this, the sun set and another day came to an end. The assembly adjourned for prayers.) The next day VASIṢṬHA continued:

After living in this manner for a long, long time, the demoness Karkaṭī was thoroughly disillusioned and repented her foolish desire to devour people, which entailed severe penance for a thousand years and the degraded existence as a needle (and cholera virus). She thus bewailed her own self-inflicted misfortune:

"Alas, where is my mountainous body and where is the form of a needle? Alas, I am lost. I have surely lost my mind and my senses! **The mind that is heading towards calamity first creates delusion and wickedness: and these themselves later expand into misfortune and sorrow.** I am never free, ever at the mercy of others. I am in the hands of others and do what they make me do. I desired to appease the goblin of a desire to devour all; but that has led to a remedy worse than the disease and a greater goblin has arisen. Surely I am a brainless fool; hence I threw away such a great and gigantic body and deliberately chose this despicable body of a virus (or a needle)."

At once Karkaṭī abandoned all wish to devour living beings, and went to the Himālayā. Standing as if on one foot, she began her penance. Karkaṭī's whole being became completely purified by this penance and she gained the highest wisdom. The energy of her penance set the Himālayā on fire, as it were. Indra the king of heaven learnt from the sage Nārada of Karkaṭī's unprecedented undertaking.

vidita parama karaṇā 'dya jātā svayam anucetana saṁvidaṁ vicārya
svamanana kalanānusāra ekastviha hi guruḥ paramo na rāghavā 'nyaḥ (74/28)

VASIṢṬHA continued:

Indra commissioned Vāyu the wind-god to find out the exact spot where Sūcikā dwelt. In the Himālayā, Vāyu saw the ascetic Sūcikā standing like another peak of the mountain. She had become almost completely dried up. When Vāyu (wind) entered her mouth, she threw it out again and again. She had withdrawn her life-force to the crown of her head and stood as a perfect yogini. Vāyu forthwith returned to heaven where he reported to Indra. Thereupon Indra went to Brahmā, and in answer to his prayer Brahmā went to where Sūcikā was engaged in penance.

In the meantime, Sūcikā had become totally pure by her penance. **She had gained direct knowledge of the supreme causeless cause of all by her own examination of the intelligence within her. Surely, direct enquiry into all the movements of thought in one's own consciousness is the supreme guru or preceptor, O Rāma, and no one else.** Brahmā said to her, "Ask a boon." She reflected within herself: "I have reached the realisation of the absolute. What shall I do with boons?"

Brahmā said: "The eternal world order cannot be set aside, O ascetic. And it decrees that you should regain your previous body, live happily for a long time and then attain liberation. You will live an enlightened life, afflicting only the wicked and the sinful, and causing the least harm — and that too only to appease your natural hunger." Sūcikā accepted what Brahmā had said and soon her needle-body grew into a mountainous body.

Karkaṭī regained her former demoniacal form. She experienced hunger; for as long as the body lasts it is subject to its own physical laws, including hunger and thirst. She heard an aerial voice say: "O Karkaṭī, approach ignorant and deluded people and awaken wisdom in them. This indeed is the only mission of enlightened beings. One whom you thus endeavour to enlighten but who fails to awake to truth is fit for your consumption. You shall incur no sin by devouring such an ignorant person."

Hearing this, Karkaṭī entered a dense forest where hill tribes and hunters dwelt. In that region there was a king known as Vikraṁ. As was his custom, this king, along with his minister, went out into the dense darkness of the night to protect his subjects by subduing robbers and dacoits. Karkaṭī saw these two men. She reflected: "Surely, these two men have come here to appease my hunger. They are ignorant and therefore a burden on earth. Such ignorant people suffer here and hereafter; suffering is the only mission in their life! Death, unto them, is a welcome release from such suffering, and it is possible that after death they will awake and seek their salvation. Ah, but, it may be that they are both wise men, and I do not like to kill wise men. For, whoever wishes to enjoy unalloyed happiness, fame and long life should by all means honour and worship good men by giving them all that they might wish to have. Let me therefore test their wisdom. If they are wise I shall not harm them. Wise men, good men, are indeed great benefactors of humanity."

saṁrambha dvāram utsṛjya samatā svacchayā dhiyā
yukttyā ca vyavahāriṇyā svārthaḥ prājñena sādhyate (78/25)

VASIṢṬHA continued:

Karkaṭī shouted: "Hey you two little worms roaming this dense forest! Who are you? Tell me quick or else I shall devour you."

The king and the minister beheld her dreadful form, and without being perturbed in the very least, the minister said to her: "O demoness, why are you so angry? To seek food is natural to all living beings; and in performing one's natural functions one need not be bad tempered. **Even selfish ends are gained by the wise by appropriate means and appropriate behaviour or action, after they give up anger and mental agitation, and resort to equanimity and clear mind.** We have seen thousands of insects like you and have dealt justly with them, for it is the duty of a king to punish the wicked and protect the good. Give up your anger, and achieve your end by resorting to tranquillity. Such indeed is appropriate conduct — whether one is able to achieve one's ambition or not, one should remain peaceful. Ask of us what you will have; for we have never turned a beggar away empty handed."

Karkaṭī greatly admired the courage and wisdom of the two men. She thought, "Let me utilise this opportunity to clear the doubts that are in my mind; for he is surely a fool who, having the company of a wise man, neglects to clear his doubts." She said to them: "If you two are men not possessed of self-knowledge, then in accordance with my inherent nature, I shall devour you both. In order to determine this I shall ask you some questions. Give me the right answers.

"O king, what is it that is one and yet is many, and in which millions of universes merge? What is it that is pure space, though it appears to be not so? What is it that is me in you and that is you in me; what is it that moves yet does not move; what is it that is a rock though conscious, and what plays wonderful tricks in empty space; what is it that is not the sun and the moon and fire and yet eternally shines; what is that atom that seems to be far and yet so near; what is it that is of the nature of consciousness and yet is not knowable; what is it that is all and yet is not any of these; what is it that, thought it is the very self of all, is veiled by ignorance and is regained after many lifetimes of intense and persistent effort; what is it that is atomic and yet contains a mountain within it, and that transforms the three worlds into a blade of grass; what is it that without ever renouncing its atomic nature appears to be bigger than the biggest mountain; what is that atom in which the entire universe rests like a seed during the cosmic dissolution?

"What is it that is responsible for the function of all the elements in the universe, though it does nothing at all; of what are the seer, the sight and the seen made; what is it that veils and reveals the threefold manifestation; in what is the apparent three-fold division of time established; what is it that comes into manifestation and vanishes alternately?"

sarvātmakatvān naivā 'sau śūnyo bhavati karhicit
yad asti na tad astiti vakttā mantā iti smṛtaḥ (10)

THE MINISTER replied:

I shall surely answer your questions, O Lady! For that to which all your questions refer is the supreme self.

That self is subtler than even space, since it has no name and cannot be described; and neither the mind nor the senses can reach it or comprehend it. It is pure consciousness. The entire universe exists in the consciousness that is atomic, even as a tree exists within the seed: but, then the universe exists as consciousness and does not exist as the universe. That consciousness exists, however, because such is the experience of all, and since it alone is the self of all. Since it is, all else is.

That self is empty like space; but it is not nothingness, since it is consciousness. It is: yet because it cannot be experienced by the mind and senses, it is not. It being the self of all, it is not experienced (as the object of experience) by anyone. Though one, it is reflected in the infinite atoms of existence and hence appears to be many. This appearance is however unreal even as 'bracelct' is an imaginary appearance of gold which alone is real. But, the self is not unreal. **It is not a void or nothingness: for it is the self of all, and it is the very self of one who says it is and of one who says (or thinks) it is not!** Moreover, its existence can be experienced indirectly just as the existence of camphor can be experienced by its fragrance. It alone is the self of all as consciousness; and it alone is the substance that makes the world-appearance possible.

In that infinite ocean of consciousness, whirlpools known as the three worlds arise spontaneously and naturally, even as whirlpools are caused by the very nature of the running water. Because this consciousness is beyond the reach of the mind and senses, it seems to be a void; but since it can be known by self-knowledge, it is not a void. On account of the indivisibility of consciousness, I am you and you are me; but the indivisible consciousness itself has become neither I nor you! When the wrong notions of 'you' and 'I' are given up, there arises the awareness that there is neither you, nor I, nor everything; perhaps it alone is everything.

The self, being infinite, moves not though moving, and yet is forever established in every atom of existence. The self does not go nor does it ever come: for space and time derive their meaning from consciousness alone. Where can the self go when all that is, is within it? If a pot is taken from one place to another the space within does not move from one place to another, for everything is forever in space.

yāvat kaṭakasaṁvittis tāvan nā 'stīva hematā
yāvac ca dṛśyatāpattis tāvan nā 'stīva sā kalā (48)

THE MINISTER continued:

The self, which is of the nature of pure consciousness, seems to be inert and insentient when it is apparently associated with inertia. In infinite space this infinite consciousness has made infinite objects appear; though all this seems to have been done, such effect being a mere fancy, nothing has been done. Hence, it is both consciousness and inertia, the doer and the non-doer.

The reality in fire is this self or consciousness: yet, the self does not burn nor is it burnt, it is the reality in all, and infinite. It is the eternal light which shines in the sun, the moon and the fire, but independent of them. It shines even when these have set: it illumines all from within all. It alone is the intelligence that indwells even trees, plants and creepers, and preserves them. That self or infinite consciousness is, from the ordinary point of view, the creator, the protector and the overlord of all; and yet from the absolute point of view, in reality, being the self of all it has no such limited roles.

There is no world independent of this consciousness: hence, even the mountains are in the atomic self. In it arises the phantasies of a moment and of an epoch: and these appear to be real time-scales, even as objects seen in a dream appear to be real at that time. Within the twinkling of an eye there exists an epoch, even as a whole city is reflected in a small mirror. Such being the case, how can one assert the reality of either duality or non-duality? This atomic self or infinite consciousness alone appears to be a moment or an epoch, near and far, and there is nothing apart from it; and these are not mutually contradictory in themselves.

As long as one sees the bracelet as a bracelet, it is not seen as gold; but when it is seen that 'bracelet' is just a word and not the reality, then gold is seen. Even so, **when the world is assumed to be real, the self is not seen:** but when this assumption is discarded, consciousness is realised. It is the all; hence real. It is not experienced; hence unreal.

What appears to be is but the jugglery of Māyā, which creates a division in consciousness into subject and object. It is as real as the dream-city. It is neither real nor unreal, but a long-standing illusion. It is the assumption of division that creates diversity, right from the creator Brahmā down to the little insect. Just as in a single seed the diverse characteristics of the tree remain at all times, even so this apparent diversity exists in the self at all times, but as consciousness.

ātmā yatnaśataprāpyo labdhe 'smin na ca kiñcana
labdhaṁ bhavati tac caitat paramaṁ vā na kiñcana (9)

KARKAṬĪ said:

I am delighted with your minister's answers, O king. Now I would like to hear your answers.

THE KING said:

Your questions, O noble lady, relate to the eternal Brahman which is pure existence. It is known when the mind-stuff is rid of all movements of thought. The extension and withdrawal of its manifestation are popularly regarded as the creation and the dissolution of the universe. It is expressed in silence when the known comes to an end, for it is beyond all expression. It is the extremely subtle middle, between the two extremes; and that middle itself has two sides. As the diversity of this universe, it seems to be divided in itself; but truly, it is undivided.

When this Brahman wishes, wind comes into being, though that wind is nothing but pure consciousness. Similarly, when sound is thought of, there is a fanciful projection of what sounds like sound. That supreme subtle atomic being is all and is nothing. By its omnipotence all this appears to be.

This self can be attained by a hundred ways and means; yet, when it is attained, nothing has been attained! It is the supreme self; yet it is nothing. One roams in this forest of saṁsāra, or repetitive history, till there is the dawn of that wisdom which is able to dispel the root-ignorance in which the world appears to be real. But the truth is that it is the infinite consciousness that perceives the universe within itself, through its own power known as Māyā.

Though the self is extremely subtle and atomic and of the essential nature of pure consciousness, by it the entire universe is wholly pervaded. This omnipresent being by its very existence inspires the world-appearance to 'dance to its tunes'. That which is thus subtler than a hundredth part of the tip of hair is yet greater than the greatest, because of its omnipresence.

The light of self-knowledge alone illumines all experiences. It shines by its own light. This inner light appears to be outside and to illumine external objects. The other sources of light are indeed non-different from the darkness of ignorance and only appear to shine. The inner light of consciousness shines for ever within and without, day and night; mysteriously, it illumines the effects of ignorance without removing the darkness of ignorance.

Within the atomic space of consciousness there exist all the experiences, even as within a drop of honey there are the subtle essences of flowers, leaves and fruits. From that consciousness all experiences expand, for the experiencing is the sole experiencer (which is consciousness). Indeed, all this infinite consciousness alone is all this: and all the hands and eyes are its own, though being extremely subtle, it has no limbs.

draṣṭā dṛśyatayā tiṣṭhan draṣṭṛtām upajīvati
satyāṁ kaṭakasaṁvittau hema kāñcanatām iva (80)

THE KING continued:

In the twinkling of an eye this infinite consciousness experiences an epoch within itself, even as in the course of a brief dream one experiences youth and old age and even death. All these objects which appear in consciousness are indeed non-different from consciousness. Therefore, though the self is neither the doer of actions nor the experiencer of experiences, it is the doer of all actions and the experiencer of all experiences: there is nothing apart from it. Within the atom of infinite consciousness the doership and the experiencer are inherent.

The world, however, has never really been created, nor does it disappear: it is regarded as unreal only from the relative point of view. From the absolute point of view it is non-different from the infinite consciousness.

Sages only speak of the inner and the outer, which are but words with no corresponding substance: it is meant to instruct the ignorant. The seer, himself remaining unseen, sees himself; and the seer does not ever become an object of consciousness. The seer is the sight only, and when the latent psychic impressions have ceased, the seer regains its pure being; when the external object is imagined, a seer has been created. If there is no subject, there is no object either: without the father there is no son. It is the subject that becomes the object. There is no object (scene) without a subject (seer). Again, the subject is subject only in relation to the object; even as it is the son that makes a man 'father'. However, because the subject (seer) is pure consciousness, he is able to conjure up the object. This cannot be the other way round: the object does not give birth to the subject. Therefore the seer alone is real, the object being hallucination; gold alone is real, the 'bracelet' is a name and a form. As long as the notion of bracelet lasts, the pure gold is not apprehended; as long as the notion of the object persists, the division between the seer and the seen also persists. But, **just as because of the consciousness in the bracelet, gold realises its goldness, the subject (seer) manifesting as the object (the seen) realises subjectivity (consciousness).** One is the reflection of the other: there is no real duality. The subject exists because of the object, and the object is but a reflection of the subject: duality cannot be if there is not one, and where is the need for the notion of 'unity' if one alone exists? When thus real knowledge is gained by means of right enquiry and understanding, only that remains which is not expressible in words.

Division is not a contradiction of unity! All this speculation concerning unity and diversity is only to overcome sorrow: that which is beyond all this is the truth, the supreme self.

mahatām eva saṁparkāt punar duḥkhaṁ na bādhate
ko hi dīpa śikhā hastas tamasā paribhūyate (82/8)

VASIṢṬHA continued:

After listening to these wise words of the king, Karkaṭī became tranquil, and her demoniacal nature left her. She said to them: "O wise men, you are both fit to be worshipped by all and to be served by all. And, I have been thoroughly awakened by your holy company. **One who enjoys the company of enlightened men does not suffer in this world, even as one who holds a candle in his hand does not see darkness anywhere."**

At the king's request Karkaṭī became a charming young woman and lived as his guest. Every night she resumed her demoniacal form and consumed the criminals and sinners sent to her by the king. During the day she continued to be a charming woman.

I told you the story because I remembered her questions, and the king's answers. In essence, even as the ramifications of the tree (with its leaves, flowers, fruits, etc.) extend from the seed in which there is no such diversification, the universe of diversity extends from the infinite consciousness.

O Rāma, by merely listening to my words you will be enlightened, there is no doubt in this. Know that the universe has arisen from Brahman and it is Brahman alone. In the scriptures words have been used in order to facilitate the imparting of instruction. Cause and effect, the self and the Lord, difference and non-difference, knowledge and ignorance, pain and pleasure — all these pairs have been invented for the instruction of the ignorant. They are not real in themselves. As long as words are used to denote a truth, duality is inevitable; however, such duality is not the truth. All divisions are illusory.

Once I asked the creator Brahmā to tell me how this universe was first created. And he gave me the following reply.

BRAHMĀ said:

My child, it is only mind that appears as all this. At the end of the previous epoch there was the cosmic night. As soon as I woke at the end of the night I offered my morning prayers and looked around, wishing to create the universe. I beheld the infinite void which was neither illumined nor dark. In my heart I saw subtle visions. There in my mind and with my mind I saw several seemingly independent universes. In them all I also saw my own counterparts — creators. In those universes I saw all kinds of beings. Looking at all this I was puzzled: 'How is it that I am seeing all these with my mind in the great void?' I thought of one of the suns in one of the solar systems and asked him the question.

**sad asaditi kalābhirātatam yat sadasadabodha vimohadāyinībhiḥ
aviratara canābhir īśvarātman pravilasatiha mano mahan
mahātman (85/39)**

THE SUN replied:

O great one, being the omnipotent creator of all this you are indeed the Lord. It is the mind alone that appears as all this ceaseless and endless creative activity, which, on account of nescience, deludes one into thinking that it is real or that it is unreal. Surely, you know the truth, Lord: yet since you commanded me to answer your query, I say this:

O Lord of lords, near the holy mountain Kailāsa in a place known as Suvarṇajaṭa, your sons had established a colony. In that place there was a holy man known as Indu, a descendant of the sage Kaśyapa. He and his wife enjoyed every blessing except an offspring. They prayed to Lord Śiva, who granted them a boon.

Very soon after this the holy man's wife gave birth to ten brilliant and radiant sons. These boys grew up into young men; they had mastered all the scriptures even when they were barely seven years of age. After a considerable time their parents abandoned their bodies and became liberated.

The ten young men were sorely distressed at the loss of their parents. One day they got together and asked themselves: "O brothers, what is the most desirable goal here, which is proper for us to aspire to and which will not lead to unhappiness? To be a king, to be an emperor, even to be Indra the god of heaven are all trivial, since even Indra rules heaven just for an hour and a half of the Creator's life-span. Ah, therefore, we think only the attainment of creatorship is the best of all lordship, for it will not come to an end for a whole epoch."

All the others heartily agreed with this statement. They said to themselves: "Well then, we should soon reach Brahmā-hood which is devoid of old age and death."

The eldest brother said: "Please do as I tell you to do. From now on contemplate as follows, 'I am Brahmā, seated on a full-blown lotus'." All the brothers thereupon began to meditate in the following manner: "I am Brahmā, the creator of the universe. The sages, as also Sarasvatī the goddess of wisdom, are within me in their personal forms. Heaven is within me, with all the celestials. Mountains, continents and oceans are within me. Demi-gods and demons are within me. The sun shines within me. Now the creation takes place. Now the creation exists. Now is the time for the dissolution. An epoch is over. The night of Brahmā is at hand. I have self-knowledge and I am liberated."

tathaiva karmakaraṇe kāmanā nāsti dhīmatāṁ
tathaiva karmasaṁtyāge kāmanā nāsti dhīmatāṁ (88/12)

THE SUN continued:

Lord, after that, still deeply contemplating on their intention to be the creators of the universe, the ten holy men stood in contemplation. Their bodies had withered away and whatever was left was consumed by wild beasts. But they continued to stand there in their disembodied state, for a long long time . . . till an epoch came to a close and there was the great scorching heat of the sun and the terrible cloud-burst which destroyed everything. The holy men still continued to stand in their disembodied state, with the sole intention of becoming the creators of the universe.

At the dawn of a new creation these men continued to stand in the same place and in the same manner and with the same intention. They became the creators. They were the ten creators whom you saw; and you saw their universes, too. Lord, I am one of the suns that shine in the universes thus created by them.

THE CREATOR asked the Sun:

O Sun, when thus the universes have been created by these ten creators, what need I do? What is there for me to do?

THE SUN replied:

Lord, you have no wishes, nor any motives of your own. Naturally there is no need for you to do anything. What benefit do you derive from creating the universe? Creation of the universe is surely a motiveless pastime to you!

Lord, creation emerges from you who are free from the least desire or motive just as the sun, without intending to shine, is reflected in a pool of water without the water intending to so reflect it. Just as the sun causes night and day to follow each other without intending to do so, even so, engage yourself in the non-volitional act of creation. For, what will you gain by abandoning your natural function?

Wise men do not desire to do anything; and wise men do not desire to abandon action either.

Lord, you are viewing this universe thus created by those holy men with your own mental eye. One beholds with physical eyes only such objects as have been created by him in his own mind — naught else. These objects which have been created by the mind are indestructible: only those objects which have been put together with material substances disintegrate. A person is made of whatever is firmly established as the truth of his being in his own mind: that he is, naught else.

mano hi jagatāṁ kartṛ mano hi puruṣaḥ paraḥ
manaḥ kṛtaṁ kṛtaṁ loke na śarīrakṛtaṁ kṛtaṁ (1)

THE SUN continued:

Lord, **the mind alone is the creator of the world; and mind alone is the supreme person. What is done by the mind is action, what is done by the body is not action.** Behold the powers of the mind: by determined thinking the sons of the holy man became creators of the universe! When one, on the other hand, thinks 'I am a little body' he becomes a mortal being. One whose consciousness is extroverted experiences pleasure and pain; on the other hand, the yogi whose vision is introverted does not entertain ideas of pain and pleasure. In this connection there is a legend which I shall narrate to you.

In the country of Magadha there was a king named Indradyumna. Ahalyā was his wife. In that place there was also a handsome young man of loose morals known as Indra. One day during a discourse the queen listened to a story of the seduction of the famed Ahalyā by Indra the king of heaven. As a result she conceived a great love for the young man Indra.

Ahalyā was distraught with love for Indra and with the help of one of her maids managed to have the young man brought to her. From then onwards Indra and Ahalyā used to meet each other in a secret house and enjoy themselves.

Ahalyā was so fond of Indra that she saw him everywhere. The very thought of him made her face radiant. As their love grew, their relationship became public, and it reached the king's ears.

The irate king, in an effort to break this relationship, punished them in numerous ways: they were immersed in ice-cold water, they were fried in boiling oil, they were tied to the legs of an elephant, they were whipped. Indra said to the king, laughingly:

"O king, the entire universe to me is nothing but my beloved. So it is to Ahalyā. Hence we are unaffected by all these. Sir, I am only mind; and mind alone is the individual. You can punish the body; but you cannot punish the mind nor bring about the least change in it. If the mind is fully saturated with something, whatever happens to the body does not affect the mind. The mind is unaffected even by boons and curses, even as the firmly established mountain is not moved by the horns of a little beast. The body does not create the mind, but the mind creates the body. The mind alone is the seed for the body: when the tree dies, the seed does not, but when the seed perishes the tree dies with it. If the body perishes the mind can create other bodies for itself."

pratibhāsam upāyāti yadyad asya hi cetasaḥ
tattat prakaṭatām eti sthairyaṁ saphalatām api (91/17)

THE SUN continued:

Lord, the king thereupon approached the sage Bharata and pleaded that he should punish the recalcitrant couple by cursing them. And, the sage pronounced a curse upon the couple. However, they said to the sage and to the king: "Alas, you are both of little understanding. By thus cursing us you have squandered the merit acquired by penance. Your curse will surely destroy our bodies, but we shall lose nothing by that. No one can destroy the minds of others." However, the sage's curse destroyed their bodies, and on leaving those bodies they were born together as animals and then as birds, and then as a human couple in a holy family. Till now, on account of the total love for each other, they are born together as husband and wife. Even the trees of the forest were inspired and infected by the supreme love and devotion of this couple.

Even the sage's curse could not bring about the mutation of the couple's mind. Even so, Lord, you cannot interfere with the creation of the ten sons of the holy man. But what do you lose if they are thus engaged in their own creation? Let them remain with the creations of their own mind! It cannot be destroyed by you, any more than the reflection in crystal can be removed.

Lord, in your own consciousness create the world as you like. In truth, the infinite consciousness, the mind (one's own consciousness) and the infinite space are all of one substance, pervaded by the infinite consciousness. Therefore regardless of what the young men have created, you can create as many worlds as you like!

BRAHMĀ said to Vasiṣṭha:

Having listened to this advice of the sun I immediately began to create the worlds as the natural expression of my own being. I requested the Sun to be my first partner in this task. Thus, he was the Sun in the creation of the young men and the progenitor of the human race in my creation, and he played this dual role efficiently. In accordance with my intentions he brought about the creation of the worlds. **Whatever appears in one's consciousness, that seems to come into being, gets established, and even bears fruits!** Such is the power of the mind. Just as the sons of the holy man gained the position of creators of the world on account of the powers of their minds, even so have I become the creator of the world. It is the mind that makes things appear here. It brings about the appearance of the body, etc. Naught else is aware of the body.

kathyate jīva nāṁnaitac cittaṁ pratanuvāsanaṁ
śānta deha camatkāraṁ jīvaṁ viddhi kramāt paraṁ (23)

THE CREATOR BRAHMĀ said:

The individualised consciousness (mind) has in it its own manifold potentialities, even as spices have taste in them. That consciousness itself appears as the subtle or ethereal body, and when it becomes gross that itself appears to be the physical or material body. **That individualised consciousness itself is known as the jīva or the individual soul, when the potentialities are in an extremely subtle state. And, when all this jugglery of the jīva ceases, that itself shines as the supreme being.** I am not, nor is there anyone in this universe, all this is nothing but the infinite consciousness. Just as the intention of the young men became manifest, all this is appearance based on infinite consciousness. The young men's intention made them feel that they were the creators: even so am I.

The pure and infinite consciousness alone thinks of itself as the jīva and as the mind and then believes itself to be the body. When this dream-like phantasy is prolonged, this long dream feels like reality! It is both real and unreal: because it is perceived it appears to be real, but because of inherent contradiction it is unreal. The mind is sentient because it is based on consciousness; when viewed as something apart from the consciousness, it is inert and deluded. When there is perception the mind takes on the role of the object of perception — but not in reality — even as when it is perceived as such, the bracelet is seen, though in truth it is gold.

Because Brahman alone is all this, even what is inert is pure consciousness; but all of us, from me down to the rock, are indefinable — neither inert nor sentient. There can be no apprehension of two completely different things: only when there is similarity between the subject and object is perception possible. Concerning what is indefinable and whose existence is not certain, 'inert' and 'sentient' are only words with no substance. In the mind, the subject is believed to be sentient and the object is said to be inert. Thus caught in delusion, the jīva hangs around. In truth, this duality itself is the creation of the mind, an hallucination. Of course, we cannot determine with certainty that such an hallucination exists, either. The infinite consciousness alone IS.

When this illusory division is not seen for what it is, there is the arising of the false egotism. But when the mind enquires into its own nature, this division disappears. There is realisation of the one infinite consciousness, and one attains great bliss.

manasaiva manas tasmāt pauruṣeṇa pumān iha
svakam eva svakenaiva yojayet pāvane pathi (28)

VASIṢṬHA asked Brahmā:

Lord, how is it possible that the sage's curse affected Indra's body and not his mind? If the body is non-different from the mind, then the curse should affect the mind too. Kindly explain to me how the mind is not thus affected — or that it is affected!

THE CREATOR BRAHMĀ replied:

Dear one, in the universe, from Brahmā to a hill, every embodied being has a twofold body. Of these the first is the mental body, which is restless and which acts quickly. The second is the body made of flesh, which does not really do anything. Of these the latter is overpowered by curses and also by boons or charms: it is dumb, powerless, weak and transient like a droplet of water on lotus-leaf, and it is entirely dependent upon fate, destiny and such other factors. Mind however, is independent, though it might seem to be dependent. When this mind confidently engages in self-effort, then it is beyond the reach of sorrow. Whenever it strives, then and there it surely finds the fruition of its striving.

The physical body achieves nothing; on the other hand, the mental body gets results. When the mind dwells constantly on what is pure, it is immune to the effects of curses. The body may fall into fire or mire, but the mind experiences only that which it contemplates. This was demonstrated by Indra. It was also demonstrated by the sage Dīrghatapā, who wished to perform a religious rite but fell into a blind well while collecting the materials for it; he performed the rite mentally and derived the fruit of actual physical performance of the rite. The ten sons of the holy man were also able to achieve Brahmā-hood by their mental effort: even I could not prevent it.

Mental and physical illness, as well as curses and 'evil eye', do not touch the mind that is devoted to the self any more than a lotus flower can split a rock into two by falling on it. Hence, **one should endeavour with the mind to make the mind take to the pure path, with the self make the self tread the path of purity.** Whatever the mind contemplates that instantly materialises. By intense contemplation it can bring about radical change within itself, to heal itself of the defective vision in which illusions were perceived as real. What the mind does, that it experiences as truth. It makes the man who is sitting in moonlight experience burning heat; and it makes one who is in burning sun experience cool comfort!

Such is the mysterious power of the mind.

eṣā jagaj jāṅgala jīrṇavallī saṁyak samāloka kuṭhārakṛttā
vallīva vikṣubdha manaḥśarīrā bhūyo na saṁrohati rāmabhadra (93/24)

VASIṢṬHA continued:

Since the absolute Brahman in its undifferentiated state pervades everything, everything is in an undifferentiated state. When that of its own accord condenses, the cosmic mind is born. In that mind there arises the intention of the existence of the different elements in their extremely subtle state; the totality of all this is the luminous cosmic person who is known as Brahmā the creator. Hence, this Creator is none other than the cosmic mind.

O Rāma, all objects and substances in this universe have emerged in Brahman the absolute, just as waves manifest in the ocean. In this uncreated universe the mind of Brahmā the creator perceives itself as the egotism, and thus does Brahmā the cosmic mind become Brahmā the creator of the universe. The power of that cosmic mind alone appears to be the diverse forces in the universe. Infinite numbers of diverse creatures manifest themselves in this cosmic mind and they are then known as diverse jīvā.

When these diverse jīvā arise in the infinite space of consciousness, seemingly composed of the elements, into each of the bodies consciousness enters through the aperture of life-force, and thence forms the seed of all bodies, both moving and unmoving. Thence, birth as individuals takes place, each individual being accidentally (like the crow alighting and a cocoanut falling) brought into contact with different potentialities whose expression gives rise to the law of cause and effect, etc., and thence to rise and fall in evolution. Desire alone is thereafter the cause of all this.

O Rāma, such is this forest known as world appearance; he who cuts its very root with the axe of investigation (enquiry) is freed from it. Some arrive at this understanding soon, others after a very long time.

O Rāma, I shall now describe to you the divisions of beings into the best, the worst and the middling, as it happened in the beginning of this cycle of creation.

The first and foremost among the creatures are born of noble practices. They are naturally good and devoted to good deeds. They reach liberation in a few lifetimes. They are full of the quality of purity and light (satva).

The middling type are the ones who are full of the quality of dynamism and desire (rajas). When such people are close enough to liberation that on their departure from this world they reach it, they have a mixture of rajas and satva.

They who even after a thousand births are still in darkness, unawakened, are known as beings of darkness (tamas). They may take a long time to reach liberation. By the will of the infinite Brahman all these beings seem to arise and then dissolve in it.

karmanāśe manonāśo manonāśo hy akarmatā
mukttasyaiṣa bhavatyeva nā 'mukttasya kadācana (95/36)

VASIṢṬHA continued:

When the cosmic mind manifested itself in the absolute Brahman, at that very instant the natural tendencies of diverse beings and their behaviour were born, and the embodied beings came to be regarded as jivā. There is no division between mind and action. Before it is projected as action it arises in the mind, with the mind itself as its 'body'. Hence, action is nothing but the movement of energy in consciousness, and it inevitably bears its own fruit. **When such action comes to an end, mind comes to an end, too; and when the mind ceases to be, there is no action. This applies only to the liberated sage, not to others.**

Mind is the only perception; and perception is movement in consciousness. The expression of this movement is action, and fruition follows this. Whatever the mind thinks of, the organs of action strive to materialise: hence, again, mind is action. However, mind, intellect, egotism, individualised consciousness, action, fancy, birth and death, latent tendencies, knowledge, effort, memory, the senses, nature, Māyā or illusion, activity and such other words are but words without corresponding reality: the sole reality is the infinite consciousness in which these concepts are conceived to exist. All these concepts have arisen when, by accidental coincidence (the crow dislodging the cocoanut), the infinite consciousness in a moment of self-forgetfulness viewed itself as the object of perception.

When thus veiled by nescience the same consciousness views diversity in an agitated state and identifies objects as such, it is known as mind. That itself when it is firmly established in the conviction of a certain perception is known as intellect (or intelligence). When it ignorantly and foolishly identifies itself as an existent separate individual, it is known as egotism. When it abandons consistent enquiry, allowing itself to play with countless thoughts coming and going, it is known as individualised consciousness (or mind-stuff).

Whereas pure movement in consciousness is karma or action without an independent doer, when it pursues the fruition of such action it is known as karma (action). When it entertains the notion 'I have seen this before' in relation to something either seen or unseen, it is known as memory. When the effects of past enjoyments continue to remain in the field of consciousness though the effects themselves are unseen, it is known as latent tendency (or potentiality). When it is conscious of the truth that the vision of division is the product of ignorance, it is known as knowledge. On the other hand, when it moves in the wrong direction towards greater self-forgetfulness and deeper involvement in false fancies, it is known as impurity. When it entertains the indweller with sensations, it is known as the senses (indriya). When it remains unmanifest in the cosmic being, it is known as nature. When it creates confusion between reality and appearance, it is known as Māyā (illusion). When it dissolves in the infinite there is liberation. When it thinks 'I am bound' there is bondage; when it thinks 'I am free' there is freedom.

yataḥ kutaścid utpannaṁ cittaṁ yat kiñcid eva hi
nityam ātma vimokṣāya yojayed yatnato 'nagha (98/1)

VASIṢṬHA continued:

Rāma, space is threefold: the infinite space of undivided consciousness, the finite space of divided consciousness and the physical space in which the material worlds exist.

The infinite space of undivided consciousness (cid ākāśa) is that which exists in all, inside and outside, as the pure witness of that which is real and of that which appears to be. The finite space of divided consciousness (citta akāśā) is that which creates the divisions of time, which pervades all beings, and which is interested in the welfare of all beings. The physical space is that in which the other elements (air, etc.) exist. The latter two are not independent of the first. In fact, the others do not exist.

O Rāma, whatever might have been the origin of the mind and whatever it might be, one should constantly direct it towards liberation through self-effort. The pure mind is free from latent tendencies, and therefore it attains self-knowledge. Since the entire universe is within the mind, the notions of bondage and liberation are also within it. In this connection there is the following legend which I heard from the creator Brahmā himself. Listen to it attentively.

There was a great forest, so large that in it millions of square miles were like the space within an atom. In it there was just one person who had a thousand arms and limbs. He was forever restless. He had a mace in his hand with which he beat himself and, afraid of the beating, he ran away in panic. He fell into a blind well. He came out of it, again beat himself and again ran away in panic, this time into a forest. He came out of it, again beat himself and again ran away in panic, this time into a banana grove. Though there was no other being to fear, he wept and cried aloud in fear. He kept running as before, beating himself as before.

I witnessed all this intuitively, and with the power of my will I restrained him for a moment. I asked him, "Who are you?" But, he was sore distressed and called me his enemy and wept aloud and then laughed aloud. Then he began to abandon his body — limb by limb.

Immediately after this, I saw another person running like the first one, beating himself, weeping and wailing. When I similarly restrained him, he began to abuse me and ran away intent on his own way of life. Like this I came across several persons. Some listened to my words and, abandoning their previous way of life, became enlightened. Some others ignored me or even held me in contempt. Some others even refused to come out of the blind well or the dense forest.

Such is the great forest, O Rāma: no one finds a sure resting place in it, whatever be the mode of life they may adopt. Even today you see such people in this world; and you yourself have seen such a life of ignorance and delusion. Because you are young and ignorant, you do not understand it.

karaṇaṁ karma kartā ca jananaṁ maraṇaṁ sthitiḥ
sarvaṁ brahmaiva nahyasti tadvinā kalpanetarā (100/30)

VASIṢṬHA continued:

O Rāma, this great forest is not far away, nor is that strange man in a strange land! The world itself is the forest. It is a great void; but this void is seen only in the light of enquiry. This light of enquiry is the 'I' in the parable. This wisdom is accepted by some and rejected by others, who continue to suffer. They who accept it are enlightened.

The person with thousands of arms is the mind with countless manifestations. This mind punishes itself by its own latent tendencies and restlessly wanders in this world. The blind well in the story is hell and the banana grove is heaven. The dense forest of thorny bush is the life of a worldly man, with the numerous thorns of wife, children, wealth, etc. hurting him all the time. The mind now wanders into hell, now into heaven and now into the world of human beings.

Even when the light of wisdom shines on the life of the deluded mind, it foolishly rejects it, considering that that wisdom is its enemy. Then it weeps and wails in distress. Sometimes it experiences an imperfect awakening and it renounces the pleasures of the world without proper understanding — such renunciation itself proves to be a great source of sorrow. But, when such renunciation arises out of the fullness of understanding, of wisdom born of enquiry into the nature of the mind, the renunciation leads to supreme bliss. Such a mind may even look at its own past notions of pleasure with puzzlement. Just as the limbs of the person as they were cut away fell down and disappeared, the latent tendencies of the person who wisely renounces the world also vanish from the mind. Behold the play of ignorance which makes one hurt oneself out of one's own volition; and which makes one run hither and thither in meaningless panic.

When one who gains wisdom preserves it for a long time and persists in the practice of enquiry, he does not experience sorrow. An uncontrolled mind is the source of sorrow; when it is thoroughly understood, the sorrow vanishes like mist at sunrise.

The absolute Brahman is omnipotent: and there is nothing which is outside of it. It is His own power or energy that pervades all things. In embodied beings, it is the cit-śakti (the power of consciousness or intelligence). It is motion in air, stability in earth, void in space, and it is the power of self-consciousness ('I am') in created beings. Yet all this is nothing but the power of the absolute Brahman. **The instruments of action, action and the doer, birth, death and existence — all this is Brahman, Nothing else is, even in imagination.** Delusion, craving, greed and attachment are non-existent; how can they exist when there is no duality? When bondage is non-existent, surely liberation is false, too.

saṅkalpajālakalanaiva jagatsamagraṁ
saṅkalpameva nanu viddhi vilāsacetyaṁ
sankalpamātramalam utsṛjya nirvikalpa
māśritya niścayam avāpnuhi rāma śāntiṁ (39)

VASIṢṬHA continued:

To illustrate this there is an interesting legend. Kindly listen to it.

A young boy asked his nanny to tell him a story, and the nanny told him the following story to which the boy listened with great attention:

Once upon a time in a city which did not exist, there were three princes who were brave and happy. Of them two were unborn and the third had not been conceived. Unfortunately all their relatives died. The princes left their native city to go elsewhere. Very soon, unable to bear the heat of the sun, they fell into a swoon. Their feet were burnt by hot sand. The tips of grass pierced them. They reached the shade of three trees, of which two did not exist and the third had not even been planted. After resting there for some time and eating the fruits of those trees, they proceeded further.

They reached the banks of three rivers; of them two were dry and in the third there was no water. The princes had a refreshing bath and quenched their thirst in them. They then reached a huge city which was about to be built. Entering it, they found three palaces of exceeding beauty. Of them two had not been built at all, and the third had no walls. They entered the palaces and found three golden plates; two of them had been broken into two and the third had been pulverised. They took hold of the one which had been pulverised. They took ninety-nine minus one hundred grams of rice and cooked it. They then invited three holy men to be their guests; of them two had no body and the third had no mouth. After these holy men had eaten the food, the three princes partook of the rest of the food cooked. They were greatly pleased. Thus they lived in that city for a long, long time in peace and joy. My child this is an extremely beautiful legend; pray remember this always, and you will grow up into a learned man.

O Rāma, when the little boy heard this he was thrilled.

What is known as the creation of the world is no more real than this story of the young boy. This world is nothing but pure hallucination. It is nothing more than an idea. In the infinite consciousness the idea of creation arose: and that is what is. O **Rāma, this world is nothing more than an idea; all the objects of consciousness in this world are just an idea; reject the error (dirt) of ideation and be free of ideas; remain rooted in truth and attain peace.**

abaddho baddha ity uktvā kiṁ śocasi mudhaiva hi
anantasyā ''tmatattvasya kiṁ kathaṁ kena badhyate (9)

VASIṢṬHA continued:

Only a fool, not a wise man, is deluded by his own ideas; it is a fool who thinks that the imperishable is perishable, and gets deluded. Egotism is but an idea based on a false association of the self with the physical elements. When one alone exists in all this as the infinite consciousness, how has what is called egotism arisen? In fact, this egotism does not exist any more than water exists in the mirage. Therefore, O Rāma, abandon your imperfect vision which is not based on fact; rest in the perfect vision which is of the nature of bliss and which is based on truth.

Enquire into the nature of truth. Abandon falsehood. **You are ever free; why do you call yourself bound and then grieve? The self is infinite; why, how and by whom is it bound?** There is no division in the self, for the absolute Brahman is all this. What then is called bondage and what is liberation? It is only in a state of ignorance that you think you experience pain, though you are untouched by pain. These things do not exist in the self.

Let the body fall or rise or let it go on to another universe; I am not confined to the body, then how am I affected by all this? The relation between the body and the self is like the relation between the cloud and wind, like the relation between lotus and the bee. When the cloud is dispersed, the wind becomes one with space. When the lotus withers, the bee flies away into the sky. The self is not destroyed when the body falls. Even the mind does not cease to be until it is burnt in the fire of self-knowledge; not to mention the self.

Death is but the veiling by time and space of the ever-present self. Only foolish people fear death.

Abandon your latent tendencies even as a bird wishing to fly into the sky breaks out of its shell. Born of ignorance, these tendencies are hard to destroy, and they give birth to endless sorrow. It is this ignorant self-limiting tendency of the mind that views the infinite as finite. However, even as sun dispels mist, enquiry into the nature of the self dispels this ignorant self-limiting tendency. In fact, the very desire to undertake this enquiry is able to bring about a change. Austerities and such other practices are of no use in this. When the mind is purified of its past by the arising of wisdom, it abandons its previous tendencies. The mind seeks the self only in order to dissolve itself in the self. This indeed is in the very nature of the mind. This is the supreme goal, Rāma: strive for this.

At this stage, another day came to a close.

tīvramandatva saṁvegād bahutvālpatva bhedataḥ
vilambanena ca ciraṁ na tu śakttim aśakttitaḥ (103/15)

VASIṢṬHA continued:

Having manifested in the infinite consciousness, the mind has by its own nature spread itself out. By its nature, again, it makes the long appear short and vice versa, and makes one's own appear to be different and vice versa. Even a little thing which it touches, it magnifies and makes its own. In the twinkling of an eye it creates countless worlds and in the twinkling of an eye it destroys them. Even as an able actor plays several roles one after the other, the mind assumes several aspects one after the other. It makes the unreal appear as real and vice versa; and on account of this it seems to enjoy and to suffer. Even that which it gets naturally it grabs with hands and feet, and as a result of this false sense of ownership, it suffers the consequences.

Time as changing seasons is able indirectly to bring about changes in the trees and plants; even so, the mind makes one thing appear to be another by its powers of thought and ideation. Therefore, even time and space and all things are under the control of the mind. **Depending upon its intensity or dullness, and upon the size (big or small) of the object created or influenced, the mind does what is to be done with some delay or much later: it is not incapable of doing anything whatsoever.**

Pray, O Rāma, listen to another interesting legend to illustrate this.

In a country known as Uttarāpāndava, in whose forests sages dwelt and whose villages were beautiful and prosperous, there reigned a king known as Lavaṇa who was a descendant of the famous king Hariścandra. He was righteous, noble, chivalrous, charitable and in every way a worthy king. His enemies had all been conquered; and their followers could not even think of him without becoming feverish with anxiety.

One day, this king went to his court and ascended the throne. After all the ministers and others had paid their homage to him, a juggler entered the court and saluted him. He said to the king: "I shall show you something wonderful!" As he waved a bunch of peacock feathers, there entered into the court a cavalier leading and exquisitely beautiful horse. He requested the king to accept it as a gift. The juggler requested the king to ride that horse and roam freely throughout the world. The king also saw the horse.

Thereupon, the king closed his eyes and sat motionless. Seeing this everyone assembled in the court became silent. Absolute peace reigned in the court, as no one dared to disturb the king's peace.

anabhyasta vivekaṁ hi deśakālavaśānugaṁ
mantrauṣadhivaśaṁ yāti mano nodāravṛttimat (105/15)

VASIṢṬHA continued:

Rāma, after some time the king opened his eyes and began to tremble as if in fear. As he was about to fall down, the ministers supported him. Dismayed to see them, the king asked: "Who are you and what are you doing to me?" The worried ministers said to him: "Lord, you are a mighty king of great wisdom and yet this delusion has overpowered you. What has happened to your mind? Only they who are attached to the little objects of this world and the false relationships of wife, children, etc., are subject to mental aberrations, not one like you, devoted to the supreme. Moreover, **only he who has not cultivated wisdom is adversely affected by spells, drugs etc., not one whose mind is fully developed.**"

Hearing this the king partly regained his composure, though upon looking at the juggler he trembled as if in fear, and said to him: "O magician, what have you done to me? You have spread a net of illusion over me. Truly, even the wise are overpowered by the jugglery of Māyā; even as, though I am still in this body, within a short period I experienced wonderful hallucinations." Turning to the members of the court the king recounted his experiences during the previous hour.

"As soon as I saw this juggler wave his bundle of peacock feathers, I jumped on the horse which stood in front of me and experienced a slight mental delusion. Then I went away on a hunting expedition. The horse led me into an arid desert where nothing lived, nothing grew, where there was no water and it was bitterly cold. I experienced great grief I spent the whole day there. Later, riding that horse again I crossed that desert and reached another which was less dreadful; I rested under a tree. The horse ran away. I rested for some time and the sun set. Frightened, I hid myself in a bush. The night was longer than an epoch.

"The day dawned. The sun rose. A little later, I saw a dark girl clad in black clothes carrying a plateful of food. I approached her and begged for food. I was hungry. She ignored me; I pursued her. At last she said "I shall give you food if you consent to marry me." I consented; survival was the first and foremost consideration then. She gave me food and later introduced me to her father who was even more dreadful to look at. Soon the three of us reached their village, which was flowing with blood and flesh. I was introduced to all as that girl's husband. I was treated by them with great respect. They entertained me with dreadful stories which were a source of pain. At a diabolical ceremony I got married to that girl."

ākruṣṭamuddharatararn ruditarn vipatsu
bhukttarn kadannamuṣitarn hatapakvaṇeṣu
kālāntararn bahu mayopahatena tatra durvāsanānigaḍa
bandhagatena sabhyāḥ (107/48)

THE KING continued:

Very soon, I had become a member of the primitive tribe. My wife gave birth to a daughter, the source of more unhappiness to me. In course of time three more babies arrived. I had become a family man in that tribe. I spent many years among this tribe, suffering the agonies of a family man with a wife and children to feed and to protect. I cut firewood and often I had to sleep under a tree at night. When the weather became cold I hid myself in a bush in order to keep warm. Pork was my staple diet.

Time rolled on and I became old. I began to trade in meat. I took the meat to the villages on the Vindhya mountains and sold the best part of it there; what could not thus be sold at a decent profit I cut up into bits and dried in a terribly filthy place. When I was afflicted with hunger I would often fight with others in the tribe for a piece of meat to eat. My body had become black as soot.

Thus, engaged in sinful activities, my mind had also become inclined towards sin. Good thoughts and feelings had taken leave of me. My heart had shed all compassion, even as a snake sheds its slough. With nets and other traps and weapons I caused untold hardship to birds and animals.

Clad only in a loin cloth I endured every inclemency of the weather. Thus I spent seven years. **Bound by the ropes of evil tendencies, I grew wild with anger and used abusive words, wept in misfortunes, and ate rotten food. Thus I lived for a long time in that place.** I drifted like a dry leaf in the wind, as if my only mission in life was eating.

There was drought in the land. The air was so hot that it seemed to waft sparks of flame. The forest caught alight. Only ashes remained. People were dying of hunger. People chased after mirages thinking there was water. They mistook pebbles to be balls of meat and began to chew on them.

Some had even begun to eat corpses. Some, while doing so, even chewed their own fingers which had been soaked in the blood of those dead bodies. Such was their demented state of starvation.

What was once a flourishing forest had been transformed into a huge crematorium. What was once a pleasure-grove resounded with the agonised cries of the dying.

Note: These two chapters are full of apt and graphic similes.

manovilāsaḥ saṁsāra iti yasyāṁ pratiyate
sarvaśaktter anantasya vilāso hi mano jagat (25)

THE KING continued:

Thus afflicted by famine many people left the country and migrated elsewhere. Some others, deeply attached to their wife and children, perished in that land. Many others were killed by wild animals.

I, too, left the country to go away along with my wife and children. At the border of the country I found the cool shade of a tree tempting and, after putting down the little children I was carrying on my shoulders, I rested under that tree for a long time.

The youngest of my children was quite small and innocent, and therefore was the dearest to my heart. With tears in his eyes he demanded food. Although I told him that there was no meat to eat, in his childish innocence he persisted in his demand, unable to bear his hunger. I said to him in despair, "All right, eat my flesh!" The innocent child said, without thinking, "Give me."

I was moved by attachment and pity. I saw that the child was unable to endure the pangs of hunger any more. I decided that the best way to end all these miseries was to end my life. I raised a pyre with the help of the timber I found nearby. And, as I ascended that pyre, I shuddered — and I found myself in this court, being hailed and greeted by all of you.

(As the king said this the juggler vanished.) The MINISTERS said:

Lord, he cannot be a juggler, for he was not interested in money, in a reward. Surely, some divine entity wished to demonstrate to you and to all of us the power of cosmic illusion. **From all this it is clear that this world-appearance is nothing but the play of the mind; the mind itself is but the play of the omnipotent infinite being.** The mind is able to fool even men of great wisdom. Else, where is the king who is well versed in all branches of learning, and where is this bewildering delusion?

Surely this is not a juggler's trick: for a juggler performs for material gain. It is really the power of illusion. Hence, the juggler vanished without looking for a reward.

VASIṢṬHA said:

Rāma, I was there in that court at that time and so I know all this first-hand. In this manner the mind veils the real nature of the self and creates an illusory appearance with many branches, flowers and fruits. Destroy this illusion by wisdom, and rest in peace.

manomātraṁ jagat kṛtsnaṁ manaḥ paryantamaṇḍalaṁ
mano vyoma mano bhūmir mano vāyur mano mahān (15)

VASIṢṬHA continued:

The impure mind sees a ghost where there is just a post and pollutes all relationship, creating suspicion among friends and making enemies of them, even as a drunken man sees that the world is revolving around him. A distressed mind turns food into poison and causes disease and death. The impure mind (laden with tendencies) is the cause for delusions (manias and phobias). One should strive to uproot these and discard them. What is man but the mind? **Mind is the whole world, mind is the atmosphere, mind is the sky, mind is earth, mind is wind; and mind is great.** Only he whose mind is foolish is called a fool: when the body loses its intelligence (for example, in death) the corpse is not said to be foolish! Mind decides the length of time: the king Lavaṇa experienced the period of less than an hour as if it were extended to a life-time.

What is more mysterious, Rāma, than that the mind is able to veil the omnipresent, pure, eternal, and infinite consciousness, making you confuse it with this inert physical body? The mind itself appears as wind in the moving element, lustre in the lustrous, solidity in the earth and void in the space.

If 'the mind is elsewhere' the taste of food that is being eaten is not really experienced. If 'the mind is elsewhere' one does not see what is right in front of oneself. The senses are born of the mind, but not the other way round.

It is only from the point of view of fools that the body and the mind are said to be quite different; in fact, they are non-different, being mind alone. Salutations to those sages who have actually realised this truth.

The sage who has realised this is not disturbed even if the body is embraced by a woman: to him it is like a piece of wood coming into contact with the body. Even if his arms are cut off, he does not experience it. He is able to convert all sorrow into bliss.

Just as an actor is able to portray in himself the character of different personalities, the mind is able to create different states of consciousness — like waking and dreaming. How mysterious is the mind which is able to make the king Lavaṇa feel that he is a primitive tribesman! The mind experiences what it itself constructs, the mind is nothing but what has been put together by thought: knowing this, do as you please.

He who does not allow his mind to roam in objects of pleasure is able to master it. Even as one who is bound to a pillar does not move, the mind of a noble man does not move from the reality: he alone is a human being, the others are worms. He attains to the supreme being by constant meditation.

yat tu cañcalatāhīnaṁ tan mano mṛtam ucyate
tad eva ca tapaḥ śāstra siddhānto mokṣa ucyate (112/8)

VASIṢṬHA continued:

Victory over this goblin known as mind is gained when, with the aid of one's own self-effort, one attains self-knowledge and abandons the craving for what the mind desires as pleasure. This can easily be achieved without any effort at all (even as a child's attention can be easily diverted) by the cultivation of the proper attitude. Woe unto him who is unable to give up cravings, for this is the sole means to one's ultimate good. By intense self-effort it is possible to gain victory over the mind; and then without the least effort the individualised consciousness is absorbed in the infinite consciousness when its individuality is broken through. This is easy and easily accomplished: they who are unable to do this are indeed vultures in human form.

Abandon your reliance on fate or gods created by dull-witted people, and by self-effort and self-knowledge make the mind no-mind. Let the infinite consciousness swallow, as it were, the finite mind, and then go beyond everything. With your intelligence united with the supreme, hold on to the self which is imperishable.

When the mind is thus conquered by remaining completely unagitated, you will consider even the conquest of the three worlds worthless. This does not involve studying the scriptures, or rising or falling — nothing but self-knowledge. Why do you consider it difficult? If this is found difficult by someone, how does he even live in this world without self-knowledge?

One who knows the deathless nature of the self is not afraid of death. Nor is he affected by separation from friends and relations. The feelings 'This is I' and 'This is mine' are the mind; when they are removed, the mind ceases to be. Then one becomes fearless. Weapons like sword generate fear; the weapon (wisdom) that destroys egotism generates fearlessness.

Towards whichever object the mind flows with intensity, in that it sees the fulfilment of its craving. Of course, there is no mind without restlessness; restlessness is the very nature of the mind. It is the work of this restlessness of the mind based on the infinite consciousness that appears as this world, O Rāma: that indeed is the power of the mind. But, **when the mind is deprived of its restlessness, it is referred to as the dead mind; and that itself is penance (tapas) as also the verification of the scriptures and liberation.**

O Rāma, mind constantly swings like a pendulum between the reality and the appearance, between consciousness and inertness. When the mind contemplates the inert objects for a considerable time, it assumes the characteristics of such inertness. When the same mind is devoted to enquiry and wisdom, it shakes off all conditioning and returns to its original nature as pure consciousness.

mā vā 'kartā bhava prājña kim akartṛtayehite
sādhyaṁ sādhyam upādeyaṁ tasmāt svastho bhavā 'nagha (7)

VASIṢṬHA continued:

The psychological tendency (or mental disposition or mental conditioning) is unreal, yet it does arise in the mind. The product of ignorance is real only to the ignorant person; to the wise, it is just a verbal expression (just as one speaks of the barren woman's son). Do not remain ignorant, O Rāma, but strive to be wise by renouncing mental conditioning.

You are not the doer of any action here, O Rāma; so, why do you assume doership? When one alone exists, who does what and how? **Do not become inactive, either; for what is gained by doing nothing? What has to be done has to be done. Therefore rest in the self.** Even while doing all the actions natural to you, if you are unattached to those actions you are truly the non-doer; if you are doing nothing and are attached to that non-doership (then you are **doing** nothing) you become the doer! When all this world is like the juggler's trick, what is to be given up and what is to be sought?

The seed of this world appearance is ignorance. This ignorance or mental conditioning is acquired by man effortlessly and it seems to promote pleasure, but in truth it is the giver of grief. It creates a delusion of pleasure only by the total veiling of self-knowledge. Thus it was able to make the king Lavaṇa experience less than an hour as if it were of several years' duration.

This ignorance or mental conditioning has but a momentary existence: yet, since it flows on, it seems to be permanent like a river. Because it is able to veil the reality, it seems to be real: but when you try to grasp it, you discover it is nothing. Yet, again, it acquires strength and firmness on account of these qualities in the world-appearance, even as a flimsy fibre when rolled into a rope acquires great strength. This conditioning seems to grow, but in fact it does not. For when you try to grasp it, it vanishes like the tip of a flame. Yet, again, even as the sky appears to be blue, this conditioning also seems to have some kind of real appearance! It is born as the second moon in diplopia, it exists like the dream-objects and it creates confusion, even as people sitting in a moving boat see the shore moving. When it is active it creates a delusion of the long dream of world-appearance. It perverts all relationships and experiences. It is this ignorance or mental conditioning that is responsible for the creation and perception of duality, and of division and the consequent confusion of perception and experience.

When this ignorance or mental conditioning is mastered by becoming aware of its unreality, mind ceases to be — even as when the water ceases to flow, the river dries up.

nā 'haṁ brahmeti saṅkalpāt sudṛḍhād badhyate manaḥ
sarvaṁ brahmeti saṅkalpāt sudṛḍhānmucyate manaḥ (23)

VASIṢṬHA continued:

O Rāma, even as darkness disappears as you turn towards light, ignorance disappears if you turn towards the light of the self. As long as there does not arise a natural yearning for self-knowledge, so long this ignorance or mental conditioning throws up an endless stream of world-appearance. Even as a shadow vanishes when it turns to see the light, this ignorance perishes when it turns towards self-knowledge.

O Rāma, from Brahmā the creator down to the blade of grass, all this is nothing but the self: ignorance is non-existent unreality. There is no second thing here known as the mind. In that self itself, the veil (that is also of itself) floats, creating the polarisation of subject-object; and the infinite consciousness itself is then known as the mind. This veil is an idea, an intention or a thought in that infinite consciousness. Mind is born of this idea or thought, and mind has to vanish with the help of an idea or thought i.e. by the coming to an end of the idea or thought.

The firm conviction that 'I am not the absolute Brahman' binds the mind; and the mind is liberated by the firm conviction that 'everything is the absolute Brahman'. Ideas and thoughts are bondage; and their coming to an end is liberation. Therefore, be free of them and do whatever has to be done spontaneously. Even as thought or idea 'sees' blueness in the sky, the mind sees the world as real.

He who does not let his mind dwell on such thoughts and ideas, by striving to be conscious of the self, enjoys peace. That which was not in the beginning does not exist even now! That which was and therefore is now, is the absolute Brahman — contemplation of this bestows peace, for that Brahman is peace. One should not contemplate anything else at any time and in any manner anywhere. One should uproot the very hope of enjoyment with one's utmost strength, and using one's utmost intelligence. Hopes and attachments seem to ramify on account of the mental conditioning which is ignorance. In this empty physical body, where is it that is called 'I'? In truth, O Rāma, 'I', 'mine', etc. have no existence at all; the one self alone is the truth at all times.

Is it not a great wonder, O Rāma, that people forget the truth that the absolute Brahman alone is, and are convinced of the existence of the unreal and non-existent ignorance? Rāma, do not let the foolish idea of the existence of ignorance take root in you; for if the consciousness is thus polluted, it invites endless suffering. Though it is unreal, it can cause real suffering! It is on account of ignorance that illusions like a mirage exist, and that one sees various visions and hallucinations (like flying in the air and flying in space) and one experiences heaven and hell. Therefore, O Rāma, give up mental conditioning which alone is responsible for the perception of duality, and remain totally unconditioned. Then, you will attain incomparable pre-eminence over all!

sarveṣu sukhaduḥkheṣu sarvāsu kalanāsu ca
manaḥ kartṛ mano bhoktṛ mānasaṁ viddhi mānavaṁ (24)

After a few minutes of deep contemplation, RĀMA asked:

Holy sage! It is indeed incredible that this non-existent nescience creates such an illusion that this non-existent world appears to be very real: pray explain to me further how this is possible. Also please tell me why the king Lavaṇa underwent all sorts of sufferings. Please tell me who or what it is that experiences all these sufferings.

VASIṢṬHA replied:

O Rāma, it is not really true that consciousness is in any way related to this body. The body has only been fancied by the consciousness as if in a dream. When consciousness, clothed as it were, by its own energy, limits itself and considers itself a jīva, that jīva, endowed with this restless energy, is involved in this world-appearance.

The embodied being who enjoys or suffers the fruits of past actions and who dons a variety of bodies is known as egotism, mind and also jīva. Neither the body nor the enlightened being undergoes suffering: it is only the ignorant mind that suffers. It is only in a state of ignorance (like sleep) that the mind dreams of the world-appearance, not when it is awake or enlightened. Hence the embodied being that undergoes suffering here is variously known as the mind, ignorance, jīva and mental conditioning, as also the individualised consciousness.

The body is insentient and hence can neither enjoy nor suffer. Nescience gives rise to heedlessness and unwisdom; hence it is nescience alone that enjoys or suffers. It is indeed the mind alone that is born, weeps, kills, goes, abuses others, etc., not the body. **In all the experiences of happiness and unhappiness, as also in all the hallucinations and imaginations, it is mind that does everything and it is mind that experiences all this: mind is man.**

I shall narrate to you the reason for the sufferings of the king Lavaṇa. Lavaṇa was a descendant of Hariścandra. Lavaṇa thought: "My grandfather performed a great religious rite and became a great man. I should also perform the same rite." He gathered the necessary materials and the religious men and he performed the rite mentally for a whole year, while sitting in his own garden.

Since he had thus successfully completed the religious rite performed mentally, he was entitled to its fruits. O Rāma, thus you see that the mind alone is the performer of all actions and hence it is also the experiencer of all happiness and unhappiness. Therefore, guide your mind along the path to salvation, Rāma.

bījajāgrat tathā jāgran mahājāgrat tathaiva ca
jāgrat svapnas tathā svapnaḥ svapna jāgrat suṣuptakaṁ
iti saptavidho mohaḥ punareva parasparaṁ (117/12)

VASIṢṬHA continued:

I myself was a witness to the scene in king Lavaṇa's court, and when they wished to know who that juggler was after he had abruptly disappeared from the court, I saw his identity through my subtle vision and found that he was a messenger of the gods. It is the tradition that Indra would send all sorts of afflictions to test the strength of anyone who engaged himself in that particular religious rite which Lavaṇa was performing mentally. The hallucinations he had were the result. The rite was performed by the mind and the hallucinations were experienced by the mind.

When the same mind is thoroughly purified, you will get rid of all duality and diversity which it creates.

Rāma, I have already narrated to you the process of cyclical creation (after the previous cosmic dissolution), and of how one comes to entertain the false notions of 'I' and 'mine'. Equipped with wisdom, he who gradually ascends the seven steps to perfection in yoga attains liberation from these.

RĀMA asked:

Holy sir, what are the seven steps you have referred to?

VASIṢṬHA replied:

O Rāma, there are seven descending steps of ignorance; and there are seven ascending steps of wisdom. I shall now describe them to you. To remain established in self-knowledge is liberation; when this is disturbed there arises egotism and bondage. The state of self-knowledge is that in which there is no mental agitation, neither distraction nor dullness of mind, neither egotism nor perception of diversity.

The delusion that veils this self-knowledge is sevenfold: seed state of wakefulness, wakefulness, great wakefulness, wakeful dream, dream, dream wakefulness and sleep. In pure consciousness, when mind and jīva exist only in name, it is the seed state of wakefulness. When notions of 'I' and 'this' arise it is known as wakefulness. When these notions get strengthened by the memory of previous incarnations, it is great wakefulness. When the mind is fully awake to its own fancies and is filled with them, it is wakeful dream. The false notions of experiences during sleep, which yet appear to be real, are dreams. In the dream wakeful state one recalls past experiences as if they are real now. When these are abandoned in favour of total inert dullness, it is sleep. These seven have their own innumerable subdivisions.

jñānabhūmiḥ śubhecchākhyā prathamā samudāhṛtā
vicāraṇā dvitīyā tu tṛtīyā tanumānasā (50)
sattvāpattiś caturthī syāt tato 'saṁsakttināmikā
padārthābhāvanī ṣaṣṭi saptamī turyagā smṛtā (6)

VASIṢTHA continued:

I shall now describe to you, O Rāma, the seven states or planes of wisdom. Knowing them you will not be caught in delusion. **Pure wish or intention is the first, enquiry is the second, the third is when the mind becomes subtle, establishment in truth is the fourth, total freedom from attachment or bondage is the fifth, the sixth is cessation of objectivity, and the seventh is beyond all these.**

'Why do I continue to be a fool? I shall seek holy men and scriptures, having cultivated dispassion' — such a wish is the first state. Thereupon one engages in the practice of enquiry (direct observation). With all these, there arises non-attachment, and the mind becomes subtle and transparent: this is the third state. When these three are practised, there arises in the seeker a natural turning away from sense-pleasures and there is natural dwelling in truth: this is the fourth state.

When all these are well practised, there is total non-attachment and at the same time a conviction in the nature of truth: this is the fifth state. Then one rejoices in one's own self, the perception of duality and diversity both within oneself and outside oneself ceases, and the efforts that one made at the inspiration of others bear fruition in direct spiritual experience.

After this there is no other support, no division, no diversity, and self-knowledge is spontaneous, natural and therefore unbroken: this is the seventh, transcendental state. This is the state of one who is liberated while living here. Beyond this is the state of one who has transcended even the body (turīyātīta).

Rāma, all these great ones who ascend these seven planes of wisdom are holy men. They are liberated and they do not fall into the mire of happiness and unhappiness. They may or may not work or be active. They rejoice in the self and do not stand in need of others to make them happy.

The highest state of consciousness can be attained by all, even by animals and by primitive men, by those who have a body and even by disembodied beings, for it involves only the rise of wisdom.

They who have reached the highest planes of consciousness are indeed great men. They are adorable; even an emperor is like a worthless blade of grass compared to them, for they are liberated here and now.

tvattā 'hantā ''tmatā tattā sattā 'sattā na kācana
na kvacid bhedakalanā na bhāvo na ca rañjanā (21)

VASIṢṬHA continued:

The self ignorantly imagines an egotistic existence, even as if gold, forgetting its goldness, might think it is a ring and weep and wail "Alas, I have lost my goldness".

RĀMA asked:

Holy sir, how can this ignorance and egotism arise in the self?

VASISTHA said:

Rāma, one should ask questions concerning the reality only, not concerning the unreal. Neither goldless ringness nor limited egotism exists in truth. When the goldsmith sells the ring he weighs out the gold: for it is gold. If one were to discuss the existence of the ringness in the ring, and the finite form in infinite consciousness, then one has to compare it with the barren woman's son. The existence of the unreal is unreal: it arises in ignorance and vanishes when enquired into. In ignorance one sees silver in the mother-of-pearl: but it cannot serve as silver even for a moment! As long as the truth that it is mother-of-pearl is not seen, the ignorance lasts. Even as one cannot extract oil from sand and even as one can obtain only gold from the ring, there are no two things in this universe: the one infinite consciousness alone shines in all names and forms.

Such indeed is the nature of this utter ignorance, this delusion and this world-process: without real existence there is this illusory notion of egotism. This egotism does not exist in the infinite self. In the infinite self there is no creator, no creation, no worlds, no heaven, no humans, no demons, no bodies, no elements, no time, no existence and no destruction, **no 'you', no 'I', no self, no that, no truth, no falsehood (none of these), no notion of diversity, no contemplation and no enjoyment.** Whatever is, and is known as the universe, is that supreme peace. There is no beginning, no middle and no end: all is all at all times, beyond the comprehension of the mind and the speech. There is no creation. The infinite has never abandoned its infinity. That has never become this. It is like the ocean, but without ocean's movement. It is self-luminous like the sun, but without activity. In ignorance, the supreme being is viewed as the object, as the world. Even as space exists in space, one with space, even so what appears to be the creation is Brahman existing in Brahman, as Brahman. The notions of far and near, of diversity, of here and there are as valid as the distance between two objects in a mirror in which a whole city is reflected.

ityevaṁ rāghavā 'vidyā mahatī bhramadāyinī
asat sattāṁ nayatyāśu saccā 'sattāṁ nayatyālaṁ (121/10)

VASIṢṬHA continued:

The day after his hallucinatory experience king Lavaṇa thought: "I should actually go to those places that I saw in the vision; perhaps they exist in reality." Immediately he set out with his retinue and proceeded in a southerly direction. Soon he came across the very scenes of his vision and the type of people whom he had seen then. He met the very people whom he knew during his existence as a tribesman. He even saw his own destitute children.

He saw there an old woman who was weeping and screaming in agony: "O my beloved husband, where have you gone, leaving us all here. I have lost my beautiful daughter who had an extraordinary stroke of luck to obtain a handsome king for her husband. Where have they all gone? Alas, I have lost all of them." The king approached her, consoled her and learnt from her that she was indeed the mother of his tribal wife! Out of compassion he gave them enough wealth to meet their needs and to help them out of the drought that had stricken the whole countryside, even as he had seen the day before. He dwelt among them for some time and then returned to his palace.

The next morning the king asked me to explain the mystery, and was fully satisfied with my answer. **O Rāma, thus the power of nescience is capable of creating a total confusion between the real and the unreal.**

RĀMA asked:

O sage, this is indeed puzzling. How can that which was seen in a dream or an hallucination be also experienced in the reality of the waking state?

VASIṢṬHA answered:

But, O Rāma, all this is ignorance! The notions of far and near, a moment and eternity, are all hallucinations. In ignorance the real appears to be unreal, and the unreal seems to be real. The individualised consciousness perceives what it thinks it perceives, on account of its conditioning. On account of ignorance, when the notion of egotism arises, at that very moment the delusion of a beginning, a middle and an end also arises. One who is thus deluded thinks that he is an animal and experiences this. All this happens on account of accidental coincidence: just as a crow flies towards a cocoanut palm and as it alights on the tree, a fruit falls down as if the crow dislodged it — though, in fact, the crow did not! Similarly, by pure coincidence and in ignorance, the unreal seems to be real.

avidyayā "tmatattvasya sambandho nopapadyate
sambandhaḥ sadṛśānām ca yaḥ sphuṭaḥ svānubhūtitaḥ (33)

VASIṢṬHA continued:

In his hypnotic state the king Lavaṇa obviously saw reflected in his own consciousness the marriage of a prince with the tribal woman, etc., and he experienced it as if it happened to him. A man forgets what he did earlier in his life even if at that time he had devoted a lot of time and energy to that action. Even so, he now thinks that he did not do what he actually did. Such discrepancies in memory are often seen.

Even as one sometimes dreams of a past incident as if it happens now, Lavaṇa experienced in his vision some past incident connected with the tribesmen. It is possible that the people in the forests on the slopes of the Vindhya experienced in their own minds the visions that appeared in the consciousness of Lavana. It is also possible that Lavaṇa and the tribesmen saw in their own minds whatever was experienced by the other. These hallucinations become reality when experienced by many, even as a statement made by very many people is accepted as true. When these are incorporated in one's life they acquire their own reality: after all what is the truth concerning the things of this world, except how they are experienced in one's own consciousness?

Nescience is not a real entity, even as oil in sand is not a real entity. **Nescience and the self cannot have any relationship: for there can be relationship only between same or similar entities — this is obvious in everyone's experience.** Thus, it is only because consciousness is infinite that everything in the universe becomes knowable. It is not as if the subject illumines the object which has no luminosity of its own, but since consciousness is all this, everything is self-luminous, without requiring a perceiving intelligence. It is by the action of consciousness becoming aware of itself that intelligence manifests itself, not when consciousness apprehends an inert object.

It is not correct to say that there is a mixture in this universe of the sentient and the inert, for they do not mix. All things are full of consciousness and when this consciousness comprehends itself there is knowledge.

One may see a relationship between a tree and a rock, though they appear to be inert: such relationship exists in their fundamental constituents which have undergone a certain kind of change to become a tree and another to become a rock. This is also seen in the sense of taste: the taste-buds in the tongue respond to the taste in the food, etc., because of their similarity in constitution.

aparijñāyamānaiṣā mahāmohapradāyinī
parijñātā tv anantākhyā sukhadā brahmadāyinī (122/29)

VASIṢṬHA continued:

All relationship is therefore the realisation of the already existing unity: it is regarded as relationship only because of the previous false and deluded assumption of a division into subject and object.

In the middle between the sight and the seen, there is a relationship which is known as the seer. When the division between the seer, the sight and the seen is abolished, that is the supreme. When the mind travels from one country to another, between them is cosmic intelligence. Be that always. Even as you do not busy yourself with the affairs of a future village, do not get tangled with the moods of your mind, but be established in truth. Regard the mind as a foreigner or a piece of wood or stone. There is no mind in infinite consciousness; that which is done by this non-existent mind is also unreal. Be established in this realisation. I have investigated the truth concerning the mind for a very long time, O Rāma, and have found none: only the infinite consciousness exists.

This seemingly endless stream of ignorance can be crossed over only by the constant company of the holy ones. From such company there arises wisdom concerning what is worth seeking and what is to be avoided. Then there arises the pure wish to attain liberation. This leads to serious enquiry. Then the mind becomes subtle because this enquiry thins out the mental conditioning. As a result of the rising of pure wisdom, one's consciousness moves in the reality. Then the mental conditioning vanishes and there is non-attachment. Bondage to actions and their fruits ceases. The vision is firmly established in truth and the apprehension of the unreal is weakened. Even while living and functioning in this world, he who has this unconditioned vision does what has to be done as if he is asleep, without thinking of the world and its pleasures. After some years of living like this, one is fully liberated and transcends all these states: he is liberated while living.

When mental conditioning is overcome and the mind is made perfectly tranquil, the illusion that deludes the ignorant comes to an end. **It is only as long as this illusion (Māyā) is not clearly understood that it generates this great delusion; but once it is clearly understood, it is seen as the infinite, and it becomes the source of happiness and the realisation of the absolute Brahman.** It is only for the sake of scriptural instruction that one speaks of the self, Brahman, etc., but in truth one alone is. It is pure consciousness, not embodied being. It is, whether one knows or not, whether one is embodied or without a body. All the unhappiness you see in this world belongs to the body; the self which is not grasped by the senses is not touched by sorrow. In the self there is no desire: the world appears in it without any wish or intention on its part. Thus, O Rāma, through my precepts the false notion of a creation and its existence has been dispelled. Your consciousness has become pure, devoid of duality.

sākāra baṭa dhānādāvaṅkurāḥ santi yukttimat
nākāre tanmahākāraṁ jagadastity ayuktikaṁ (1/33)

RĀMA asked:

It has been said that this universe remains in a seed-state in the supreme being, to manifest again in the next epoch: how can this be and are they who hold this view to be regarded as enlightened or ignorant?

VASIṢṬHA continued:

They who say that this universe exists in a seed-state after the cosmic dissolution are those who have firm faith in the reality of this universe! This is pure ignorance. O Rāma. It is a totally perverted view which deludes both the teacher and the hearer. The seed of a plant contains the future tree: this is because both the seed and the sprout are material objects which are capable of being apprehended by the senses and the mind. But, that which is beyond the reach of the mind and the senses — how can that be the seed for the worlds? In that which is subtler than space, how can there exist the seed of the universe? When that is so, how can the universe emerge from the supreme being?

How can something exist in nothing? And if there is something called the universe in it, how is it not seen? How can a tree spring out of the empty space in a jar? How can two contrary things (Brahman and the universe) co-exist: can darkness exist in the sun? **It is appropriate to say that the tree exists in the seed, because both these have appropriate forms. But in that which has no form (Brahman) it is inappropriate to say that this cosmic form of the world exists.** Hence, it is pure foolishness to assume that there exists a causal relationship between Brahman and the world: the truth is that Brahman alone exists and what appears to be the world is that alone. It is as real as a dream-vision; for it is produced out of nothing by no one with no instruments on nothing.

Rāma, if the universe existed in a seed-state in the absolute Brahman during the cosmic dissolution, then it would need a co-operative cause for its manifestation after the dissolution. To assume that the universe manifested without such co-operative causation is to assume the existence of a barren woman's daughter. At the conclusion of the cosmic dissolution, there arose the Creator of the universe who was nothing more than a memory. The thoughts that arose from that memory constitute this world appearance, which is no more real than a pie in the sky; for the memory from which the thoughts sprang has itself no valid basis. When there is no-one to remember, how can memory exist?

Millions of universes appear in the infinite consciousness (cid ākāśa) like specks of dust in a beam of light streaming into a room through a hole in the roof. In one small atom all the three worlds appear to be, with all their components like space, time, action, substance, day and night. In that there are other atoms in which there are such world-appearances, just as there is a figure in an uncarved marble slab and that figure (which is marble) has a figure in its limbs, and so on ad infinitum.

manaḥ sarvam idaṁ rāma tasmin antaś cikitsite
cikitsito vai sakalo jagaj jālamayo bhavet (4/5)

VASIṢṬHA continued:

O Rāma, the only way to cross this formidable ocean of world-appearance is the successful mastery of the senses. No other effort is of any use. When one is equipped with the wisdom gained by the study of the scriptures and the company of sages, and has his senses under control, he realises the utter non-existence of all objects of perception.

Rāma, mind alone is all this: and when that is healed this jugglery of world-appearance is also healed. This mind alone, by its thinking faculty, conjures up what is known as the body: no body is seen where the mind does not function! Hence, the treatment of the psychological illness known as perception of objects is the best of all treatments in this world. The mind creates delusion, the mind produces ideas of birth and death; and, as a result of its own thoughts, it is bound and it is liberated.

RĀMA asked:

O Holy sage, kindly tell me: how does this enormous universe exist in the mind?

VASIṢṬHA replied:

O Rāma, it is like the universes created by the brāhmaṇa boys. Again, it is like the hallucinations suffered by the king Lavaṇa. There is another illustration. It is the story of the sage Śukra which I shall presently narrate to you.

A long time ago the sage Bhṛgu was performing intense penance on the peak of a mountain. His son Śukra was a young man at that time. While the father sat motionless in meditation, the young son attended to the father's needs. One day this young man beheld in the sky a beautiful flying nymph. His mind was disturbed with desire for her; so was her mind disturbed when she saw the radiant young Śukra.

Intensely overcome by desire for the nymph, Śukra closed his eyes and (mentally) pursued her. He reached heaven. There he saw the radiant celestial beings, gods and their consorts, the celestial elephant and horses. He saw the creator Brahmā himself, as also the other deities who govern this universe. He saw the siddhā (perfected beings). He listened to celestial music. He visited the celestial gardens in heaven. Finally, he saw the king of heaven, Indra himself, seated in all his majesty, waited upon by incomparably beautiful nymphs. He saluted Indra. Indra got up from his throne and greeted the young sage Śukra and begged him to stay in heaven for a long time. Śukra also consented to do so.

vividha janmadaśāṁ vividhāśayaḥ samanubhūya śarīraparamparāḥ sukham atiṣṭhad asau bhṛgunandano varanadīsutaṭe dṛḍhavṛkṣavat (8/29)

VASIṢṬHA continued:

Śukra had completely forgotten his previous identity. After spending some time in the court of Indra, Śukra roamed the heaven and soon discovered the whereabouts of the nymph he had seen. When they looked at each other they were overcome by desire for each other, for wish-fulfilment is the characteristic of heaven.

Śukra wished for the darkness of night to envelop the pleasure-garden where he met the nymph. So it was dark. Śukra then entered the beautiful rest house in that garden: the nymph followed. She pleaded, "Great one, I am tormented by desire for you. Only the dull-witted deride love, not the wise ones. Even the lordship of the three worlds is nothing compared to the delight of the company of the loved one. Hence, pray, give me shelter in your heart." So saying, she collapsed on his chest.

Śukra spent a very long time with that nymph, roaming at will in heaven. He lived with that nymph for a period equal to eight world-cycles.

After this length of time, as if his merit had been exhausted, Śukra fell from heaven, along with that nymph. When their subtle bodies fell on earth, they became dew-drops which entered food-grains which were eaten by a holy brāhmana, from whom his wife received their essence. Śukra became their son. He grew up there. The nymph had become a female deer, and Śukra begot through her a human child. He became greatly attached to his son. Worries and anxieties caused by this child soon aged Śukra, and he died longing for pleasures.

On account of this Śukra became the ruler of a kingdom in the next birth, and he died to that embodiment longing for a life of austerity and holiness. In the next birth he became a holy man. **Thus, after passing from one embodiment to another and enduring all manner of destinies Śukra practised intense austerity, standing firm on the bank of a river.**

Thus contemplating while seated in front of his father, Śukra spent a long time. His body had become extremely emaciated. In the meantime the restless mind created scene after scene of successive life-spans, birth and death, ascent to heaven and descent to earth and the peaceful life of a hermit. He was so immersed in these that he regarded them as the truth. The body had been reduced to skin and bone, for it had been assailed by the inclemencies of every type of weather. It appeared terribly frightening even to look at. Yet, it was not consumed by carnivorous beasts, as it stood right in front of the sage Bhṛgu who was engaged in deep meditation, and as Śukra himself had endowed it with psychic strength through the practice of yoga discipline.

svayam ūrdhvaṁ prayāty agniḥ svayaṁ yānti payāṁsy adhaḥ
bhokttāraṁ bhojanaṁ yāti sṛṣṭiṁ cā 'py antakaḥ svayaṁ (29)

VASIṢṬHA continued:

After a hundred celestial years of contemplation the sage Bhṛgu got up from his seat. He did not see his son, Śukra, in front of him, but saw the dried up body. The body appeared hideous, an abode of worms which, dwelling in the eye-sockets, had multiplied very fast indeed. Deeply concerned with what he saw and without really reflecting over the natural course of events, Bhṛgu was filled with rage and resolved to curse Time for causing the untimely death of his son.

Time (or Death) instantly approached the sage in physical form. Time had a sword in one hand and a noose in the other. He had impenetrable armour. He had six arms and six faces. He was surrounded by a host of his servants and messengers. He was radiant with the flames of destruction that emanated from his body and from the weapons he held in his hands.

Calmly and in an unfaltering voice, TIME thus addressed Bhṛgu:

O Sage, how is it that such a wise sage as you are, contemplates such unworthy conduct? Wise men are not upset even when they are offended; yet, you have lost your balance of mind even though no one has offended you! You are indeed an adorable person, and I am one of those who strictly adhere to the appropriate mode of behaviour; hence I salute you — not with any other motive.

Do not waste your merit in useless exhibition of your power to curse! Know that I am unaffected even by the fires of cosmic dissolution; how childish of you to hope to destroy me with your curse!

I am Time: and I have destroyed countless beings, even the gods who preside over this universe. Holy one, I am the consumer and you are our food: this indeed is ordained by nature. This relationship is not based on mutual likes or dislikes. **Fire by its very nature flames upward and water naturally flows down: food seeks the consumer and created objects seek their end.** This is how it has been ordained by the Lord: in the self of all, the self dwells as itself. To the purified vision there is neither a doer nor an enjoyer; but to the unpurified vision which sees division, such a division seems to exist.

You are indeed a knower of truth and you know there is neither doership nor non-doership here. Creatures come and go like flowers on trees, their causation is naught else than conjecture. All these are attributed to time. This can be considered real or unreal. For, when the surface of the lake is agitated, the reflection of the moon seems to be agitated. This can be considered both true and false.

kartavyaṁ eva niyataṁ kevalaṁ kāryakovidaiḥ
suṣuptivṛttim āśritya kadācittvaṁ na nāśaya (39)

TIME continued:

Do not give way to anger, O sage: that is surely the path to disaster. For what will be will be. Realise this truth. We are not swayed by vanity; we are naturally inclined to the fulfilment of our natural functions. Such indeed is the nature of wise ones. **What has to be done has to be done by wise men here, remaining ego-less and unselfish as if in deep sleep: do not let this be violated.**

Where is your wisdom, your greatness and your moral courage? O sage, though you know the path to blessedness, why do you act like a fool? Surely you know that the ripe fruit falls to the ground; ignoring this, why do you think of cursing me?

Surely, you know that everyone has two bodies, the one physical and the other mental. The physical body is insentient and seeks its own destruction; the mind is finite but orderly — but that mind is disturbed in you! The mind makes the body dance to its tunes, bringing about successive changes in it, like the child playing with mud. Mental actions alone are actions; its thoughts cause bondage and its own pure state is liberation. It is the mind that creates the body with all its limbs. Mind itself is both the sentient and the insentient beings; all this endless diversity is nothing but mind. Mind itself in its function as determination is known as the intellect and in its function as identification is known as the ego-sense. The physical body is only physical matter; yet the mind deems it as its own. Yet, if the mind turns towards the truth it abandons its identification with the body and attains the supreme.

O sage, while you were engaged in contemplation your son went far, far away in his own fancy. He left here the body which was 'the son of Bhṛgu' and rose up to the heaven. There in heaven he enjoyed the celestial nymphs. In course of time, when his merit had been exhausted by such enjoyment, he fell down on earth like a ripe fruit, along with the nymph. He had to leave his celestial body in heaven. He fell on earth to be born with a physical body. Here on earth he had to undergo a series of births. He was, successively, a brāhmaṇa boy, a king, a fisherman, a swan, again a king, a great yogi with psychic powers, a celestial demi-god, the son of a sage, a king again, and again the son of a sage, and on account of evil deeds he became a hunter, a king, and then as worms and plants, a donkey, a bamboo, a deer in China, a snake, a bird, and once again a demi-god, and now once again he has become the son of a brāhmaṇa known as Vasudeva. He is well read in the scriptures and is at present engaged in penance on the bank of the holy river Samaṅga.

nanu vijñāta saṁsāra gatayo vayam āpadāṁ
saṁpadāṁ caiva gacchāmo harṣāmarṣa vaśam vibho (13)

VASIṢṬHA continued:

Encouraged by Time (Yama), the sage Bhṛgu thereupon entered into the eye of wisdom in order to behold the life of his son. In an instance he saw in his own intelligence the entire story of his son's transmigration. Wonderstruck at what he saw, he re-entered his own body.

Completely devoid of all attachment to his son, BHṚGU said:

Lord, you are indeed the knower of the past, present and future, whereas we are of little understanding. The world-appearance which though unreal appears to be real, deludes even the heroic man of wisdom. Surely, all this is within you, and only you know the true form of this phantom created by the imaginations of the mind.

This son of mine is not dead: yet, taking him to be dead I became agitated. I thought that my son had been taken away from me before his time arrived. **Lord, though we understand the course of earthly events we are moved to joy and sorrow by what we consider as good fortune and misfortune.**

In this world anger impels man to do what should not be done, but tranquillity enables one to do what should be done. As long as there exists the delusion of world-existence, so long the distinction between appropriate and inappropriate action is valid. It is inappropriate that we should be agitated by your natural function, which is to cause the apparent death of beings here.

By your grace I have seen my son again, and I realise that mind alone is the body. It is the mind alone that conjures up this world-vision.

TIME said:

Well said, O sage; truly mind is the body; it is the mind that 'creates' the body by mere thoughts, just as the potter makes a pot. It creates new bodies and brings about the destruction of what exists, and all this by mere wish. It is surely obvious that within mind exist the faculties of delusion (or hallucination), dreaming and irrational thought, which create a pie in the sky. Even so it creates the appearance of the body within itself; but the ignorant man with a gross physical vision sees the physical body as different from and independent of the mind.

The three worlds (of waking, dream and sleep) are nothing but the expression of the faculties of the mind: this expression can be considered neither real nor unreal. When the mind conditioned by the perception of diversity 'sees', it sees the diversity.

nā 'sti bandho na mokṣo 'sti tanmayastviva lakṣyate
grastaṁ nityam anityena māyāmayam aho jagat (11/63)

TIME continued:

The mind itself gets involved in this world-appearance by entertaining countless notions (like 'I am weak, unhappy, foolish, etc.'). When the understanding arises that all this is but the false creation of the mind, I am what I am — then the peace of the supreme arises in one's consciousness.

The mind is like the vast ocean with infinite variety of creatures within it, on the surface of which ripples and waves of different sizes rise and fall. The small wave thinks it is small; the big one that it is big. The one that is broken by the wind thinks it has been destroyed. One thinks it is cold, another that it is warm. But all the waves are but the water of the ocean. It is indeed true to say that there are no waves in the ocean; the ocean alone exists. Yet, it is also true that there are waves!

Even so, the absolute Brahman alone exists. Since it is omnipotent, the natural expression of its infinite faculties appears as the infinite diversity in this universe. Diversity has no real existence except in one's own imagination. 'All this is indeed the absolute Brahman' — remain established in this truth. Give up all other notions. Even as the waves, etc. are non-different from the ocean, all these things are non-different from Brahman. Even as in the seed is hidden the entire tree in potential, in Brahman there exists the entire universe for ever. Even as the multicoloured rainbow is produced by sunlight, all this diversity is seen in the one. Even as the inert web emanates from the living spider, this inert world-appearance has sprung from the infinite consciousness.

Even as the silk-worm weaves its cocoon and thus binds itself, the infinite being fancies this universe and gets caught in it. Even as an elephant effortlessly breaks loose from the post to which it is tied, the self liberates itself from its bondage. For, the self is what it considers itself to be. In fact, there is neither bondage nor liberation for the Lord. I do not know how these notions of bondage and liberation have come into being! **There is neither bondage nor liberation, only that infinite being is seen: yet the eternal is veiled by the transient, and this is indeed a great wonder (or a great illusion).**

Though revolving thus in the wheel of ignorance and delusion, when one steps on to the wisdom concerning the supreme truth he is instantly redeemed.

Come, let us go to where your son is engaged in penance, after momentarily enjoying the pleasures of the heaven.

(Saying thus, Yama (Time) caught hold of Bhṛgu and led him away . . . . While the sage Vasiṣṭha said this the eighth day came to a close and the asssembly dispersed.)

jñasyā 'jñasya ca dehasya yāvad dehamayaṁ kramaḥ
lokavad vyavahāro 'yaṁ sakttyā 'sakttyā 'thavā sadā (15/35)

VASIṢṬHA continued:

O Rāma, the sage Bhṛgu and the deity presiding over Time proceeded towards the bank of the river Samaṅga. There, the sage Bhṛgu saw his son who had another body and whose nature was different from what it was before, who was of a peaceful disposition and whose mind was established in the tranquillity of enlightenment. Seeing the two radiant beings standing in front of him, Śukra (the son of Bhṛgu) greeted them appropriately and seated them on a rock. In soft and sweet words, he said: "O divine beings, I am truly blessed to behold both of you!" The sage Bhṛgu said to him: "Recollect yourself, for you are not an ignorant person!" Śukra was instantly awakened to the memory of his previous existence, which he beheld with his eyes closed for a brief period.

Śukra said: "Behold, I have passed through countless embodiments and through countless experiences of pain and pleasure, wisdom and delusion. I have been a cruel king, a greedy trader and a wandering ascetic. There is no pleasure that I have not enjoyed, no action I have not performed, no unhappiness or happiness I have not endured. Now I wish for nothing, nor do I wish to avoid anything: let nature take its course. Come father, let us go to where the previous body stands, dried up."

Soon they arrived at the place where the body of Śukra, the son of Bhṛgu, lay in an advanced condition of decay. Looking at this, Śukra wailed: "Ah, look at this body which was admired and adored by even celestial nymphs; it is now the abode of worms and vermin. O body! You are now known as a corpse and you are truly frightening me. Even wild beasts are afraid of your dreadful appearance. Totally devoid of sensations, this body remains in a state of utter freedom from thoughts and ideas. Freed from the goblin of the mind, it remains unaffected by even natural calamities. Rid of the frolics of the restless monkey known as mind, this tree of the body has fallen uprooted. It is indeed good fortune that I am able to see this body, liberated from sorrow, in this dense forest."

Śukra (now known as Vasudeva) bemoaned only that body which was born of Bhṛgu because all the other bodies were the hallucinations of this original body, which was that of Śukra, the son of sage Bhṛgu. **Whether one is wise or ignorant, as long as the body lasts its functions continue unaltered according to its nature. And the embodied person functions as it is appropriate in the world, either attached or unattached.** The difference between the two lies in their mental dispositions; in the case of the wise these are liberating and in the case of the ignorant these are binding. As long as there is the body, so long shall pain be painful and pleasure pleasant: but the wise are not attached to either. Rejoicing in joy and suffering in suffering, the great ones appear to behave like the ignorant, though in fact they are enlightened. The wise behave appropriately in society though inwardly they are free of all need to conform.

matputro 'yam iti sneho bhṛgum apy aharat tadā
paramātmiyatā dehe yāvad ākṛtibhāvinī (16/18)

VASIṢṬHA continued:

Hearing the young ascetic Vasudeva mourning the fate of his previous body, Time (or Death) intervened and said to Sukra: "O son of Bhṛgu! Abandon this body of yours and re-enter your other body. At the end of the epoch you will give up that body, never to become embodied again." Having said this, Time vanished at that very place.

Thereupon, Śukra did so. At that very moment the body of Vasudeva fell down and became a corpse. The sage Bhṛgu sprinkled the body of Śukra with holy water, uttering sacred hymns which had the power to revive that body. Instantly, that body became youthful and radiant as it was before.

Śukra got up from the meditative posture and fell prostrate at Bhṛgu's feet. Bhṛgu was delighted to see his son thus resurrected from the dead. **The feeling of affection at the thought, 'This is my son', overcame even the sage Bhṛgu; this is natural as long as there is body-consciousness.** Both Bhṛgu and Śukra then performed the funeral rites of the body of the brāhmaṇa boy Vasudeva; for thus do the men of wisdom honour social customs and traditions.

Both of them then shone with the radiance of the sun and the moon. In course of time, Śukra became the spiritual preceptor of the demons; and his father, Bhṛgu, became one of the sages of highest wisdom.

Such is the story of the sage Śukra who, on account of his infatuation with a nymph, wandered in countless wombs.

RĀMA asked:

Holy sir, why does not the wish of others materialise as the wish of Śukra materialised in his ascent to heaven, etc.?

VASIṢṬHA replied:

Śukra's mind was pure, since that was his first embodiment; that mind was not loaded with the impurities of other previous embodiments. That mind is pure in which all cravings are in a state of quiescence. Whatever that pure mind wishes, that materialises. What happened in this respect to Śukra is possible for everyone else.

Śukra had been taught by his father, Bhṛgu, concerning the succession of births, and this teaching had conditioned Śukra's mind which conjured up the expansion of such conditioning. Only when the mind is totally purified of all conditioning does it regain its utter purity; that pure mind experiences liberation.

dṛśyaṁ paśyan svamātmānaṁ na draṣṭā saṁprapaśyati
prapañcākrānta saṁvitteḥ kasyodeti nijā sthitiḥ (27)

VASIṢṬHA continued:

The diversity that is seen in this creation, O Rāma, is but an appearance of diversity. Evolution or involution has the one infinite consciousness as its source and as its goal. During evolution there seems to be an apparent diversity in the one infinite consciousness, in accordance with the notions that appear in that consciousness. Some of these notions intermingle, thus producing infinite variety in this diversity. Some do not thus intermingle. But, in fact, all these notions appear in every atom of existence and these atoms exist independent of one another. The totality is known as the absolute Brahman.

Each individual sees only those objects which are rooted in his own mind. When the ideas in the mind do not bear fruits there is a change in the mind; there follows a succession of births to suit these psychological changes. It is this psychological connection that creates the conviction in the reality of birth and death, and in the reality of the body. When this conviction is given up there is the cessation of embodiment.

O Rāma, the tree in a seed grows out of it after destroying the seed: but Brahman creates this world without destroying itself. Hence it is impossible to compare the incomparable Brahman with anything whatsoever; whereas the tree, etc. are definable material substances, Brahman is nameless and formless being. It is Brahman alone that becomes what appears to be of a different nature; yet, from another point of view, it does not so become, for it is eternal and changeless.

When the self is seen as an object, the seer is not seen (realised); as long as the objective universe is perceived one does not realise the self. When you see the mirage as water you do not perceive the rising hot air; but, when you perceive the hot air, you do not see water in the mirage! When one is truth, the other is not.

It is only when the division between the seer and the seen is given up, only when the two are 'seen' as of one substance, that the truth is realised. There is no object which is totally of a different nature from the subject. Nor can the subject (self) be seen as if it were an object! There is no division in such a vision.

citrāmṛtaṁ nāmṛtameva viddhi citrānalaṁ nānalameva viddhi
citrāṅganā nūnamanaṅganeti vācā vivekastv aviveka eva (18/69)

VASIṢṬHA continued:

Each jiva experiences within itself whatever and however it has given rise to within itself with the help of its own life-force. O Rāma, behold with the eye of your inner wisdom the truth that in every atom of existence there are countless world-appearances. This world-appearance is but a long dream. This dream-like appearance is yet true during the period of the dream itself.

Within every atom is the potential experience of every kind. Therefore, give up all your notions of diversity or unity. Time, space, action (or motion) and matter are all but different aspects of the one infinite consciousness. The rare few realise that the world-appearance seen within themselves is illusory, except as the one infinite consciousness which alone is ever true. On account of this consciousness the world appears in the jiva: and there are jīvā within jīvā, ad infinitum. It is when one thus experiences the truth, that he is freed from illusion. At the same time one's craving for pleasure is thinned out. This is the only proof of wisdom. **A painted pot of nectar is not nectar, nor a painted flame fire, and a painting of a woman is not a woman: wise words are mere words (ignorance) not wisdom,** unless they are substantiated by the absence of desire and anger.

They who contemplate the absolute Brahman, become Brahman. Hence one should resort to that which is not limited, conditioned or finite. By contemplating the form of the nymph, Śukra was bound; and when he realised the purity of his self which is infinite consciousness, he was instantly liberated.

RĀMA asked:

Holy sir, pray tell me of the true nature of the waking and dreaming states.

VASIṢṬHA said:

That state which endures is known as the waking state; and that which is transient is the dream state. During the period of even the dream, it takes on the characteristics of the waking state; and when the waking state is realised to be of a fleeting nature, it gets the characteristic of dream. The two are the same. That consciousness which is awake even in deep sleep and which is also the light that shines in waking and dreaming, is the transcendental consciousness, turīya.

When again the seeds of ignorance and delusion expand, there arises the first thought — which is the thought 'I am'. Then one perceives thought-forms within the mind in dreams. At this time the external sense-organs do not function, but the inner senses function and there is perception within oneself. This is the dream state. When the life-force again activates the sense-organs, once again there is wakefulness.

śūnya eva kusūle tu siṁho 'stīti bhayaṁ yathā
śūnya eva śarīre 'ntar baddho 'smīti bhayaṁ tathā (21/49)

RĀMA asked:

Lord, how does the mind ever get tainted?

VASIṢṬHA replied:

It is a beautiful question, Rāma, but this is not the proper time to ask: when you have listened to what I have to say, you will surely find the answer to this question with the utmost clarity. That the mind is impure is the experience of everyone who strives for liberation. Depending upon one's particular point of view, everyone describes it differently.

Just as air coming into contact with different flowers takes on their scent, so mind entertaining different notions takes on those moods, creates bodies suitable to them and, as the energy activating the senses, enjoys the fruition of its own notions. It is the mind, again, that provides the fuel for the functioning of the organs of action. Mind is action and action is mind — the two are like the flower and its scent. The conviction of the mind determines the action and the action strengthens the conviction.

Mind is everywhere devoted to dharma, wealth, pleasure and freedom: but everyone has a different definition of these and is convinced that that definition is the truth.

Rāma, bondage is none other than the notion of an object. This notion is Māyā, ignorance, etc. It is the cataract that blinds one to the sun of truth. Ignorance raises a doubt; doubt perceives — that perception is perverted. **In darkness when one approaches even a lion's empty cage, he is afraid. Even so, one ignorantly believes he is imprisoned in this empty body.** The notions of 'I' and 'the world' are but shadows, not truth. Such notions alone create 'objects': these objects are neither true nor false. Therefore Rama, abandon the notions of 'I' and 'this' and remain established in the truth.

It is only when the mind has become devoid of all attachment, when it is not swayed by the pairs of opposites, when it is not attracted by objects and when it is totally independent of all supports, that it is freed from the cage of delusion. When all doubt comes to rest and when there is neither elation nor depression, then the mind shines like the full moon.

When the impurities of the mind have ceased to be, there arise in the heart all the auspicious qualities, and there is equal vision everywhere. Even as darkness is dispelled by the rising sun, the world-illusion is dispelled when the sun of infinite consciousness arises in the heart. Such wisdom as is capable of gladdening the hearts of all beings in the universe, manifests and expands. In short, he who has known that which alone is worth knowing transcends all coming and going, birth and death. When there is absence of egoism there is no confusion in the mind, and that mind functions naturally. Just as waves rise and fall in the ocean, the worlds arise and vanish: this deludes the ignorant, but not the wise.

mayi sarvaṁ idaṁ protaṁ sūtre maṇiganā iva
cittaṁ tu nā 'haṁ eveti yaḥ paśyati sa paśyati (31)

VASIṢṬHA continued:

O Rāma, he sees the truth who sees the body as a product of deluded understanding and as the fountain source of misfortune, and who knows that the body is not the self.

He sees the truth who sees that in this body pleasure and pain are experienced on account of the passage of time and the circumstances in which one is placed, and that they do not pertain to him.

He sees the truth who sees that he is the omnipresent infinite consciousness which encompasses within itself all that takes place everywhere at all times.

He sees the truth who knows that the self, which is as subtle as the millionth part of the tip of a hair divided a million times, pervades everything.

He sees the truth who sees that there is no division at all between the self and the other, and that the one infinite light of consciousness exists as the sole reality.

He sees the truth who sees that the non-dual consciousness which indwells all beings is omnipotent and omnipresent.

He sees the truth who is not deluded into thinking that he is the body which is subject to illness, fear, agitation, old age and death.

He sees the truth who sees that all things are strung in the self as beads are strung on a thread, and who knows 'I am not the mind'.

He sees the truth who sees that all this is Brahman, neither 'I' nor 'the other'.

He sees the truth who sees all beings in the three worlds as his own family, deserving of his sympathy and protection.

He sees the truth who knows that the self alone exists and that there is no substance in objectivity.

He is unaffected who knows that pleasure, pain, birth, death, etc., are all the self only.

He is firmly established in the truth who feels: "What should I acquire, what should I renounce, when all this is the one self?"

Salutations to that abode of auspiciousness who is filled with the supreme realisation that the entire universe is truly Brahman alone, which remains unchanged during all the apparent creation, existence and dissolution of the universe.

ajñasyeyam anantānāṁ duḥkhānāṁ kośamālikā
jñasya tviyam anantānāṁ sukhānāṁ kośamālikā (23/18)

VASIṢṬHA continued:

Rāma, he who treads the superior path, though he dwells in this body which functions as the potter's wheel does by past momentum, is untainted by the actions that might be performed. In his case, the body exists for his pleasure and for the liberation of his soul; he does not experience unhappiness in it.

To the ignorant, this body is the source of suffering; but to the enlightened man, this body is the source of infinite delight, and when its life-span comes to an end he does not regard it as a loss at all. And, since it transports him in this world in which he roams freely and delightfully, the body is regarded as a vehicle of wisdom. The body does not subject the wise man to the temptations of lust and greed, nor does it allow ignorance or fear to invade him. The embodied being comes lightly into contact with the body while it lasts but is untouched by it once it is gone, even as air touches a pot which exists, but not one that does not exist.

The wise man who is rid of all doubts, in whom there is no image of self, reigns supreme in the body. Therefore one should abandon all cravings for pleasure and attain wisdom. Only the mind that has been well disciplined really experiences happiness. The captive king, when freed, is delighted with a piece of bread; the king who has not been subjected to captivity does not enjoy as much, even should it be the annexation of another kingdom. Hence, the wise man grinds his teeth and strives to conquer his mind and senses: such conquest is far greater than conquest of external foes.

O Rāma, in the great empire known as dreadful hell, evil actions roam like mighty elephants in rut. The senses which are responsible for these actions are equipped with a formidable magazine of cravings. Hence, these senses are hard to conquer. These ungrateful senses destroy the body — their own abode and support.

However, one who is equipped with wisdom is able to restrain craving without injuring the being, even as a noose restrains the elephant without harming its being. The bliss enjoyed by the wise man who has his senses under control is incomparably superior to the enjoyment of a king who rules over a city built with brick and mortar. The former's intelligence grows in clarity as his craving for sense-pleasure is worn out. However, the craving disappears completely only after the supreme truth has been seen.

To the wise, the mind is an obedient servant, good counsellor, able commander of the senses, pleasing wife, protecting father and trustworthy friend. It impels him in good actions.

yasyā 'ntar vāsanā rajjvā grathibandhaḥ śarīriṇaḥ
mahānapi bahujño 'pi sa bālenā 'pi jīyate (27/20)

VASISTHA continued:

O Rāma, be established in truth and live in freedom in a mindless state. Behave not like the demons Dāma, Vyāla and Kaṭa, whose story I shall presently narrate to you.

In the netherworld there was a mighty demon known as Saṁbara. He was a past-master in the art of magic. He created a magic city. He was a terror to the gods of heaven. When he was asleep or away from his city, the gods took advantage of the situation and killed his army. Enraged, the demon invaded heaven. The gods, afraid of his magic powers, hid themselves. He could not find them. In order to protect his forces, the demon created three other demons: Dāma, Vyāla and Kaṭa.

These three had had no previous incarnation and hence they were free from every type of mental conditioning. They had no fear, doubt or other predispositions; they did not flee before the enemy, they were not afraid of death; they did not know the meaning of war, victory or defeat. In fact, they were not independent jīvā at all; they were merely the robot-like working projections of the demon Saṁbara.

The demon Saṁbara despatched his invulnerable army, protected by the three new invincible but unarmed demons, to fight the gods. A fierce hand-to-hand fight ensued. The three principal demons looked for the principal gods, but they could not be found. The demons went back to Saṁbara to report to him. The gods prayed to the creator Brahmā, (who appeared before them at once) and begged him to find a way to destroy the three demons.

BRAHMĀ said:

O gods, Saṁbara cannot be killed now. It is wise for you to retreat from battle. In due course, on account of their engagement in this war, the ego-sense will arise in the three demons. Then they will be subjected to psychological conditioning and develop latent tendencies. Just now, they are utterly devoid of the ego-sense and its adjuncts (conditioning and tendencies).

They in whom the ego-sense ('me') and its counterpart (the tendencies) do not exist, know neither desire nor anger. They are invincible. **He who is bound by the ego-sense ('me') and by the conditioning of the mind, even if he is regarded as a great man or a man of great learning, can be defeated even by a child.** In fact, the notions of 'I' and 'mine' are the eager receptacles of sorrow and suffering. He whose mind is conditioned can be defeated: in the absence of such conditioning even a mosquito becomes immortal.

naikaṭhyātiśayād yad vad darpaṇaṁ bimbavad bhavet
abhyāsātiśayāt tadvat te sāhaṅkāratāṁ gatāḥ (29/6)

VASIṢṬHA continued:

Brahmā concluded: "Do what you can to create in the demons the feelings of 'I' and 'mine'. Since they are ignorant creatures of the demon Saṁbara they will easily fall for this bait. Then they can be easily defeated by you all."

Having said thus, the creator Brahmā vanished. The gods rested in their abodes for a while, in preparation for a fresh onslaught on the demons. The renewed fighting between the armies of the gods and the demons was even more fierce than the previous one.

The continued involvement in fighting generated in the three demon leaders the basic notion of 'I am'. **Even as a mirror reflects an object held close to it, one's behaviour reflects as the ego-sense in one's consciousness.** However, if this behaviour is 'held at a distance' from consciousness and there is no identification with such behaviour, the ego-sense does not arise.

Once this ego-sense arose, there quickly followed the desire for the prolongation of life in the body, acquisition of wealth, health, pleasure, etc. These desires greatly debilitated their personality. Then there arose confusion in their minds, which in turn gave rise to the feelings of 'This is mine' and 'This is my body'. All these inevitably resulted in inefficiency and inability to do their own work. They were greatly attached to eating and drinking. Objects gave them feelings of pleasure and thus robbed them of their freedom. With the loss of freedom, their courage also went and they experienced fear. They were terribly worried at the very thought, "We shall die in this war".

The gods took advantage of this situation and began to attack these demons. The three demons who were possessed by fear of death fled. When the demon army saw that their invincible protectors had fled before the invading gods, they were thoroughly demoralised; the demons fell by the thousands.

When the demon Saṁbara heard that his army had been routed by the gods, he was furious. Referring to the three invincible demons, Dāma, Vyāla and Kaṭa, he demanded: "Where have they gone?" Afraid of his wrath, these three demons took refuge in the nethermost world.

Though the demons Dāma, Vyāla and Kaṭa were really free from the cycle of birth and death, on account of their ego-sense they had to be subjected to birth and death. After a number of incarnations in different sub-human species, they now live as fish in a lake in Kashmir.

cidākāśo 'ham ityeva rajasā rañjitaprabhaḥ
svarūpam atyajanneva virūpam api buddhyate (32/31)

RĀMA asked:

O holy sage, pray tell me when and how the three demons will attain liberation.

VASIṢṬHA replied:

Rāma, when they listen to the narration of their story and are reminded of their own essential nature as pure consciousness, they will be liberated.

In course of time there will arise a city named Adhiṣṭhāna in the middle of the country known as Kashmir. In the centre of that city there will be a hill whose peak will be known as Pradyumna. On top of that hill there will be a skyscraper. In a corner of that building the demon Vyāla will be born as a sparrow.

In that building a king known as Yaśaskar will reside. The demon Dāma will be born as a mosquito and reside in a hole in one of the pillars of that palace.

Elsewhere in that city there will be a palace known as Raṭnāvalī-vihāra which will be inhabited by the state minister known as Narasiṁha. The demon Kaṭa will be born as a bird (myna) and live in that palace.

One day that minister, Narasiṁha, will recite the story of the three demons — Dāma, Vyāla and Kaṭa. Listening to it, the myna will be enlightened. It will recall that its original personality was but a magical creation of the demon Saṁbara; this recollection will free it from the magic of Śaṁbara. The demon Kaṭa will thus attain liberation.

Other people will recount this story and the sparrow will also attain liberation after listening to it. Thus will the demon Vyāla attain liberation.

In the same way, the mosquito-demon Dāma will also listen to this story and will also attain liberation.

Such is the story, O Rāma, of Dāma, Vyāla and Kaṭa, who, on account of their ego-sense and their cravings, fell into hell. All this is nothing more than the play of ignorance and delusion. All these notions of 'I' and 'you', O Rāma, are unreal. That you and I are seen to be real entities does not alter the truth; even if a dead person appears before you now, he is still dead!

In fact, it is the pure consciousness that entertains the impure notion of 'I am', playfully as it were, and without ever renouncing its essential nature as consciousness, experiences the distorted image of itself within itself. Even though this distorted image is truly unreal, the ego-sense ('I am') believes it to be real and gets deluded.

ācāracārucaritasya viviktavṛtteḥ
saṁsārasaukhyaphaladuḥkhadaśāsvagṛdhnoḥ
āyuryaśāṁsi ca guṇāś ca sahaiva lakṣmyā
phullanti mādhavalatā iva satphalāya (60)

VASIṢṬHA continued:

O Rāma, they who are established in the state of liberation, as pointed out by the scriptures, surely cross this ocean of world-appearance as their consciousness flows towards the self. But they who are caught in the net of polemics, which are only productive of sorrow and confusion, forfeit their own highest good. Even in the case of the path shown by the scriptures, only one's direct experience leads one along the safest way to the supreme goal.

What else is left of a greedy man except a handful of ashes? But, he who looks upon the world as less valuable than a blade of grass never comes to grief. He who has fully realised the infinite is protected by cosmic deities. Hence, one should not set foot on the wrong path even in times of great distress. He who has earned a good reputation through a virtuous life gains whatever has not been gained and is rid of misfortune. Only he can be considered a human being who is not complacent with his own virtue, who is devoted to the teaching he has heard and who strives to tread the path of truth: others are animals in human disguise. He who is filled with the milk of human kindness is surely the abode of the lord Hari (who is said to dwell in the ocean of milk).

Whatever has to be enjoyed has already been enjoyed, whatever has to be seen has been seen: what else is there new in this world which a wise man should seek? Hence, one should be devoted to one's duty as ordained by the scriptures, having given up all craving for pleasure. Adore the saints: this will save you from death.

Adhering to the injunctions of the scriptures one should patiently wait for perfection which comes in its own time. Arrest the downward trend by studying this holy scripture for liberation. Enquire constantly into the nature of truth, knowing that 'this is but a reflection'. Do not be led by others; only animals are led by others. Wake up from the slumber of ignorance. Wake up and strive to end old age and death.

Wealth is the mother of evil. Sense-pleasure is the source of pain. Misfortune is the best fortune. Rejection by all is victory. **Life, honour and noble qualities blossom and attain fruition in one whose conduct and behaviour are good and pleasant, who is devoted to seclusion and who does not crave for the pleasures of the world which lead to suffering.**

aham artho 'parijñātaḥ paramārthāṁbare malaṁ
parijñāto 'ham arthas tu paramātmāṁbaraṁ bhavet (24)

VASIṢṬHA continued:

O Rāma, every zealous effort is always crowned with fruition. Hence, do not abandon right effort. Weigh the worthiness of the end result. You will surely discover that self-knowledge alone is capable of utterly destroying all pain and pleasure. Hence, zealous effort should be directed towards self-knowledge alone. Get rid of all notions of objectivity created by the pleasure-seeking desire within you. Is there any happiness which is untainted by unhappiness?

Both the absence of restraint and the practice of restraint are indeed one in the absolute Brahman and there is no real division between them; yet, the practice of restraint bestows great joy and auspiciousness upon you. Hence, resort to self restraint and give up ego-sense.

Thus have I explained to you in a thousand ways the essential unreality of the world-as-an-object-of-perception. It is nothing but the pure space of consciousness. When in accordance with its own nature it closes and opens its eyes, as it were, there is what is known as dissolution and creation of the universe.

When it is not rightly understood, the 'I' appears to be an impure notion in the infinite consciousness; but, when the 'I' is rightly understood, its meaning is seen as the infinite consciousness. When this truth is revealed to one with a pure mind, his ignorance is at once dispelled; but others cling to their own false notion like a child clinging to the notion of the existence of a ghost.

When the 'I' as a separate entity is thus known to be false, how can one believe in the other notions (of heaven, hell etc.) that are related to it? Craving for heaven and even for liberation arises in one's heart only as long as the 'I' is seen as an entity. As long as the 'I' thus remains, there is only unhappiness in one's life. And, this notion of the 'I' cannot be got rid of except through self-knowledge.

However, the higher form of 'I-ness' which gives rise to the feeling 'I am one with the entire universe, there is nothing apart from me', is the understanding of the enlightened person. Another type of 'I-ness' is when one feels that the 'I' is extremely subtle and atomic in nature and therefore different from and independent of everything in this universe: this, too, is unobjectionable, being conducive to liberation. But the 'I-ness' that has been described earlier on is one which identifies the self with the body: this is to be abandoned firmly. By the persistent cultivation of the higher form of 'I-ness', the lower form is eradicated.

Then one may either engage oneself in all activity or remain in seclusion: there is no fear of downfall for him.

śrūyatāṁ jñānasarvasvaṁ śrutvā caivā 'vadhāryatāṁ
bhogecchāmātrako bandhas tattyāgo mokṣa ucyate (35/3)

VASIṢṬHA continued:

O Rāma, after Saṁbara had been deserted by the three demons Dāma, Vyāla and Kaṭa, he realised that they had foolishly entertained egoistic notions and had thus come to grief. Hence, he resolved to create more demons, but this time with self-knowledge and wisdom, so that they might not fall into the same trap of ego-sense.

Saṁbara thereupon created by his own magic power three more demons known as Bhīma, Bhāsa and Dṛḍha. They were omniscient, they were endowed with self-knowledge, they were full of dispassion, and sinless. They regarded the whole universe as of no more value than a blade of grass.

They began to fight with the army of the gods. In spite of fighting for a considerable time, the ego-sense did not arise in them. Whenever the ego-sense raised its head, they subdued it with self-enquiry ('Who am I?'). They were therefore free from fear of death; devoid of the feeling 'I did this', they did the work allotted to them by the master Saṁbara. The army of the gods was quickly defeated by them. The gods fled to Lord Viṣṇu for refuge. At his command, they took up their abode in another region.

After this, Lord Viṣṇu himself had to fight with the demon Saṁbara: slain by the Lord the demon instantly reached the abode of Viṣṇu. Lord Viṣṇu also liberated the three demons Bhīma, Bhāsa and Dṛḍha, who, when the body fell, became enlightened, as they had no ego-sense.

O Rāma, the conditioned mind alone is bondage; and liberation is when the mind is unconditioned. The conditioning of the mind drops away when the truth is clearly seen and realised; and when the conditioning has ceased one's consciousness is made supremely peaceful, as when the flame of a lamp is put out. To realise that 'The self alone is all this, whatever one may think of anywhere' is clear perception. 'Conditioning' and 'mind' are but words without corresponding truth: when the truth is investigated they cease to be meaningful — this is clear perception. When this clear perception arises, there is liberation.

Dāma, Vyāla and Kaṭa illustrate the mind that is conditioned by the ego-sense; Bhīma, Bhāsa and Dṛḍha illustrate the mind that is free from conditioning or ego-sense. O Rāma, do not be like the former, but be like the latter. That is the reason why I narrated this story to you, my dear and highly intelligent disciple. O Rāma, they are the true heroes who have brought under control the mind which is dominated by ignorance and delusion. Such control of the mind is the only way by which one can remedy the sufferings of this world-appearance (or cycle of birth and death) and the endless chain of tragedy. **I shall declare to you the quintessence of all wisdom: listen and let it perfume your whole life. Bondage is the craving for pleasure; and its abandonment is liberation.**

yena śabdaṁ rasaṁ rūpaṁ gandhaṁ jānāsi rāghava
so 'yamātmā paraṁ brahma sarvam āpūrya saṁsthitaḥ (37/7)

RĀMA asked:

Lord, the infinite consciousness is transcendental; pray, tell me how this universe exists in it.

VASIṢṬHA replied:

O Rāma, this universe exists in the infinite consciousness just as future waves exist in a calm sea; non-different in truth but with the potentiality of an apparent difference. The infinite consciousness is unmanifest, though omnipresent, even as space, though existing everywhere, is unmanifest. Just as the reflection of an object in crystal can be said to be neither real nor entirely unreal, one cannot say that this universe which is reflected in the infinite consciousness is real or unreal. Again, just as space is unaffected by the clouds that float in it, this infinite consciousness is unaffected and untouched by the universe that appears in it. Just as light is not seen except through the refracting agent, even so the infinite consciousness is revealed through these various bodies. It is essentially nameless and formless, but names and forms are ascribed to its reflections. Consciousness reflecting in consciousness shines as consciousness and exists as consciousness; yet, to one who is ignorant (though considering oneself as wise and rational) there arises the notion that there has come into being and there exists something other than this consciousness.

This consciousness is not created, nor does it perish; it is eternal and the world-appearance is superimposed on it, even as waves in relation to the ocean. In that consciousness, when it is reflected within itself, there arises the 'I am' notion which gives rise to diversity. As space, the same consciousness enables the seed to sprout; as air, it draws the sprout, as it were; as water, it nourishes it; as earth, it stabilises it; and as light, the consciousness itself reveals the new life. It is the consciousness in the seed that in due course manifests as the fruit.

Thus, this world-appearance comes and goes as the very nature of the infinite consciousness. Being non-different from the infinite consciousness this world-appearance has a mutual causal relationship with it — arises in it, exists in it and is absorbed in it. Though like the deep ocean it is not agitated, yet it is agitated like the waves appearing on the surface. Even as one who is intoxicated sees himself as another person, this consciousness, becoming conscious of itself, considers itself as another.

This self, the supreme Brahman, which permeates everything, is that which enables you to experience sound, taste, form and fragrance, O Rāma. It is transcenddental and omnipresent; it is non-dual and pure. In it there is not even a notion of another. All these diversities like existence and non-existence, good and evil, are vainly imagined by ignorant people. It matters not whether this imagination is said to be based on the not-self or the self itself.

ajñasyā 'rdhaprabuddhasya sarvaṁ brahmeti yo vadet
mahānarakajāleṣu sa tena viniyojitaḥ (39/24)

VASIṢṬHA continued:

O Rāma, the sense of doership (the notion 'I do this') which gives rise to both happiness and unhappiness, or which gives rise to the state of yoga, is fictitious in the eyes of the wise; to the ignorant, however, it is real. This notion arises when the mind, spurred by the predisposition, endeavours to gain something; the resultant action is then attributed to oneself. When the same action leads to the experience of its fruition, the notion 'I enjoy this' arises. The two notions are in truth the two faces (phases) of the same notion. The wise man, even while acting in this world, is not interested in the fruits of those actions. He lets actions happen in his life, without attachment to those actions; and whatever be the results of those actions, he regards them as non-different from his own self. But such is not the attitude of one who is immersed in the mental states.

Whatever the mind does, that alone is action: hence, the mind alone is the doer of actions, not the body. The mind alone is this world-appearance; this world-appearance has arisen in it and it rests in the mind. When the objects as well as the experiencing mind have become tranquil, consciousness alone remains.

The wise declare that the mind of the enlightened is neither in a state of bliss nor devoid of bliss, neither in motion nor static, neither real nor unreal, but between these two propositions. His unconditioned consciousness blissfully plays its role in this world-appearance as if in a play. He does not even entertain the notion of liberation, nor that of bondage. He sees the self and self alone.

O Rāma, the absolute Brahman being omnipotent, his infinite potencies appear as this visible universe. All the diverse categories like reality, unreality, unity, diversity, beginning and end, exist in that Brahman.

RĀMA asked:

Lord, Brahman is free from sorrow; and yet that which has emerged from it is the universe which is full of sorrow. How is this possible?

VĀLMĪKI said: Hearing this question, Vasiṣṭha contemplated thus for a while: "Obviously, Rāma's understanding is not efficient because there is impurity in his mind. If the mind is pure, then it instantly comprehends the truth. Hence, it is said that **he who declares 'All this is Brahman' to one who is ignorant or half-awakened, goes to hell.** A wise teacher should encourage his students first to be established in self-control and tranquillity. Then the student should be properly examined before the knowledge of the truth is imparted to him." Then,

VASIṢṬHA said:

You will discover the truth for yourself whether Brahman is free from sorrow or not. Or, I shall help you understand this in course of time.

brahma cid brahma ca mano brahma vijñānavastu ca
bṛahmārtho brahma śabdaś ca brahma cid brahma dhātavaḥ (29)

VASIṢṬHA continued:

O Rāma, this entire creation of world-appearance is but an accidental manifestation of the intention of the omnipotent conscious energy (cit-śakti) of the infinite consciousness or Brahman. The intention itself condenses and thus gives rise in the mind to the substance thus intended. Immediately the mind reproduces the substance as if in the objective field. At this stage there is a notion of this creation having factually abandoned its fundamental and true nature as the infinite consciousness.

This infinite consciousness apparently sees within itself a pure void: and the conscious energy (cit-śakti) thereupon brings space into existence. In that conscious energy there arises an intention to diversify: this intention itself is then regarded as the creator Brahmā, with his retinue of other living creatures. Thus have all the fourteen worlds appeared in the space of infinite consciousness, with their endless variety of beings — some immersed in dense darkness, some very close to enlightenment and others fully enlightened.

In this world, O Rāma, among the many species of living beings only the human beings are fit to be instructed into the nature of truth. Even among these human beings many are obsessed by sorrow and delusion, hate and fear. All this I shall presently deal with in great detail.

But all this talk about who created this world and how it was created is intended only for the purpose of composing scriptures and expounding them: it is not based on truth. Modifications arising in the infinite consciousness or organisation of the cosmic being do not really take place in the Lord, though they appear to do so. There is naught but the infinite consciousness, even in imagination! To think of that being the creator and the universe as the created, is absurd: when one lamp is kindled from another there is no creator-creature relationship between them. Fire is one. Creation is just a word, it has no corresponding substantial reality.

Consciousness is Brahman, the mind is Brahman; the intellect is Brahman, Brahman alone is the substance. Sound or word is Brahman and Brahman alone is the component of all substances. All indeed is Brahman; there is no world in reality.

Just as when the dirt is removed, the real substance is made manifest; just as when the darkness of the night is dispelled, the objects that were shrouded by the darkness are clearly seen; even so when ignorance is dispelled, truth is realised.

kuto jāteyam iti te rāma mā 'stu vicāraṇā
imāṁ katham ahaṁ hanmityeṣā te 'stu vicāraṇā (41/32)

RĀMA asked:

Lord, how could there be even an intention to diversify in the infinite consciousness?

VASIṢṬHA said:

O Rāma, you will see the beauty of the truth in my statements when you attain the vision of truth. Descriptions of creation etc. are given in the scriptures for the purpose of instructing disciples. When you realise that which is indicated by the words, then naturally you will abandon the jugglery of words. In the infinite consciousness itself there is neither an intention nor the veil of delusion. But, that itself is before you as the world.

This can be realised only when ignorance comes to an end. Ignorance will not cease except with the help of instruction which rests in the use of these words and descriptions. This ignorance seeks to destroy itself and hence seeks the light of true knowledge. Weapons are destroyed by other weapons, dirt cleans dirt, poison cures poison and enemies are destroyed by other enemies: even so this Māyā rejoices when it is destroyed! The moment you become aware of this Māyā, it vanishes.

This ignorance will not go away without self-knowledge. And, self-knowledge arises only when the scriptures are studied deeply. Whatever may be the origin of this ignorance, surely, even that exists in the self. Hence, **O Rāma, do not enquire into 'How has this ignorance arisen', but enquire into 'How shall I get rid of it'.** When this ignorance or Māyā has ceased to be, then you shall know how it arose. You will realise that this ignorance is not a real entity.

I shall again declare to you the way in which the one infinite consciousness has come to appear as the jīva and all the rest of it. You see in the ocean that it is tranquil in places and agitated in other places. Even so, the infinite consciousness seems to embrace diversity in some places, though it in itself is non-dual. It is natural for the omnipotent infinite consciousness to manifest in all its infinite glory.

The manifestation of the omnipotence of infinite consciousness enters into an alliance with time, space and causation, which are indispensable to the manifestation. Thence arose the infinite names and forms. But all these apparent manifestations are in reality non-different from the infinite consciousness. That aspect of this infinite consciousness which relates itself to the manifestation of the names and forms and thus to time, space and causation is known as the 'knower of the field', or the witness consciousness. The body is the field; that which knows this field inside out and in all its aspects is the knower of the field or witness consciousness. This witness consciousness becomes involved in the latent predispositions and develops the ego-sense. The foolish person then abandons all right thinking or enquiry into the truth and voluntarily embraces ignorance as bliss.

viharanti jagat kecin nipatanty utpatanti ca
kandukā iva hastena mṛtyunā 'viratam hataḥ (43/25)

VASISTHA continued:

This incidental manifestation of the power of the infinite consciousness appears as the millions of species of beings in this universe. These countless beings are caught up in their own mental conditioning. They are found in every country and in every place in the universe, and they are in every conceivable kind of situation.

Some of them are part of the new creation in this epoch, others are more ancient. Some have incarnated just a couple of times, others have had countless incarnations. Some are liberated. Others are sunk in dreadful suffering. Some are celestials, some are demi-gods, and others are the deities presiding over this manifest universe. Some others are demons, others are goblins. Some are members of the four castes of human beings, and others are members of primitive uncivilised tribes.

Some of them are in the form of herbs and grass; others appear as roots, fruits and leaves. Some are in the form of creepers, and some are living as flowers. Some are the kings and their ministers clad in royal robes; others are clad in rags and bark of trees, either because they are anchorites or they are beggars.

Some are snakes and others are insects; others are animals like lions, tigers, etc. Some are birds, others are elephants and donkeys.

Some are prosperous; others are in adverse circumstances. Some are in heaven, others are in hell. Some are in the region of the stars, others are in holes of dying trees. Some live amongst liberated sages; others are already liberated sages who have risen above body-consciousness. Some are endowed with enlightened intelligence; some are extremely dull.

O Rāma, just as in this universe there are countless beings of various species, in other universes, too, there are similar beings, with different bodies suited to those universes.

But, all of them are bound by their own mental conditioning. **These beings roam this universe sometimes uplifted, sometimes degraded; and death plays with them as with a ball.** Bound to their own countless desires and attachments and limited by their own mental conditioning, they migrate from one body to another. They will continue to do so, till they perceive the truth concerning their own self which is infinite consciousness. After attaining this self-knowledge, they are liberated from delusion and they do not return to this plane of birth and death any more.

(As the sage said this, the ninth day came to an end, and the assembly dispersed.)

asadidam akhilaṁ mayā sametaṁ tviti vigaṇayya viṣāditā 'stu mā te
sadiha hi sakalaṁ mayā sametaṁ tviti ca vilokya viṣāditā 'stu mā te (45/50)

VASIṢṬHA continued:

That which was non-existent in the beginning, and that which shall cease to be in the end, is not real in the middle (in the present), either. That which exists in the beginning, and in the end, is the reality in the present, too. **See that 'all this is unreal, including myself' and there will be no sorrow in you: or, see that 'all this is real, including myself' and sorrow will not touch you either.**

Knowing that the entire universe, including one's wealth, wife, son, etc., are nothing but the creation of the jugglery of the mind, one does not grieve when they are lost, nor does one feel elated when they prosper. If an unreal appearance has vanished, what does one lose? If it is utterly unreal, then how can it even be destroyed? On the other hand, it may be proper to feel unhappy when they prosper; for such prosperity may intensify one's ignorance. Hence, that which generates attachment and craving in the fool, generates detachment and cool indifference in the wise.

The nature of the wise person is not to desire for those experiences which one does not effortlessly obtain, and to experience those which have already arrived.

If one is able to wean the mind away from craving for sense-pleasure by whatever means, one is saved from being drowned in the ocean of delusion. He who has realised his oneness with the entire universe, and who has thus risen above both desire 'for' and desire 'against', is never deluded.

Therefore, O Rāma, realise that self or infinite consciousness which permeates and therefore transcends both the unreal and the real; and, then, neither grasp nor give up whatever is inside or outside. The wise sage who is established in such self-knowledge is free from any sort of colouring or mental conditioning or self-limitation: he is like the sky or space which is totally free from being tainted by anything that happens within it.

O Rāma, in this ocean of ignorant mental conditioning, he who has found the raft of self-knowledge is saved from drowning; he who has not found that raft is surely drowned. Therefore, O Rāma, examine the nature of the self with an intelligence as sharp as the razor's edge; and then rest established in self-knowledge. All the powers that are inherent in the mind and by which the world has been brought into being are found in the infinite consciousness. Hence the sages have declared that the mind is omnipotent.

Live as the sages of self-knowledge live. They know the infinite consciousness and the world-appearance: hence, they do not relish nor renounce activity in this world. You too have attained self-knowledge, Rāma, and you are at peace.

kriyāviśeṣabahulā bhogaiśvarya hatāśayaḥ
nā 'pekṣante yadā satyaṁ na paśyanti śaṭhās tadā (1)

VASIṢṬHA continued:

O Rāma, they who are busy with the diverse affairs in this world in pursuit of pleasure and power do not desire to know the truth which they obviously do not see. He who is wise, but who has not completely controlled the pleasure-seeking tendencies of his senses, sees the truth and sees the illusion. And, he who has clearly understood the nature of the world and of the jīva and who has firmly rejected the world-appearance as the reality, is liberated and is not born again. The ignorant strive for the welfare of the body and not of the self: be not like the ignorant, O Rāma, but be wise.

To illustrate this I shall now narrate to you an interesting legend. In the country known as Magadha, which had an abundance of pleasure gardens, there lived a sage by name Dāsūra. He was engaged in breathtaking penance. He was a great ascetic who had no interest at all in worldly pleasures; and he was learned, too.

He was the son of another sage known as Śaraloma. But as ill luck would have it, he lost both his parents when he was young. The deities of the forest took pity on this orphan who was inconsolable in his grief, and they said to him:

"O wise boy! You are the son of a sage; why do you weep like an ignorant fool? Do you not know the evanescent nature of this world appearance? Young one, such is the very nature of this world-appearance: things come into being, exist for a while and are then destroyed. Whatever being there appears to be, from the relative point of view, (even if that being is called Brahmā, the creator) is subject to this inevitable end. There is no doubt about this. Hence, do not grieve over the inevitable death of your parents."

The young man's sorrow was ameliorated. He got up and performed the funeral rites of his parents. Then he began to lead a rigorously religious life, hemmed in on all sides with do's and dont's. Since he had not yet realised the truth he was immersed in the performance of the rituals with all their injunctions and prohibitions. All this created in him a feeling that the whole world is full of impurities. He sought to live in an unpolluted place. A tree-top, he decided! Wishing to live on a tree-top he performed a sacred rite during which he cut off and offered his own flesh into the sacred fire. Soon the fire deity himself appeared before him and announced, "You will surely attain the wish which has already appeared in your heart."

After accepting the ascetic's worship, Fire disappeared.

jñānaṁ tvam evā 'sya vibho kṛpayopadiśā 'dhunā
ko hi nāma kule jātaṁ putraṁ maurkhyeṇa yojayet (51/28)

VASIṢṬHA continued:

The sage then saw in front of him a huge Kadamba tree which had a majestic appearance. It seemed to wipe with its hands (its foliage) the tears (raindrops) of his beloved sky. It had actually covered the space between heaven and earth with the thousands of its arms (branches) and it stood like the cosmic form of the Lord, with the sun and the moon for his eyes. Laden with flowers, it rained them on the holy and divine sages who traversed the sky, and the bees that dwelt on it sang a song of welcome to those sages. (The detailed description of the tree is graphic and beautiful. — S.V.)

The sage ascended this tree, which stood like a pillar linking heaven and earth. He sat on the topmost branch of the tree. For a brief moment he let his eyes roam in all the directions. He had a vision of the cosmic being. (The detailed description of what he saw, given in chapter 50, is also interesting — S.V.)

Because he had taken his abode on the Kadamba tree he had come to be known as Kadamba-dāśūra. He commenced his austerities sitting on the top of that tree. He had been accustomed to the ritualistic performances enjoined in the Vedā, and so he engaged himself in their performance, but this time mentally. Yet, such is the power of such mental performance that it purified the sage's mind and heart, and he attained pure wisdom.

One day he beheld in front of him a nymph clad in flowers. She was extremely beautiful. The sage asked her: "O beautiful lady, with your radiance you can overpower even Cupid. Who are you?" She replied: "Lord, I am a deity of the forest. In this world nothing is unattainable to one who resorts to the presence of an enlightened sage like you. I have just been to attend a festival in the forest, where I met several other goddesses of the forest, each one of them with her offspring. I was the only one among them who had no children. Hence, I am unhappy. However, when you are in this forest why should I be unhappy? Grant me a son or I shall reduce myself to ashes." The sage picked up a creeper, and handing it to her said: "Go. Just as this creeper will produce flowers in a month, you too, will give birth to a son." The grateful goddess went away.

She returned to the sage after twelve years with the son of that age. She said: "Lord, this is your son. And, I have instructed him in all branches of learning. I **pray that you may instruct him in self-knowledge: for who will let one's son grow into a fool?"** The sage accepted to do so and the goddess went away. From that day the sage began to instruct the young man in all branches of self-knowledge.

jayati gacchati valgati jṛmbhate sphurati bhāti na bhāti bhāsuraḥ
suta mahāmahimā sa mahīpatiḥ patirapāmiva vātarayākulaḥ (29)

VASIṢṬHA continued:

During this period I was myself going over that very tree and heard the sage's instructions to his son.

DĀŚŪRA said:

I shall illustrate with a story what I wish to say concerning this world. There lives a mighty king name Khottha who is capable of conquering the three worlds. The deities presiding over the worlds faithfully honour his commands. No one can even catalogue his innumerable deeds which were productive of both happiness and unhappiness. His valour could not be challenged by anyone using any weapon whatsoever, or even by fire, any more than one can hit space with a fist. Even Indra, Viṣṇu and Śiva could not equal him in his enterprises.

This king had three bodies, which had completely engulfed the worlds: and they were respectively the best, the middling and the least. This king arose in space and got established in space. There the king built a city with fourteen roads and three sectors. In it were pleasure gardens, beautiful mountain peaks for sports and seven lakes with pearls and creepers in them. In it there were two lights which were hot and cold and whose light never diminished.

In that city the king created several types of beings. Some were placed above, others in the middle and yet others below. Of them some were long-lived and others short-lived. They were covered with black hair. They had nine gates. They were well ventilated. They had five lamps, three pillars, and white supporting wooden poles. They were soft with clay-plastering. All this was created by the Māyā or illusory power of the king.

Here, the king besports himself, with all the ghosts and goblins (which are afraid of enquiry or investigation) that had been created to protect the mansions (the different bodies). When he thinks of moving he thinks of a future city and contemplates migrating to it. Surrounded by the ghosts he runs fast to the new abode after leaving the previous one, and occupies the new city built in the fashion of a magic creation. In that again, when he contemplates destruction, he destroys himself. Sometimes he wails, "What shall I do? I am ignorant, I am miserable". Sometimes he is happy, at others pitiable.

Thus he lives and conquers, goes, talks, flourishes, shines and does not shine: my son, thus this king is tossed in this ocean of world-appearance.

asat sat sadasat sarvaṁ saṅkalpādeva nā 'nyataḥ
saṅkalpaṁ sadasaccaivamiha satyaṁ kimucyatāṁ (45)

DĀŚŪRA continued:

Thus has been illustrated the creation of the universe and of man. Khottha, who arose in the great void, is none but a notion or an intention. This notion arises in the great void of its own accord and dissolves in the great void of its own accord, too. The entire universe and whatever there is in it is the creation of this notion, or intention, and naught else. In fact, even the trinity (Brahmā, Viṣṇu and Śiva) are the limbs of that notion. That intention alone is responsible for the creation of the three worlds, the fourteen regions and the seven oceans. The city built by the king is nothing but the living entity, with his different organs and their characteristics. Of the different kinds of beings thus created, some (the gods) are in a higher region and the others are in lower realms.

Having built this imaginary city, the king placed it under the protecting care of ghosts: these ghosts are the ahaṁkāra (ego-principle). The king thenceforth sports in this world, in this body. In a moment he sees the world in the waking state; and after some time he abruptly shifts his attention to the world within which he enjoys in his dreams. He moves from one city to another, from one body to another, from one realm to another.

After many such peregrinations he develops wisdom, getting disillusioned with these worlds and their pleasures, and reaches the end of his wandering by the cessation of all notions.

In one moment he seems to enjoy wisdom, whilst the very next moment he is caught up in pleasure-seeking, and in an instant his understanding gets perverted, just as in the case of a little child. These notions are either like dense darkness (and give rise to ignorance and births in the lower orders of creation) or pure and transparent (and give rise to wisdom, drawing one close to the truth) or impure (and give rise to worldliness). When all such notions cease, then there is liberation.

Even if one engages oneself in every other sort of spiritual endeavour, even if one has the gods themselves as one's teachers, and even if one were in heaven or any other region, liberation is not had except through the cessation of all notions. **The real, the unreal and the admixture of these two are all but notions and naught else; and notions themselves are neither real nor unreal. What then shall we call real in this universe?** Hence, my son, give up these notions, thoughts and intentions. When they cease, the mind naturally turns to what is truly beyond the mind — the infinite consciousness.

mā saṅkalpaya saṅkalpaṁ bhāvaṁ bhāvaya mā sthitau
etāvataiva bhāvena bhavyo bhavati bhūtaye (54/12)

DĀŚŪRA continued:

My son when, in the infinite consciousness, the consciousness becomes aware of itself as its own object, there is the seed of ideation. This is very subtle. But soon it becomes gross and fills the whole space, as it were. When consciousness is engrossed in this ideation it thinks the object is distinct from the subject. Then the ideation begins to germinate and to grow. Ideation multiplies naturally by itself. This leads to sorrow, not to happiness. There is no cause for sorrow in this world other than this ideation.

Do not entertain ideas. Do not hold onto the notion of your existence. For it is only by these that the future comes into being. There is no cause for fear in the destruction of all ideation. When there is no thought, notion or ideation ceases. My son, it is easier to cease to entertain notions, than it is to crush a flower that lies on the palm of your hand. The latter demands effort; the former is effortless.

Already as the notions weaken, one is less affected by happiness and unhappiness, and knowledge of the unreality of the objects prevents attachment. When there is no hope, there is neither elation nor depression. The mind itself is the jīva when it is reflected in consciousness; and mind itself builds castles in the air, stretching itself, as it were, into the past, the present and the future. It is not possible to comprehend the ripples of ideation, but this much can be said: sense-experiences multiply them, and when these are given up, they cease to be. If these notions are real, like the blackness of coal, then you cannot remove them; but that is not so. Hence they can be destroyed.

VASIṢTHA continued:

Hearing the sage's words, I descended upon that Kadaṁba tree. For a considerable time the three of us discussed self-knowledge, and I awakened in them the supreme knowledge. Then I took leave of them and went away. O Rāma, this is meant to illustrate the nature of the world-appearance, and therefore, this story is as true as the world itself!

Even if you believe that this world and yourself are real, then be it so: rest firmly in your own self. If you think that this is both real and unreal, then adopt the appropriate attitude to this changing world. If you believe that the world is unreal, then be firmly established in the infinite consciousness. Similarly, whether you believe that the world has had a creator or not, let it not cloud your understanding.

O Rāma, you may feel, 'I am not the doer, I do not exist' (or 'I am the doer and I am everything'), or enquire into the nature of the self ('Who am I') and realise 'I am not any of this that is attributed to me'. Rest established in the self which is the highest state of consciousness, in which the best among the holy men who know of this state ever dwell.

yadi tvam ātmanā "tmānam adhigacchasi taṁ svayaṁ
etat praśnottaraṁ sādhu jānāsyatra na saṁśayaḥ (15)

RĀMA asked:

Holy sage, how does this unreal world exist in the absolute Brahman: can snow exist in the sun?

VASIṢṬHA said:

Rāma, this is not the right time for you to ask this question, for you will not be able to comprehend the answer now. Love stories are uninteresting to a little boy. Every tree bears its fruits in due season: and my instruction will also bear fruit in good time. **If you seek your self with the self by your own self effort you will clearly find the answer to your question.** I discussed the question of doership and non-doership in order that the nature of the mental conditioning or ideation may become evident.

Bondage is bondage to these thoughts and notions: freedom is freedom from them. Give up all notions; even those of liberation. First, by the cultivation of good relationships like friendship, give up tendencies and notions which are gross and materialistic. Later, give up even such notions as friendship, even though continuing to be friendly, etc. Give up all desires and contemplate the nature (or notion) of cosmic consciousness. Even this is within the realm of ideation or thought, hence give this up in due course. Rest in what remains after all these have been given up. And, renounce the renouncer of these notions. When even the notion of the ego-sense has ceased you will be like the infinite space. He who has thus renounced everything from his heart is indeed the supreme Lord, whether he continues to live an active life or whether he rests in contemplation all the time. To him neither action nor inaction is of any use. O Rāma, I have examined all the scriptures and investigated the truth; there is no salvation without the total renunciation of all notions or ideas or mental conditioning.

This world of diverse names and forms is composed of the desirable and the undesirable! For these people strive, but for self-knowledge no one strives. Rare are the sages of self-knowledge in the three worlds. One may be an emperor of the world or the king of heaven; but all these are only composed of the five elements! It is a pity that people indulge in such colossal destruction of life for these petty gains. Shame on them. None of these engages the attention of the sage, because he is equipped with self-knowledge. He is established in that supreme seat to which the sun and the moon have no access (the suṣumnā?). Hence, the sage of self-knowledge is not enamoured of the gains or the pleasures of the entire universe.

kiṁ karomi kva gacchāmi kiṁ gṛhṇāmi tyajāmi kiṁ
ātmanā pūritaṁ viśvaṁ mahākalpāṁbunā yathā (58/5)

VASIṢṬHA continued:

In this connection, O Rāma, I remember an inspiring song sung by the son of the preceptor of the gods, Kaca. This Kaca was established in self-knowledge. He lived in a cave on the mount Meru. His mind was saturated with the highest wisdom and hence it was not attracted by any of the objects of the world composed of the five elements. Feigning despair, Kaca sang this meaningful song. Pray listen to this.

KACA said:

What shall I do? Where shall I go? What shall I try to hold? What shall I renounce? This entire universe is permeated by the one self. Unhappiness or sorrow is the self. Happiness is the self, too. All desires are but empty void. Having known that all this is the self, I am freed from all travail. In this body, within and without, above and below, everywhere — here and there — there is only the self and self alone, and there is no non-self. The self alone is everywhere; everything exists as the self. All this is truly the self. I exist in the self as the self. I exist as all this, as the reality in all everywhere. I am the fullness. I am the self-bliss. I fill the entire universe like the cosmic ocean.

Thus he sang. And he intoned the holy word OṀ which resounded like a bell. He had merged his entire being in that holy sound. He was neither inside anything nor outside anything. This sage remained in that place totally absorbed in the self.

RĀMA asked:

When the mind regains the state of the Creator himself by the destruction of all notions, how does the notion of the world arise in it?

VASIṢṬHA continued:

O Rāma, the first-born Creator on arising from the womb of the infinite consciousness uttered the sound 'Brahmā': hence he is known as Brahmā, the creator. This Creator first entertained the notion of light, and light came into being. In that light he visualised his own cosmic body, and this came into being — from the brilliant sun to the diverse objects that fill the space. He contemplated the same light as of infinite sparks, and all these sparks became diverse beings. Surely, it is the cosmic mind alone that has become this Brahmā and all the other beings. Whatever this Brahmā created in the beginning is seen even today. After creating the universe by his own thought-force, the Creator rested — rested in his own self in deep meditation. From there on, created beings acquired the character of the things with which they associated. By associating with the good they became good, and those who associated with the worldly became worldly. Thus one gets bound to this world-appearance: and thus one is liberated too.

yaiva cid bhuvanābhogabhūṣaṇe vyomni bhāskare
dharāvivarakośasthe saiva citkīṭakodare (61/18)

VASIṢṬHA continued:

After the creation of the world-appearance the living beings that arose in the ocean of infinite consciousness like waves and ripples entered into the physical space; and when the elements like air, fire, water and earth were evolved they became involved in them. Then the cycle of birth and death began to revolve.

The jīvā come down, as it were, riding the rays of the moon, and enter into the plants and herbs. They become the fruits, as it were, of those plants. Then they are ready to incarnate. The subtle notions, ideas and mental conditioning are dormant even in the unborn being; at birth, the veil that covered them is removed.

Some of these beings are born pure and enlightened (sātvika). Even in their own previous births they had turned away from the lure of sensual pleasures. But the nature of the others who are born merely to perpetuate the cycle of birth and death, is a mixture of the pure, the impure and the dark. There are others whose nature is pure with just a slight impurity; they are devoted to the truth and are full of noble qualities. Other people are enveloped by the darkness of ignorance and stupidity — they are like rocks and hills!

Those beings in whom purity is preponderant with just a slight impurity (the rājasa-sātvika people) are ever happy, enlightened and do not grieve nor despair. They are unselfish like trees, and like them, they live to experience the fruition of past actions without committing new ones. They are desireless. They are at peace within themselves and they do not abandon this peace even in the worst calamities. They love all, and look upon all with equal vision. They do not drown in the ocean of sorrow.

By all means one should avoid drowning in the ocean of sorrow and engage oneself in the enquiry into the nature of the self: 'Who am I, how has this world-illusion arisen?' One should thus abandon egoism in the body and attraction to the world. Then one will realise that there is no division in space, whether or not a building stands in space. **The same consciousness that shines in the sun also dwells as the little worm that crawls in a hole on this earth.**

O Rāma, one who is wise and who is capable of enquiring into the nature of truth should approach a good and learned person and study the scripture. This teacher should be free from craving for pleasure and he should also have had direct experience of the truth; and with his help, one should study the scripture and by the practice of the great yoga, one can reach the supreme state. It is by emulating the example of the holy ones that one makes progress towards the supreme state.

Rāma, only a person who is intelligent like you, who is good natured and equal visioned like you, and who sees only what is good, is entitled to the vision of wisdom which I have described here. Rāma, you are already a liberated being: live like one!

**yad yad rāghava saṁyāti mahājana saparyayā
dinaṁ tad iha sālokaṁ śeṣāstv andhā dinālayaḥ (4/12)**

VĀLMĪKI said:

The people listened to sage Vasiṣṭha's words of wisdom with total attention. In the evening the congregation was given leave to retire for the day. When the assembly had thus dispersed, Vasiṣṭha gave leave to the princes, Rāma and his brothers, to retire for the day. When night fell all except Rāma retired to bed. But Rāma could not sleep.

RĀMA contemplated the illuminating words of the sage Vasiṣṭha thus:

What exactly are the means that the sage Vasiṣṭha has prescribed for the conquest of the senses and the mind, which are surely the sources of sorrow. It is impossible to abandon enjoyment of pleasure, and it is not possible to end sorrow without abandoning such enjoyment; this indeed is a problem. But, since the mind is the crucial factor in all this, surely if the mind once tastes the supreme peace, freed of all world-illusion, it will not abandon that and run after sense-pleasure.

O, when will my mind rest in the infinite even as a wave is re-absorbed in the ocean? When will I be free from all craving? When will I be blessed with equal vision? When will I be rid of this terrible fever of worldliness? O my intellect, you are my friend: contemplate the teachings of sage Vasiṣṭha in such a way that we shall both be saved from the miseries of this worldly existence.

When the day dawned, Rāma and the others got up and performed their morning religious functions. Soon after this all of them entered the assembly and took up their respective places.

Opening the day's proceedings, DAŚARATHA said:

O blessed Lord, we feel highly elevated by the words of supreme wisdom that you uttered yesterday. Our deluded belief in the reality of this world-appearance is also provided with a powerful challenge. **O Rāma, only that day on which such sages are worshipped can be regarded as fruitful; the other days are of darkness.** This is your best opportunity: enquire and learn from the sage that which is worth learning.

RĀMA said to Vasiṣṭha:

O Lord, giving up sleep I have spent the whole night meditating upon your enlightening words, endeavouring to see the truth that the words point to. Thus have I enshrined that truth in my heart. Who will not bear your teachings on his head, knowing that they confer the highest bliss on him? At the same time, they are extremely sweet to hear, they promote every type of auspiciousness and they bring us the incomparable experience.

Hence, O Lord, I pray: resume your most excellent discourse.

he janā aparijñāta ātmā vo duḥkhasiddhaye
parijñātastv anantāya sukhāyopaśamāya ca (23)

VASIṢṬHA said:

O Rāma, kindly listen to this discourse on the dissolution of the universe and the attainment of supreme peace.

This seemingly unending world-appearance is sustained by impure (rājasa) and dull (tāmasa) beings, even as a superstructure is sustained by pillars. But it is playfully and easily abandoned by those who are of a pure nature, even as the slough is effortlessly abandoned by a snake. They who are of a pure (sātvika) nature and they whose activities (rajas) are based on purity and light (satva) do not live their life mechanically, but enquire into the origin and the nature of this world-appearance. When such enquiry is conducted with the help of the right study of scriptures and the company of holy ones, there arises a clear understanding within oneself in which the truth is seen, as in the light of a lamp. Not until this truth is perceived by oneself for oneself through such enquiry is the truth seen truly. O Rāma, you are indeed of a pure nature: therefore, enquire into the nature of the truth and the falsehood, and be devoted to the truth. That which was not in the beginning and which will cease to be after a time, how can that be regarded as truth? That alone can be regarded as truth which has always been and which will always be.

Birth is of the mind, O Rāma: and growth is mental, too. And when the truth is clearly seen, it is mind that is liberated from its own ignorance. Hence, let the mind be led along the path of righteousness by the prior study of the scriptures, company of the holy ones and the cultivation of dispassion. Equipped with these one should resort to the feet of a master (guru) whose wisdom is perfected. By faithfully adhering to the teachings of the master, one gradually attains to the plane of total purity.

O Rāma, behold the self by the self through pure enquiry, even as the cool perceives the entire space. One is tossed over the waters of this illusory world-appearance like a piece of straw only as long as one does not get into the secure boat of self-enquiry. Even as particles of sand floating in water settle down when the water is absolutely steady, the mind of the man who has gained the knowledge of the truth settles down in total peace. Once this knowledge of the truth is gained, it is not lost: even if a piece of gold has lain in a heap of ashes, the goldsmith finds no problem in seeing it. When the truth has not been known, there may be confusion: but once it is known there can be no confusion. **Ignorance of the self is the cause of your sorrow: knowledge of the self leads to delight and tranquillity.**

yathā rajobhir gaganaṁ yathā kamalam ambubhiḥ
na lipyate hi saṁśliṣṭair dehair ātmā tathaiva ca (31)

VASIṢṬHA continued:

Resolve the confusion between the body and the self, and you will be at peace at once. Even as a nugget of gold fallen into mud is never spoiled by the mud, the self is untainted by the body. With uplifted arms I proclaim, "The self is one thing and the body is another, even as the water and the lotus", but no one listens to me! As long as the inert and insentient mind pursues the path of pleasure, so long this darkness of world illusion cannot be dispelled. But, the moment one awakens from this and enquires into the nature of the self, this darkness is dispelled at once. Hence, one should constantly endeavour to awaken the mind which dwells in the body in order that one may go beyond the process of becoming — for such becoming is fraught with sorrow.

Even as the sky is not affected by the dust particles floating in it, the self is unaffected by the body. Pleasure and pain are falsely imagined to be experienced by oneself, even as one falsely thinks that 'the sky is polluted by dust'. In fact, pleasure and pain are neither of the body nor of the self which transcends everything: they belong only to ignorance. Their loss is no loss. Neither pleasure nor pain belong to anyone: all indeed is the self which is supreme peace and infinite. Realise this, O Rāma.

The self and the world are neither identical nor are they different (dual). All this is but the reflection of the truth. Nothing but the one Brahman exists. 'I am different from this' is pure fancy: give it up, O Rāma.

The one self perceives itself within itself as the infinite consciousness. Therefore, there is no sorrow, no delusion, no birth (creation) nor creature: whatever is, is. Be free from distress, O Rāma. Be free of duality; remain firmly established in the self, abandoning even concern for your own welfare. Be at peace within, with a steady mind. Let there be no sorrow in your mind. Rest in the inner silence. Remain alone, without self-willed thoughts. Be brave, having conquered the mind and the senses. Be desireless, content with what comes to you unsought. Live effortlessly, without grabbing or giving up anything. Be free from all mental perversions and from the blinding taint of illusion. Rest content in your own self. Thus, be free from all distress. Remain in an expansive state in the self, like the full ocean. Rejoice in the self by the self, like the blissful rays of the full moon.

kecittvakarmaṇi ratā viratā api karmaṇaḥ
narakānnarakaṁ yānti duḥkhād duḥkhaṁ bhayādbhayaṁ (6/3)

VASIṢṬHA continued:

O Rāma, he who knows that all the activities merely happen because of the mere existence of consciousness — even as a crystal reflects the objects around it without intending to do so — is liberated. They who, even after taking this human birth, are not interested in such non-volitional activity, go from heaven to hell and from hell to heaven again.

Some there are who are devoted to inaction, having turned away from or suppressed all action; they go from hell to hell, from sorrow to sorrow, from fear to fear. Some are bound by their tendencies and intentions to the fruits of their own actions; and they take birth as worms and vermin, then as trees and plants, then as worms and vermin again. Others there are who know the self; blessed indeed are they for they have carefully enquired into the nature of the mind and overcome all cravings: they go to higher planes of consciousness.

He who has taken birth for the last time now, is endowed with a mixture of light (satva) and a little impurity (rajas). Right from birth he grows in holiness. The nobler type of knowledge enters into him with ease. All the noble qualities like friendliness, compassion, wisdom, goodness and magnanimity seek him and take their abode in him. He performs all appropriate actions, but is not swayed if their results appear to be gain or loss; nor does he feel elated or depressed. His heart is clear. He is much sought after by the people.

Such a one who is full of all the noble qualities, seeks and follows an enlightened master, who directs him along the path of self-knowledge. He then realises the self which is the one cosmic being. Such a liberated one awakens the inner intelligence, which has been asleep so far: and this awakened intelligence instantly knows itself to be the infinite consciousness. Becoming constantly aware of the inner light, such a blessed one instantly ascends into the utterly pure state.

Such is the normal course of evolution, O Rāma. However, there are exceptions to this rule. In the case of those who have taken birth in this world, two possibilities exist for the attainment of liberation. The first is: treading the path indicated by the master, the seeker gradually reaches the goal of liberation. The second is: self-knowledge literally drops into one's lap, as it were, and there is instant enlightenment.

I shall narrate to you an ancient legend which illustrates the second type of enlightenment. Please listen.

upaśamasukhamāharet pavitraṁ suśamavataḥ śamameti sādhucetaḥ praśamitamanasaḥ svake svarūpe bhavati sukhe sthitiruttamā cirāya (18)

VASIṢṬHA continued:

O Rāma, there is a great monarch whose vision is unlimited, who rules over the Videha territory: he is known as Janaka. To those who seek his aid, he is a cornucopia. In his very presence the heart-lotuses of his friends blossom: he is like unto a sun for them. He is a great benefactor to all good people.

One day he went to a pleasure-garden where he roamed freely. While he was thus roaming he heard the inspiring words uttered by certain holy, perfected ones.

Thus did the PERFECTED SAGES sing:

We contemplate that self which reveals itself as the pure experience of bliss when seer (the experiencer) comes into contact with the object (the experience), without a division or conceptualisation.

We contemplate the self in which the objects are reflected non-volitionally, once the divided experience (predicate) of subject-object and the intention or volition that created this division have ceased.

We contemplate that light that illumines all that shines, the self that transcends the twin concepts of 'is' and 'is not' and which therefore is 'in the middle' of the two sides, as it were.

We contemplate that reality, in which everything exists, to which everything belongs, from which everything has emerged, which is the cause of everything and which is everything.

We contemplate the self which is the very basis of all language and expression, being the alpha and the omega, which covers the entire field from 'a' to 'ha' and which is indicated by the word 'aham' ('I').

Alas, people run after other objects, foolishly giving up the Lord who dwells in the cave of one's own heart.

He who, having known the worthlessness of the objects still remains bound at heart to them, is not a human being!

One should strike down every craving with the rod of wisdom, whether that craving has arisen or is about to rise in the heart.

One should enjoy the delight that flows from peace. The man whose mind is well-controlled is firmly established in peace. When the heart is thus established in peace, there arises the pure bliss of the self without delay.

arajjureva baddho 'ham apaṅko 'smi kalaṅkitaḥ
patito 'smyupariṣṭho 'pi hā mamātman hatā sthitiḥ (16)

VASIṢṬHA continued:

Having heard the words of the sages, king Janaka became terribly depressed. With the utmost expedition he retraced his steps to the palace. Quickly dismissing all his attendants he sought the seclusion of his own chamber. In a mood of intense anguish,

KING JANAKA said to himself:

Alas, alas, I am helplessly swinging like a stone in this world of misery. What is the duration of a life-span in eternity? Yet, I have developed a love for it! Fie on the mind. What is sovereignty even during a whole lifetime? Yet, like a fool, I think I cannot do without it! This life-span of mine is but a trivial moment — eternity stretches before and after it. How shall I cherish it now?

Ah, who is that magician who has spread this illusion called the world and thus deluded me? How is it that I am so deluded? Realising that what is near and what is far is all in my mind, I shall give up the apprehension of all external objects. Knowing that all the busy-ness in this world leads only to endless suffering, what hope shall I cherish for happiness? Day after day, month after month, year after year, moment after moment, I see happiness comes to me bearing sorrow, and sorrow comes to me again and again!

Whatever is seen or experienced here is subject to change and destruction: there is nothing whatsoever in this world which the wise would rely on. They who are exalted today are trodden under foot tomorrow: O foolish mind, what shall we trust in this world?

Alas, I am bound without a cord; I am tainted without impurity; I am fallen, though remaining at the top. O my self, what a mystery! Even as the ever-brilliant sun suddenly faces a cloud floating in front of him, I find this strange delusion mysteriously floating towards me. Who are these friends and relatives, what are these pleasures? Even as a boy seeing a ghost is frightened, I am deluded by these fanciful relatives. Knowing such relatives as cords that bind me to this old age, death, etc., I still cling to them. Let these relatives continue or perish: what is it to me? Great events and great men have come and gone, leaving just a memory behind: on what shall one place reliance even now? Even gods and the trinity have come and gone a million times: what is permanent in this universe? It is vain hope that binds one to this nightmare known as world-appearance. Fie on this wretched condition.

kākatālīyayogena saṁpannāyāṁ jagatsthitau
dhūrtena kalpitā vyarthaṁ heyopādeyabhāvanā (49)

KING JANAKA continued:

I am like an ignorant fool deluded by the goblin known as the ego-sense which creates the false feeling 'I am so-and-so'. Knowing full well that Time has trampled under foot countless gods and trinities, I still entertain love for life. Days and nights are spent in vain cravings, but not in the experience of the bliss of infinite consciousness. I have gone from sorrow to greater sorrow, but dispassion does not arise in me.

What shall I regard as excellent or desirable, seeing that whatever one cherished in this world has passed away, leaving one miserable. Day by day people in this world grow in sin and violence, hence day by day they experience greater sorrow. Childhood is wasted in ignorance, youth is wasted in lusting after pleasures and the rest of one's life is spent in family worries: what does a stupid person achieve in this life.

Even if one performs great religious rites, one may go to heaven — nothing more. What is heaven? Is it on earth or in the netherworld, and is there a place which is untouched by affliction? Sorrow brings happiness, and happiness brings sorrow on its shoulders! The pores of the earth are filled by the dead bodies of beings; hence it looks solid.

There are beings in this universe whose winking is of the duration of an epoch. What is my life-span in comparison? Of course there appear to be delightful and enduring objects in this world, but they bring with them endless worries and anxieties! Prosperity is truly adversity, and adversity may be desirable, depending upon their effect upon the mind. Mind alone is the seed for this delusion of world-appearance; it is the mind that gives rise to the false sense of 'I' and 'mine'.

In this world which appears to have been created even as the fruit of cocoanut palm might appear to have been dislodged by a crow which coincidentally happens to alight on the tree at that moment, sheer ignorance generates feelings like 'this I should have' and 'this I should reject'. It is better to spend one's time in seclusion or in hell than to live in this world-appearance.

Intention or motivation alone is the seed for this world-appearance. I shall dry up this motivation! I have enjoyed and suffered all kinds of experiences. Now I shall rest. I shall not grieve anymore. I have been awakened. I shall slay this thief (the mind) who has stolen my wisdom. I have been well instructed by the sages: now I shall seek self-knowledge.

sthite manasi niṣkāme same vigataarañjane
kāyāvayavajau kāryau spandāspandau phale samau (28)

VASIṢṬHA continued:

Seeing the king thus seated engrossed in deep contemplation, his body-guard respectfully approached him and said: "Lord, it is time to consider your royal duties. Your Majesty's handmaiden awaits your pleasure, having prepared your perfumed bath. The holy priests await your arrival in the bath chamber to commence the chanting of the appropriate hymns. Lord, arise and let what has to be done be done; for noble men are never unpunctual or negligent."

Ignoring the bodyguard's words, KING JANAKA continued to muse:

What shall I do with this court and the royal duties when I know that all these are ephemeral? They are useless to me. I shall renounce all activities and duties, and remain immersed in the bliss of the self.

O mind, abandon your craving for sense-pleasures so that you may be rid of the miseries of repeated old age and death. Whatever be the condition in which you hope to enjoy happiness, that very condition proves to be the source of unhappiness! Enough of this sinful, conditioned, pleasure-seeking life. Seek the delight that is natural and inherent in you.

(Seeing that the king was silent, the bodyguard became silent too.)

What shall I seek to gain in this universe — on what eternal truth in this universe shall I rest with confidence? What difference does it make if I am engaged in ceaseless activity or if I remain idle? Nothing in this world is truly enduring in any case. Whether active or idle, this body is impermanent and ever-changing. When the intelligence is rooted in equanimity, what is lost and how?

I do not long for what I do not have, nor do I desire to abandon what has come to me unsought. I am firmly established in the self; let what is mine be mine! There is nothing that I should work for, nor is there any meaning in inaction. Whatever is gained by action or by inaction is false. **When the mind is thus established in desirelessness, when it does not seek pleasure, when the body and its limbs perform their natural functions, action and inaction are of equal value or meaning.** Hence, let the body engage itself in its natural functions; without such activity, the body will disintegrate. When the mind ceases to entertain the notions 'I do this', 'I enjoy this', in regard to the actions thus performed, action becomes non-action.

citta cañcala saṁsāra ātmano na sukhāya te
śamamehi śamāc chāntaṁ sukhaṁ sāram avāpyate (5)

VASIṢṬHA continued:

Reflecting thus, king Janaka rose from his seat as the sun rises on the horizon, and began to engage himself in the royal duties, without any attachment to them. Having abandoned all concepts of the desirable and the undesirable, freed from all psychological conditionings and intention, he engaged himself in spontaneous and appropriate action — as if in deep sleep, though wide awake. He performed the day's tasks, including the adoration of the holy ones; and at the conclusion of the day he retired to his own seclusion to spend the night in deep meditation, which was easy and natural to him. His mind had naturally turned away from all confusion and delusion, and had become firmly established in equanimity: and when he rose in the morning

KING JANAKA thus reflected in his own mind:

O unsteady mind! This worldly life is not conducive to your true happiness. Hence, reach the state of equanimity. It is in such equanimity that you will experience peace, bliss and the truth. Whenever you create perverse thinking in yourself out of your wantonness, it is then that this world illusion begins to expand and spread out. It is when you entertain desire for pleasures that this world illusion sprouts countless branches. It is thought that gives rise to this network of world-appearance. Hence, abandon this whim and fancy and attain to equanimity. Weigh in the balance of your wisdom the sense-pleasures on one side and the bliss of peace on the other. Whatever you determine to be the truth, seek that. Give up all hopes and expectations, and freed from the wish to seek or to abandon, roam about freely. Let this world-appearance be real or unreal, let it arise or set; but, do not let its merits and demerits disturb your equanimity. For at no time do you have a real relationship with this world-appearance: it is only because of your ignorance that such a relationship has appeared in you. O mind, you are false, and this world-appearance is also false; hence there is a mysterious relationship between you two — like the relationship between the barren woman and her son. If you think that you are real and that the world is unreal, how can a valid relationship exist between the two? On the other hand, if both are real, where then is the justification for exultation and sorrow? Hence, abandon sorrow and resort to deep contemplation. There is naught here in this world which can lead you to the state of fullness. Hence, resolutely take refuge in courage and endurance, and overcome your own waywardness.

prajñayeha jagat sarvaṁ samyagevā 'ṅga dṛśyate
samyag darśanamāyānti nā ''pado na ca sampadaḥ (38)

VASIṢṬHA continued:

Having reached the understanding already described, Janaka functioned as the king and did all that was necessary, without getting befuddled and with a great strength of mind and spirit. In fact, he moved about as if he were continually in a state of deep sleep.

The light of self-knowledge (cid-ātmā) arose in his heart, free from the least taint of impurity and sorrow, even as the sun rises on the horizon. He beheld everything in the universe as existing in cosmic power (cid-śakti). Endowed with self-knowledge, he saw all things in the self which is infinite. Knowing that all that happens happens naturally, he neither experienced elation nor suffered depression, and remained in unbroken equanimity. Janaka had become a liberated one while still living (jīvanmukta). Remaining forever in the consciousness of the infinite, he experienced the state of non-action, even though he appeared to others to be ever busy in diverse actions.

Janaka attained whatever he did by dint of his own enquiry. Similarly, one should pursue the enquiry into the nature of truth till one reaches the very limits of such enquiry.

Self-knowledge or knowledge of truth is not had by resorting to a guru (preceptor) nor by the study of scripture, nor by good works: it is attained only by means of enquiry inspired by the company of wise and holy men. One's inner light alone is the means, naught else. When this inner light is kept alive, it is not affected by the darkness of inertia.

Whatever sorrows there may be that seem to be difficult to overcome are easily crossed over with the help of the boat of wisdom (the inner light). He who is devoid of this wisdom is bothered even by minor difficulties. The effort and the energy that are directed by the people in worldly activities should first be directed to the gaining of this wisdom. One should first destroy the dullness of wit which is the source of all sorrow and calamities and which is the seed for this huge tree of world-appearance.

Wisdom or the inner light is like the legendary precious stone, O Rāma, which bestows on its owner whatever he wishes to have. When one's intelligence and understanding are properly guided by this inner light, one reaches the other shore; if not, one is overcome by obstacles.

Defects, desires and evils do not even approach that man of wisdom whose mind is undeluded. **Through wisdom (in the inner light) the entire world is clearly seen as it is; neither good fortune nor misfortune even approach one who has such clear vision.** The darkness of ego-sense which veils the self is dispelled by wisdom (inner light). He who seeks to be established in the highest state of consciousness, should first purify his mind by the cultivation of wisdom or by the kindling of the inner light.

dhāvamānam adhobhāge cittaṁ pratyāhared balāt
pratyāhāreṇa patitam adho vārīva setunā (30)

VASIṢṬHA continued:

O Rāma, thus do enquire into the nature of the self, even as Janaka did. Neither god, nor rites and rituals (or any action) nor wealth nor relatives are of any use in this; to those who are afraid of the world-illusion only self-effort as self-enquiry is capable of bringing about self-knowledge. This ocean of world-appearance can be crossed only when you are firmly established in supreme wisdom, when you see the self with the self alone and when your intelligence is not diverted or coloured by sense-perceptions.

Thus have I narrated to you how king Janaka attained self-knowledge as if by an act of grace which caused the knowledge to drop from heaven, as it were. When the limited and conditioned feeling 'I am so-and-so' ceases, there arises consciousness of the all-pervading infinite. Hence, O Rāma, like Janaka, you too abandon in your heart the false and fanciful notion of the ego-sense. When this ego-sense is dispelled the supreme light of self-knowledge will surely shine in your heart. He who knows 'I am not', 'Nor does the other exist', 'Nor is there non-existence', and whose mental activity has thus come to a standstill, is not engrossed in acquisitiveness. O Rāma, there is no bondage here other than craving for acquisition and the anxiety to avoid what one considers undesirable.

They in whom the twin-urges of acquisition and rejection have come to an end do not desire anything nor do they renounce anything. The mind does not reach the state of utter tranquillity till these two impulses (of acquisition and rejection) have been eliminated. Even so, as long as one feels 'this is real' and 'this is unreal', his mind does not experience peace and equilibrium. How can equanimity, purity or dispassion arise in the mind of one who is swayed by thoughts of 'this is right', 'this is wrong', 'this is gain', 'this is loss'? When there is only one Brahman (which is forever one and the many) what can be said to be right and what wrong?

Desirelessness (absence of all expectations), fearlessness, unchanging steadiness, equanimity, wisdom, non-attachment, non-action, goodness, total absence of perversion, courage, endurance, friendliness, intelligence, contentment, gentleness, pleasant speech — all these qualities are natural to one who is free from the instincts of acquisition and rejection: and even those qualities are non-intentional and spontaneous.

One should restrain the mind from flowing downward, even as the flow of a river is blocked by the construction of a dam. Cut down the mind with the mind itself. Having reached the state of purity, remain established in it right now. Rooted in equanimity, doing whatever happens to be appropriate in all situations and not even thinking about what has thus befallen you unsought, live a non-volitional life here. Such is the nature of the Lord who may therefore be said to be both the doer and the non-doer of all actions here.

cetyena rahitā yaiṣā cit tad brahma sanātanaṁ
cetyena sahitā yaiṣā cit seyaṁ kalanocyate (53)

VASIṢṬHA continued:

You are the knower of all — the self. You are the unborn being, you are the supreme Lord; you are non-different from the self which pervades everything. He who has abandoned the idea that there is an object of perception which is other than the self, is not subjected to the defects born of joy and grief. He is known as a yogi. He who is confirmed in his conviction that the infinite consciousness alone exists, is instantly freed from the thoughts of pleasure and is therefore tranquil and self-controlled.

They who are well versed in the scriptures declare that the fictitious movement of energy in consciousness is known as mind. And the expressions of the mind (like the hissing of the snake) are known as thoughts or ideas. **Consciousness minus conceptualisation is the eternal Brahman the absolute; consciousness plus conceptualisation is thought.** A small part of it, as it were, is seated in the heart as the reality. This is known as the finite intelligence or individualised consciousness. However, this limited consciousness soon 'forgot' its own essential conscious nature and continued to be, but inert. It then became the thinking faculty with reception and rejection as its inherent tendencies.

Then this inner intelligence is not awakened, it does not really know or understand anything: and what appears to be known through the thoughts is of course not the reality. These thoughts themselves derive their value from consciousness. On account of this borrowed intelligence, thought is able to know a minute fragmented fraction of this cosmic consciousness. The mind blossoms fully only when the light of the infinite shines upon it. Otherwise, though appearing to be intelligent, thought is unable to contemplate anything really, even as the granite figure of a dancer does not dance even when requested to do so. Can a battle-scene painted on a canvas generate the roar of fighting armies? Can a corpse get up and run? Does the figure of the sun carved on a rock dispel darkness? Similarly, what can the inert mind do? The mind appears to be intelligent and active only because of the inner light of consciousness.

Ignorant people misconstrue the movement of life-force to be the mind: but in fact it is nothing more than the prāṇa or life force. But, in the case of those whose intelligence is not fragmented or conditioned by thoughts, it is surely the radiance of the supreme being or self.

The intelligence that identifies itself with certain movements of life-force in the self (by entertaining notions of 'this am I', 'this is mine') is known as the jīva or the living soul. Intelligence, mind, jīva, etc., are names which are used even by wise men: such entities are not real, however, from the absolute point of view. In truth, there is no mind, no intelligence, no embodied being: the self alone exists at all times. Because it is extremely subtle it seems not to exist, though it exists.

prāṇaśaktau niruddhāyāṁ mano rāma vilīyate
dravyacchāyā 'nu tad dravyaṁ prāṇarūpaṁ hi mānasaṁ (83)

VASIṢṬHA continued:

A thought arising in the supreme being is known as individual consciousness; when this consciousness is freed from thought and individualisation, there is liberation. The seed or the sole cause for this world-appearance is but the arising of a thought in the infinite consciousness, which gave rise to the limited finite individual consciousness. When consciousness thus moved away from its utterly quiescent state and became tainted as it were, from thought, the thinking faculty arose and, with it, the mind thought of the universe.

O Rāma, by the control of the life-force the mind is also restrained; even as the shadow ceases when the substance is removed, the mind ceases when the life-force is restrained. It is because of the movement of the life-force that one remembers the experiences one had elsewhere; it is known as mind because it thus experiences movements of life-force. The life-force is restrained by the following means: by dispassion, by the practice of prāṇāyāma (breath-control), by the practice of enquiry into the cause of the movement of the life-force, by the ending of sorrow through intelligent means and by direct knowledge or experience of the supreme truth.

It is possible for the mind to assume the existence of intelligence in a stone. But the mind does not possess the least intelligence. Movement belongs to the life-force which is inert: intelligence or the power of consciousness belongs to the self which is pure and eternally omnipresent. It is the mind that fancies a relationship between these two factors: but such fancy is false and hence all knowledge that arises from this false relationship is also false. This is known as ignorance, Māyā or cosmic illusion, which gives rise to the dreadful poison known as world-appearance.

This relationship between the life-force and consciousness is imaginary; if it is not so imagined there can be no world-appearance! The life-force by its association with consciousness becomes conscious and experiences the world as its object. But all this is as unreal as the experience of a ghost by a child: the movement within the infinite consciousness alone is the truth. Can this infinite consciousness be affected by any finite factor? In other words, can an inferior entity overwhelm a superior one? Hence, O Rāma, in truth there is no mind or finite consciousness. When this truth is clearly understood, that which was falsely imagined as the mind comes to an end. It appeared to be because of imperfect understanding; when this misunderstanding ceases, the mind also ceases to be.

jaḍatvān niḥsvarūpatvāt sarvadaiva mṛtaṁ manaḥ
mṛtena māryate lokaś citreyaṁ maurkhyacakrikā (13/100)

VASIṢṬHA continued:

This mind is inert and not a real entity: hence it is forever dead! Yet, beings in this world are killed by this dead thing: how mysterious is this stupidity!! The mind has no self, no body, no support and no form; yet, by this mind is everything consumed in this world. This is indeed a great mystery. He who says that he is destroyed by the mind which has no substantiality at all, says in effect that his head was smashed by the lotus petal. To say that one can be hurt by the mind which is inert, dumb and blind is like saying that one is roasted by the heat of the full moon. The hero who is able to destroy a real enemy standing in front of him is himself destroyed by this mind which is found to be non-existent when its existence is enquired into. It is indeed strange that this unreal and false non-entity is sought to be strengthened by living beings.

This world conjured up by the non-existent mind is also destroyed by another equally non-existent mind. This illusory world-appearance is none other than the mind. He who is unable to understand the true nature of the mind is also unfit for being instructed in the truth expounded in the scripture. Such a mind is full of fear. It is afraid of the melodious sound of the veena and it is even afraid of a sleeping relative. It is frightened by hearing someone shout aloud and flees that spot. The ignorant man is completely overcome by his own deluded mind.

My teachings are not meant for those, O Rāma, whose intelligence has been silenced by a firm faith in the reality of this illusory world, and the consequent striving for the pleasures of this world. What foolish man will endeavour to show a colourful forest to one who refuses to see? Who will strive to educate that man whose nose has been eaten away by leprosy, in the delicate art of distinguishing different perfumes? Who will instruct the drunkard in the subtleties of metaphysics? Who will make enquiries concerning village affairs from a corpse lying in the crematorium? If a fool does just this, who can dissuade him from such foolish attempts? Even so, who can instruct that ignorant person who finds it difficult to govern the mind which is dumb and blind?

What indeed is the jīva (individual soul) but a word which has befuddled the intelligence of people? Even the finite or individualised consciousness is an unreal fancy: what can it do! Seeing the fate of the ignorant people who are suffering because the mind that they have fancied into existence veils the truth which alone exists, I am filled with pity.

In this world fools are born only to suffer and perish. Every day millions upon millions of mosquitoes are killed by the wind; from the smallest ant to the greatest of divinities, all are subject to birth and death. Every moment countless beings die and countless others are born, totally regardless of whether people like it or not, whether they rejoice or grieve. Hence, it were wiser neither to grieve nor to rejoice over the inevitable.

adṛśyaivā 'tti māṁsāsthirudhirādi śarīrakāt
manobilavilīnaiṣā tṛṣṇa vanaśuni nṛṇāṁ (15/8)

VASIṢṬHA continued:

O Rāma, they who behave like beasts cannot be instructed, for they are being led like animals by the rope of their own mind. Hence, the wise man does not attempt to teach those who have not overcome their own mind and are therefore miserable in every way. On the other hand, the wise do endeavour to remove the sorrow of those who have conquered their mind and who are therefore ripe to undertake self-enquiry.

When objectivity arises in your consciousness, the latter becomes conditioned and limited: that is bondage. When objectivity is abandoned, you become mindless: that is liberation. In the middle between the self as the seer and the world as the seen, you are the seeing (sight): always remain in this realisation. Between the experiencer and the experience you are the experiencing: knowing this remain in self-knowledge.

When, abandoning this self you think of an object, then you become the mind (subject) and thus become the subject of unhappiness. That intelligence which is other than self-knowledge is what constitutes the mind: that is the root of sorrow. When it is realised that all this is but the self, there is no mind, no subject, no object and no thinking. When you think 'I am the jīva' etc. the mind arises, and with it sorrow. When you know 'I am the self; the jīva and such other things do not exist', the mind ceases to be and there is supreme bliss.

When the self, self-forgetfully, identifies itself with the objects seen and experienced and is thus impurified, there arises the poison of craving. This craving intensifies delusion. Whatever terrible sufferings and calamities there are in the world are all the fruits of cravings, O Rāma. **Remaining unseen and subtle, this craving is yet able to consume the very flesh, bone and blood of the body.** In a moment it seems to subside, the next moment it is in an expanded state.

When this craving has ceased, one's life-force is pure and all divine qualities and virtues enter one's heart. The river of craving flows only in the heart of the unwise person. Even as an animal falls into a trap (a blind well) on account of its craving for food (the bait), a man following the trail of his craving falls into hell. Craving makes one cringe, yet it is on account of craving that the sun shines on earth, the wind blows, the mountains stand and the earth upholds living beings; all the three worlds exist only on account of craving. All the beings in the three worlds are bound by the rope of craving, hard to break. Therefore, O Rāma, give up craving by giving up thinking or conceptualisation. The mind cannot exist without thinking or conceptualisation. First let the images of 'I', 'you' and 'this', not arise in the mind, for it is because of these images that hopes and expectations come into being. Ego-sense is the source of all sins. Cut at the very root of this ego sense with the sword of wisdom of the non-ego. Be free from fear.

sarvatra vāsanātyāgo rāma rājīvalocana
dvividhaḥ kathyate tajjñair jñeyo dhyeyaś ca mānada (6)

RĀMA said:

Lord, you instruct me to abandon the ego-sense and the craving that it gives rise to. If I abandon the ego-sense, then surely I should also give up this body and all that is based on the ego-sense. For, the body and the life-force rest on the support of the ego-sense. When the root (the ego-sense) is cut, then the tree (the body, etc.) will fall. How is it possible for me to abandon the ego-sense and yet live?

VASIṢṬHA replied:

Rāma! The abandonment of all notions, conditioning and conceptualisation is said to be of two kinds: one is based on knowledge or direct realisation and the other is based on contemplation. I shall describe them to you in detail.

One should become aware of one's deluded notion in which one thinks 'I belong to these objects of the world and my life depends upon them. I cannot live without them and they cannot exist without me, either.' Then by profound enquiry, one contemplates 'I do not belong to these objects, nor do these objects belong to me.' Thus abandoning the ego-sense through intense contemplation, one should playfully engage oneself in the actions that happen naturally, but with the heart and mind ever cool and tranquil. Such an abandonment of the ego-sense and the conditioning is known as the contemplative egolessness.

When there is knowledge or direct experience of the non-dual truth, one abandons the ego-sense and conditioning and entertains no feeling of 'This is mine' even with regard to the body. This is known as direct realisation of egolessness.

He is liberated even while living who playfully abandons the ego-sense through the contemplative method. He who uproots this ego-sense completely by the direct experience is established in equanimity; he is liberated. Janaka and others like him follow the contemplative method. Others who have the direct experience of egolessness are one with Brahman and have risen beyond body consciousness. However, both of them are liberated and both have become one with Brahman.

He is considered a liberated sage who is not swayed by the desirable and the undesirable, who lives in this world and functions though inwardly totally untouched by the world, as if in deep sleep.

(As the sage Vasiṣṭha said this, another day came to an end. The assembly dispersed.)

bhāvādvaitam upāśritya sattādvaitamayātmakaḥ
karmādvaitamanādṛtya dvaitādvaitamayo bhava (17-29)

VASIṢṬHA continued:

The desire that arises in the course of one's natural functions devoid of craving is that of a liberated sage. But that desire which is bound up with craving for external objects is conducive to bondage. However, when all ego based notions have ceased in one's heart, the attention that is directed naturally is also the nature of the liberated sage. That which is afflicted by contact with external objects is the craving conducive to bondage; the non-volitional desire which is unaffected by any object is liberation. That desire which existed even before contact with the objects, exists even now and for ever: it is natural, therefore sorrowless and free from impurity. Such a desire is regarded by the wise as free from bondage.

'I want this to be mine.' When such a craving arises in one's heart, it gives rise to impurity. Such a craving should be abandoned by a wise person by all means at all times. Give up the desire that tends to bondage and the desire for liberation too. Remain still like the ocean. Knowing that the self is free from old age and death, let not these disturb your mind. When the whole universe is realised as illusory, craving loses its meaning.

The following four types of feelings arise in the heart of man: (1) I am the body born of my parents, (2) I am the subtle atomic principle, different from the body, (3) I am the eternal principle in all the diverse perishable objects in the world, and (4) the 'I' as also the 'world' are pure void like space. Of these the first is conducive to bondage and the others to freedom.

Once the realisation that 'I am the self of all' has arisen, one does not again fall into error or sorrow. It is this self alone which is variously described as the void, nature, Māyā, Brahman, consciousness, Śiva, Puruṣa, etc. That alone is ever real; there is naught else. **Resort to the understanding of non-duality, for the truth is non-dual; however, action involves duality and hence functions in apparent duality — thus, let your nature partake of both duality and non-duality.** The reality is neither duality (for it is the mind that creates division) nor unity (for the concept of unity arises from its antithesis of duality). When these concepts cease, the infinite consciousness alone is realised to be the sole reality.

The liberated sage who is disinterested in the events of the past, present and future looks at the state of the world with amusement. We are unable to expound the philosophy of the fools who have not controlled their own minds and who are immersed in the mire of sense-pleasure. They are only interested in sexual pleasures and in the acquisition of material wealth. We are also unable to expound the path of rituals and routines which bestows all kinds of rewards in the shape of pain and pleasure.

madhyasthadṛṣṭayaḥ svasthā yathāprāptārtha darśinaḥ
tajjñāstu preṣakā eva sākṣidharme vyavasthitāḥ (20/40)

VASIṢṬHA continued:

O Rāma, in this connection there is an ancient legend which I shall narrate to you.

In the continent known as Jambūdvīpa, on the bank of the river Vyoma Gaṅgā, there lived a holy man named Dīrghatapā who had two sons named Puṇya and Pāvana. Puṇya had reached full enlightenment, but Pāvana, though he had overcome ignorance, had not yet reached full enlightenment and hence he had semi-wisdom. With the inexorable passage of invisible and intangible time, the sage Dīrghatapā abandoned the body and reached the state of utter purity. Using the yogic method she had learnt from him, his wife too followed him. At this sudden departure of the parents, Pāvana was sunk in grief and wailed aloud inconsolably. Puṇya, on the other hand, performed the funeral ceremonies but remained unmoved by the bereavement. He approached his grieving brother, Pāvana.

PUṆYA said: Brother, why do you bring this dreadful sorrow upon yourself? The blindness of ignorance alone is the cause of this torrential downpour of tears from your eyes. Our father has departed from here along with our mother to that state of liberation or the highest state, which is natural to all beings and is the very being of those who have overcome the self. You have ignorantly bound yourself to the notions of 'father' and 'mother'; and yet you grieve for those who are liberated from such ignorance!

Brother, enquire within yourself — this body is inert and is composed of blood, flesh, bones, etc.; what is the 'I' in it? If you thus enquire into the truth, you will realise that there is nothing which is 'you' nor anything which is 'I'. What is called Puṇya or Pāvana is but a false notion. However, if you still think 'I am', then in the incarnations past you have had very many relatives. Why do you not grieve for their death? You had many swan-relatives when you were a swan, many tree-relatives when you were a tree, many lion-relatives when you were a lion, many fish-relatives when you were a fish. Why do you not weep for them? You were a prince, you were a donkey, you were a peepul tree and then a banyan tree. You were a brāhmaṇa, you were a fly and also a mosquito, you were an ant. You were a scorpion for half a year, you were a bear, and now you are my brother. In these many other embodiments you have taken birth again and again countless times.

Even so, I have had very many embodiments. I see them all, and your embodiments too, through my subtle intelligence which is pure and clear-visioned. I was a bird, a crane, a frog, a tree, a camel, a king, a tiger — and now I am your elder brother. In all these embodiments there were countless relatives. Whom shall I mourn? Considering this, I do not grieve. Abandon the notion of the world which arises in your mind as the 'I'. You have no unhappiness, no birth, no father, no mother: you are the self and naught else. **The sages perceive the middle path, they see what is at the moment, they are at peace, they are established in witness consciousness.**

Thus instructed by his brother, Pāvana was awakened. Both of them remained as enlightened beings, endowed with wisdom and direct realisation.

tameva bhukttavirasaṁ vyāpāraugham punaḥ punaḥ
divase divase kurvan prājñaḥ kasmānna lajjate (22/33)

VASIṢṬHA continued:

Craving is the root of all sorrow, O Rāma: and the only intelligent way is to renounce all cravings completely and not to indulge in them. O Rāma this indeed is the Brahman-state — pure, free from craving and from illness. The mind attains fulfilment only by utter dispassion, not by filling it with desires and hopes. To those who are devoid of any attachment or craving, the three worlds are as wide as the footprint of a calf and a whole world-cycle is but a moment. Hence, for restoring peace to the mind, remove the disturbing cause — which is hope or craving.

Or, O Rāma, bring about a transmutation of the mind even as king Bali did. I shall narrate to you the story of Bali.

The demon-king Bali, son of Virocana, ruled over Pātāla region. The Lord of the universe, Śrī Hari, himself was the protector of this king; hence, even the king of heaven, Indra, adored him. By the heat of the very radiance of this king Bali, the oceans got dried up, as it were. His eyes were so powerful that by a mere look he could move mountains. Bali ruled for a very long time over the nether world.

In course of time, intense dispassion overcame king Bali and he began to enquire thus: "How long should I rule over this nether world; how long shall I wander in the three worlds? What shall I gain by ruling over this kingdom? When all that is in the three worlds is subject to destruction, how can one hope to enjoy happiness through all this?

"Again and again, **the same disgusting pleasures are experienced and the same acts are repeated day after day in this world: how is it that even a wise man is not ashamed of this?** The same day and the same night, again and again, life in this world revolves like a whirlpool. Doing all this every day, how can one reach that state in which there is cessation of this repetitive existence? How long should we continue to revolve in this whirlpool, and of what use is it?"

While he was thus reflecting he remembered:

Ah I remember what my father Virocana once told me. I had asked him: "Father, what is the destination of this world-appearance or repetitive existence? When will it come to an end? When will the delusion of the mind cease? Gaining what shall one attain total satisfaction, seeing what shall one seek naught else? I see that it is impossible to attain this by means of experience of the worldly pleasures or actions. For they only aggravate the delusion! Pray, tell me the means by which I shall rest forever in supreme peace."

eka evā 'sti sumahāms tatra rājā mahādyutiḥ
sarvakṛt sarvagaḥ sarvaḥ sa ca tūṣṇīm vyavasthitaḥ (6)

VIROCANA said to Bali:

My son, there is a vast realm wide enough to engulf the three worlds. In it there are no lakes, no oceans, no mountains, no forests, no rivers, no earth, no sky, no winds, no moon, no gods, no demons, no demi-gods, no vegetation, no heaven, no high and low, no words; not me, nor the gods like Viṣṇu. **Only one is there, and that is the supreme light. He is omnipotent, omnipresent, he is all — and he remains silent, as if inactive.** Prompted by him (the king) his minister does everything — what has not been he brings about and what is, he alters. This minister is incapable of enjoying anything; he does not know anything: though ignorant and insentient he does everything for the sake of his master, the king. The king remains alone, established in peace.

BALI asked:

Father, what is that realm which is free from psychosomatic illnesses? Who is that minister and who is that king? The story is wonderful and unheard of. Kindly explain all this to me in detail.

VIROCANA replied:

All the gods and demons put together and even a force many times their strength cannot even challenge the minister. He is not Indra the king of the gods, nor the god of death, nor the god of wealth, nor a god, nor a demon whom you can easily conquer. Though it is believed that the god Viṣṇu killed the demons, it was indeed this minister who destroyed them. In fact, even the gods like Viṣṇu were overpowered by him and made to take birth here. Cupid derives his power from this minister. Anger derives its power from him, too. It is because of his wish that there is unceasing conflict between good and evil here.

This minister can only be defeated by his own master, the king; by no-one else. When in due course of time there arises such a wish in the heart of the king, this minister can be easily defeated. He is the most powerful in all the three worlds; and the three worlds are but his exhalation! If you have the ability to conquer him, then indeed, you are a hero.

When the minister arises the three worlds are manifested, even as the lotus blossoms when the sun rises. When he retires, the three worlds become dormant. If you can conquer him, with your mind utterly one-pointed and completely free of delusion and ignorance, then you are a hero. If he is conquered, then all the worlds and everything in them are conquered. If he is not conquered, then nothing is conquered, even if you think you have conquered this or that in this world.

Hence, my son, in order to attain absolute perfection and eternal bliss, strive with all your might and in every possible manner, whatever be the difficulties and obstacles, to conquer that minister.

viṣayān prati bhoḥ putra sarvāneva hi sarvathā
ạnāsthā paramā hyeṣā sā yukttir manaso jaye (17)

BALI asked:

Father, by what effective means can that powerful minister be conquered?

VIROCANA replied:

Though this minister is almost invincible, my son, I shall tell you how to conquer him. He is overcome in a moment if one grasps him by means of intelligent action; in the absence of such intelligent action, he burns everything like a venomous snake. One who approaches him intelligently, plays with him as one plays with a child and playfully subdues him; such a one beholds the king and is established in the supreme state. For, once the king is seen, the minister comes completely under one's control; and when the minister is under one's control, the king is seen clearly. Until the king is seen, the minister is not really conquered; and until the minister is conquered, the king is not seen! When the king is not seen the minister plays havoc and spreads sorrow; when the minister is not conquered the king remains unseen. Therefore, one's intelligent practice has to be simultaneously two-fold: to behold the king and to subdue the minister. By intense self-effort and steady practice you can gain both these, and then you will enter that region and never again experience sorrow. That is the region inhabited by holy men who are forever established in peace.

My son I shall now make all this explicit to you! The region I have referred to is the state of liberation, which is the end of all sorrow. The king there is the self who transcends all other realms and states of consciousness. The minister is the mind. It is the mind that has made all this world, as pots from clay. When the mind is conquered, everything is conquered. Remember that the mind is almost invincible, except through intelligent practice.

BALI asked:

Father, kindly tell me what intelligent practice will enable me to conquer the mind.

VIROCANA replied:

The very best intelligent means by which the mind can be subdued is complete freedom from desire, hope or expectation in regard to all objects at all times. It is by this means that this powerful elephant (the mind) can be subdued. This means is both very easy and extremely difficult, my son; it is very difficult for one who does not engage himself in serious practice, but very easy for one who is earnest in his effort. Just as there is no harvest without sowing, the mind is not subdued without persistent practice. Hence, take up this practice of renunciation. Until one turns away from sense-pleasure here, one will continue to roam in this world of sorrow. Even a strong man will not reach his destination if he does not move towards it. No one can reach the state of total dispassion without persistent practice.

avaśyaṁ bhavitavyākhyā sveha yā niyatikriyā
ucyate daivaśabdena sā naraireva netaraiḥ (27)

VIROCANA continued:

Only by right exertion can dispassion be attained; there is no other means. People talk of divine grace or fate; but in this world we perceive the body, not a god. **When people speak of god they imply what is inevitable; what is beyond their control and the events of natural order.** Even so, whatever brings about total equanimity and the cessation of joy and sorrow is also referred to as divine grace. Divine grace, natural order and right self-exertion all refer to the same truth; the distinction is due to wrong perception or illusion.

Whatever the mind conceives of through right self-exertion comes to be in its fruition, and when the mind apprehends such fruition there is experience of joy etc. The mind is the doer, and whatever it conceives of, the natural order (niyati) creates and manifests. The mind is also able to run counter to the natural order; hence it may even be said that mind is the prompter of the natural order.

Even as wind moves in space, the jīva (the individual) functions in this world, doing what has to be done within the natural order though such action appears to be selfish or egotistic. Prompted by nature, he seems to move or stand still — both of which are mere expressions or false superimpositions, even as the movement of trees on a mountain-top makes it look as if the peak is swaying.

Hence, as long as there is mind there is neither god nor a natural order; when the mind has ceased to be, let there be whatever is!

BALI asked:

Lord, tell me how the cessation of craving for pleasure can be firmly established in my heart.

VIROCANA said:

My son, self-knowledge is the creeper that yields the fruit of cessation of craving for pleasure. It is only when the self is seen that the highest form of dispassion becomes firmly rooted in the heart. Hence, one should simultaneously behold the self through intelligent enquiry, and thereby get rid of the craving for pleasure.

When he intelligence is still unawakened one should fill two quarters of the mind with enjoyment of pleasure, one part with study of scriptures and the other with service of the guru. When it is partially awakened, two parts are given over to the service of the guru and the others get one part each. When it is fully awakened, two parts are devoted to service of the guru and the other two to the study of scriptures, with dispassion as the constant companion.

deśakrameṇa dhanam alpavigarhaṇena
tenā 'ṅga sādhujanamarjaya mānapūrvaṁ
tatsaṅgamottha viṣayādyavahelaṇena
saṁyag vicāravibhavena tavā ''tmalābhaḥ (51)

VIROCANA continued:

Only when one is filled with goodness is one qualified to listen to the exposition of the highest wisdom. Hence, one should constantly endeavour to educate the mind with purifying knowledge and nourish it with the inner transformation brought about by the study of scriptures. When the mind has thus been transformed, it is able to reflect the truth without distortion. Then without delay one should endeavour to see the self. These two — self-realisation and cessation of craving — should proceed hand in hand, simultaneously.

True dispassion does not arise in one by austerity, charity, pilgrimage, etc., but cnly by directly perceiving one's own nature. There is no means for direct self-realisation except right self-exertion, hence one should give up dependence upon a god or fate, and by right self-exertion firmly reject the seeking of pleasure. When dispassion matures, the spirit of enquiry arises in oneself. The spirit of enquiry strengthens dispassion; the two are interdependent, even as the ocean and the clouds are. These two and also self-realisation are all intimate friends and always exist together.

Hence, first of all one should abandon all dependence on extraneous factors (like god) and, grinding one's teeth with intense self-exertion, cultivate dispassion. One may, however, earn wealth without violating local traditions and customs and without defying one's relatives, etc. One should utilize this wealth to acquire the company of good and holy men endowed with noble qualities. Such company of holy men generates dispassion. Then there arises the spirit of enquiry, knowledge and the study of scriptures. By stages, one reaches the supreme truth.

My son, when you turn completely away from the pursuit of pleasure you attain to the supreme state through the means of enquiry. When the self is completely purified you will be firmly established in the supreme peace. You will never again fall into the mire of conceptualisation, which is the cause of sorrow. Though you continue to live you will remain freed from all hopes and expectations. You are pure! Salutations to you, O embodiment of auspiciousness!!

In accordance with the prevailing social tradition, acquire a little wealth; and with that acquire the company of saints, and adore them. By their company you will gain contempt for the objects of pleasure. And by right enquiry you will gain self-knowledge.

bhavyo 'si cettadetasmāt sarvamāpnoṣi niścayāt
no cettad bahvapi prokttaṁ tvayi bhasmani hūyate (26/12)

VASIṢṬHA continued:

Bali said to himself: "Luckily, I remembered all that my father said to me. Now that craving for pleasure has ceased in me, I shall give up everything and with my mind completely withdrawn from the pursuit of pleasure, I shall remain happily established in the self. This universe is but the creation of the mind: what is lost by abandoning it?" Having thus resolved, Bali contemplated the guru of the demons, Śukra. On account of the infinite consciousness he was established in, Śukra was omnipresent and knew that his disciple needed his presence. Instantly he materialised his body in front of king Bali.

BALI asked Śukra: Lord, it is the reflection of your own divine radiance that prompts me to place this problem before you. I have no desire for pleasure and I wish to learn the truth. Whom am I? Who are you? What is this world? Please tell me all this!

ŚUKRA replied: I am on my way to another realm, O Bali: but I shall give you in a few words the very quintessence of wisdom. Consciousness alone exists, consciousness alone is all this, all this is filled with consciousness. I, you and all this world, are but consciousness. **If you are humble and sincere you will gain everything from what I have said; if not, an attempt at further explanation will be like pouring oblations into a heap of ashes.**

After Śukra left, BALI reflected thus: What my preceptor said to me was indeed correct and appropriate. Surely, all that is is consciousness and there is naught else. If consciousness did not recognise a mountain, would it exist as a mountain? Consciousness itself is all this. It is indeed on account of that consciousness that I am able to come into contact with the objects and experience them, not because of the body itself. Since consciousness exists one without a second, who is my friend and who is my enemy? Even hate and other such qualities are but modifications of consciousness. Hence, again, there is neither hate nor attachment, neither mind nor its modifications — since the consciousness is infinite and absolutely pure, how can perversions arise in it. Consciousness is not its name, it is but a word! It has no name. I am the eternal subject free from all object and predicate. I am that consciousness in which the craving for experience has ceased. Movement of energy in one substance is neither loss nor gain. When consciousness alone is everything, thoughts or its expansions do not make that consciousness expand or contract. Hence, I shall continue to be active till I reach absolute quiescence in the self.

Having thus reflected, Bali, uttering the sacred word OM and contemplating its subtle significance, remained quiet. Freed from all doubts, from perception of objects and without division between thinker, thought and thinking (meditator, meditation and the object of meditation), with all intentions and concepts quietened, Bali remained firmly established in the supreme state with a mind in which all movement of thought had ceased, like a lamp in a windless place. Thus he lived for a considerable time.

na kiñcidapi kartavyaṁ yadi nāma mayā 'dhunā
tat kasmānna karomīdaṁ kiñcit prakṛtakarma vai (29/18)

VASIṢṬHA continued:

All the demons (followers or subjects of the king Bali) rushed to the palace and surrounded the king, who was seated in deep contemplation. Unable to understand the mystery, they thought of their preceptor, Śukra. They beheld Śukra in front of them. ŚUKRA saw that Bali was in a superconscious state. He said to the demons, with a smile radiating joy:

It is indeed wonderful, O demons, that this king Bali has attained such perfection by dint of his own resolute enquiry. Let him remain established in his own self. The mental activity that gives rise to the perception of the world has ceased in him: hence do not try to talk to him. When the dark night of ignorance comes to an end the sun of self-knowledge arises. Such is his state now. In course of time he himself will come out of that state when the seed of world-perception begins to sprout in his consciousness. Hence, go about doing your work as before. He will return to world-consciousness in a thousand years from now.

VASIṢṬHA continued:

Hearing this the demons returned to their posts of duty and carried on the work of the realm. After a thousand celestial years of such contemplation, king Bali was awakened by the music of the celestials and divinities. A supernatural light that radiated from him illumined the entire city.

Even before the demons could reach him again, BALI reflected thus:

It was indeed a wondrous state in which I remained for a brief moment. I shall continue to remain in that state. What have I to do with the affairs of the external world? Supreme peace and bliss reign in my own heart now. (In the meantime, the demons rushed to where he sat. After looking at them, BALI continued to reflect thus:)

I am consciousness and in me there does not exist any perversion. What is there for me to acquire or to abandon? What fun! I long for liberation, but who has bound me, when and how! Why do I long for liberation then? There is no bondage and no liberation. What shall I gain by meditation or by not meditating? Freed from delusion of meditation and non-meditation, let be what has to be: there is neither gain nor loss to me. I do not desire either meditation or non-meditation, neither joy nor non-joy, I do not desire the supreme being or the world. I am neither alive nor dead, I am neither real nor unreal. Salutations to myself, the infinite being! Let this world be my kingdom, I shall be what I am; let this world be not my kingdom, I shall be what I am. What have I to do with meditation and what have I to do with the kingdom? Let be what has to be. I belong to none and none belongs to me. **There is absolutely nothing that has to be done by what is known as me; then why should I not do that action which is natural?**

Having thus reflected, the king Bali turned his radiant gaze towards the assembled demons, as the sun gazes upon a lotus.

yeṣu yeṣu pradeśeṣu mano majjati bālavat
tebhyas tebhyaḥ samāhṛtya taddhi tattve niyojayet (29/54)

VASIṢṬHA continued:

King Bali thereafter ruled the kingdom, doing everything spontaneously without premeditation. He worshipped the brāhmaṇā, gods and the holy ones. He treated his relatives with deference. He rewarded his servants amply and gave in charity more than what they who sought it had expected. He fondly sported with the womenfolk.

Thus have I told you the story of king Bali, O Rāma. Gain such a vision as he had and enjoy supreme felicity. You are the light of consciousness, O Rāma; in you are the worlds rooted. Who is your friend and who is other? You are the infinite. In you are all the worlds strung like beads of a rosary. That being which thou art is neither born nor does he die. The self is real; birth and death are imaginary. Enquire into the nature of all the illnesses that beset life and live without craving. You are the light and the Lord, Rāma, and this world appears to be in that light. It has no real and independent existence. Formerly, you had repeatedly entertained the wrong notions of the desirable and the undesirable: give up these too. Then you will enjoy equanimity, and the wheel of birth will come to a halt. **In whatever the mind tends to sink, retrieve it from it and direct it towards the truth.** Thus will the wild elephant of the mind be tamed.

O Rāma, I shall narrate to you another story which illustrates the path to enlightenment which is free from obstacles. In the nether world there was a mighty demon-king known as Hiraṇyakaśipu. He had wrested the sovereignty of the three worlds from Indra (Hari?). He ruled the three worlds. He had many sons. Among them was the famous Prahlāda who shone like a brilliant diamond among jewels.

The demon-king, who thus enjoyed the lordship of the three worlds, the blessing of a mighty army and good children, became proud and arrogant. His aggressive ways and his rule of terror greatly worried the gods. In answer to their prayer, the lord Hari assumed the form of Narasiṁha and destroyed the demon-king and his family.

PRAHLĀDA, whose life had been spared, mused:

Who is there to help us now? The very seeds of the demon families have been destroyed by Hari. The gods, who used to bow down humbly to the feet of my father, have occupied our realm. My own relatives, the demons, who were strong and powerful once, are weak and timid. The gods have taken back the wish-fulfilling tree. Even as the demons delighted to look at the faces of the goddesses before, the gods delight to look at the demonesses now. The demi-goddesses and others who enjoyed life in the inner apartments of the demons have escaped and gone away to the forests of the mount Meru and live like birds of the forest. My own mothers (the queens) are the very images of grief. Alas, my father's fan serves Indra now. By the grace of Hari, we have been subjected to incomparable and inexpressible adversity, the very thought of which makes us miserable and desperate.

avisṇuh pūjayan visṇum na pūjāphalabhāgbhavet
visṇurbhūtvā yajed visṇumayam visṇuraham sthitah (31/40)

PRAHLĀDA continued to muse:

It is Viṣṇu that protects the whole universe and upholds it. He alone is the refuge of all beings in this world, therefore by all means one should take refuge in him — there is no other way. From this very moment I shall also be devoted to Viṣṇu and live as if filled with his presence.

However, one who is not Viṣṇu does not derive any benefit by worshipping Viṣṇu. One should worship Viṣṇu by being Viṣṇu. Hence I am Viṣṇu. He who is known as Prahlāda is none other than Viṣṇu: there is no duality. Who can be my enemy and who can challenge me now? Since I am Viṣṇu, he who is hostile to me has surely reached the end of his life-span. These demons who stand in front of me find it difficult or impossible to endure the dazzling brilliance that radiates from me. And those gods are really singing my own praises, as I am Viṣṇu. He am I and I salute him.

VASIṢṬHA continued:

Having thus transfigured himself into the very image of Viṣṇu, Prahlāda mentally worshipped Viṣṇu with all the materials ordained by tradition and scriptural injunctions. After this he also worshipped Viṣṇu with external rites and rituals. Upon completion of this worship, Prahlāda rejoiced. From that time, Prahlāda worshipped Viṣṇu in that manner every day. Seeing him and following his example, all the demons in the kingdom also became staunch devotees of Viṣṇu. The gods in heaven were bewildered. They approached Viṣṇu and asked him.

THE GODS said:

Lord, what is this mystery? The demons are your traditional enemies. That they should turn into your devotees appears to be unreal and a trick. Where is the diabolical nature of the demons; and where is devotion to you which arises only during the last incarnation of a jīva? Surely, the qualities of a being are always in accordance with the fundamental nature of that being. To hear that these demons have become your devotees overnight is almost painful. If it were said that they had gradually evolved into higher states of being, cultivated good qualities and then become your devotees, we could very well understand it. But that someone who has been of wicked disposition has all at once become your devotee, is incredible.

THE LORD replied:

O gods, do not suffer doubt and despair. Prahlāda has become my devotee. This is indeed his last birth and he deserves to be liberated now. The seeds of his ignorance have been burnt; he will not be born anymore. It is meaningless and painful to hear that a good man has become evil minded. It is appropriate and good to hear that one who has had no good qualities has become good. Prahlāda's change is for your good.

tribhuvanabhavanābhirāmakośaṁ sakalakalaṅkaharaṁ paraṁ prakāśaṁ aśaraṇaśaraṇaṁ śaraṇyamīśaṁ harimajamacyutamīśvaraṁ prapadye (33/19)

VASIṢṬHA continued:

After thus reassuring the gods, Viṣṇu disappeared and the gods became friendly towards Prahlāda.

Every day Prahlāda thus worshipped the lord Viṣṇu by thought, word and deed. As the immediate fruit of such worship, all the noble qualities like wisdom and dispassion grew in him. Lord Viṣṇu went to where Prahlāda was worshipping him. Seeing that lord Viṣṇu himself had come to the palace,

PRAHLĀDA prayed: **I take refuge in the Lord in whom the three worlds rejoice, who is the supreme light which destroys the darkness of every kind of ignorance and impurity, who is the refuge of the helpless destitute, who alone is the Lord whose refuge is worth seeking, the unborn, the surest security.** You are radiant like the blue lotus or the blue jewel, your body is blue like the zenith of the clear winter sky — I take refuge in you.

THE LORD said: O Prahlāda, you are an ocean of good qualities and you are indeed the jewel among the demons. Ask of me any boon of your choice which is conducive to the cessation of the sorrow of birth.

PRAHLĀDA said: Lord, you are the indweller of all beings and you grant the fruition of all our wishes. Pray, grant me that boon which you consider to be limitless and infinite.

THE LORD said: Prahlāda, may you be endowed with the spirit of enquiry till you rest in the infinite Brahman, so that all your delusions might come to an end and you may attain the highest fruit (blessing). (Having said this, the Lord disappeared.)

PRAHLĀDA contemplated: The Lord had commanded "Be continually engaged in enquiry"; hence, I shall engage myself in enquiry into the self. Surely, I am not this world which is outside and which is inert, composed of trees, shrubs and mountains. Nor am I the body which was born on account of the movement of the life-breath, and which seems to live for a very brief moment. I am not sound (word or name or expression) which is apprehended by the inert substance known as the ear, which is but a momentary movement of air and which is devoid of form and devoid of existence. I am not the sense or experience of touch, which is also momentary and which is able to function only on account of the infinite consciousness. Nor am I the sense of taste based on the ever changing and restless tongue ever devoted to its objects. I am not the sense of sight (or form) which too is momentary and which is but a perversion of the understanding of the seer. Nor am I the sense of smell, which is an imaginary creation of the nose and which has an indeterminate form. I am peace beyond thought.

ā idānīṁ smṛtaṁ satyam etattad akhilaṁ mayā
nirvikalpacidābhāsa eṣa ātmā 'smi sarvagaḥ (19)

PRAHLĀDA continued to contemplate:

Ah, I now recollect the truth that I am the self which is omnipresent, in which there is no conceptualisation. It is by that self that all the senses and their experiences are made possible for it is the inner light. It is because of that inner light that these objects acquire their apparent substantiality. It is thanks to that inner light of consciousness, which is utterly free from all modifications, that the sun is hot, the moon is cool, the mountain is heavy and water is liquid. It is the cause of all the effects that manifest as this creation, but it is itself uncaused.

I salute this self which is its own light, free from duality of knower and known, subject and object. In it exist all things of this universe; and into it they enter. When thought of by this consciousness, these things seem to come into being; when thought of as non-existent, they reach their end. Thus, all these infinite objects appear in the limitless space of consciousness. They appear to grow and they appear to diminish, even as a shadow seems to grow and to diminish in the light of the sun.

This self or inner light of consciousness is unknown and unseen: it is attained by those who have purified their heart. But by the holy ones it is seen in the supremely pure cosmic space (dimension) of consciousness. This self exists in an undivided state in the three worlds.

The one self, which is the sole experiencing, is therefore the experiencer in all: hence the self is said to have a thousand hands and a thousand eyes. With this beauteous body of the sun, this self which is 'I' roams the space as also in the body of air. I am woman, I am man, I am the youth, I am the senile old man; and on account of embodiment, I am apparently born here. From the ground of the infinite consciousness I raise trees and plants, being present in them as their very essence. Even as clay in the hands of a playful child, this world-appearance is pervaded by me for my own delight.

This world exists in me, the self or infinite consciousness, even as a reflection seems to exist in a mirror. I am the fragrance in flowers. I am the light in radiance and even in that light I am the experience. Whatever mobile and immobile beings exist in this universe, I am their supreme truth or consciousness free from conceptualisation. I am the very essence in all things in the universe. Just as butter exists in milk and liquidity exists in water, even so as the energy of consciousness I exist in all that exists.

This world appearance of the past, the present and the future exists in the infinite consciousness without the distinction of objectivity. This omnipresent, omnipotent cosmic being is the self which is indicated by the 'I'.

bhāvenā 'bhāvamāśritya bhāvastyajati duḥkhatāṁ
prekṣya bhāvamabhāvena bhāvastyajati duṣṭatāṁ (99)

PRAHLĀDA continued to contemplate:

Truly, it was but the infinite consciousness that existed: how has this finite, limited ego-sense arisen in it, without any justification and support? What has given rise to the delusion which expresses itself in statements like 'This is you' and 'This I am'? What is this body and what is bodilessness, who lives and who is it that dies? Surely, my ancestors were of little understanding in that they abandoned this infinite consciousness and roamed this little earth. What comparison is there between the vision of the infinite and this fearful vanity known as worldly glory, which is full of dreadful desires and cravings? This vision of the infinite consciousness is pure and is of the nature of supreme peace: and it is surely the very best among the visions that are possible in this universe. The sovereignty of the world, as also all things in the three worlds, exists in consciousness: why do people not experience the truth that there is nothing outside of consciousness?

Everything, everywhere and at all times is easily obtained through consciousness, which is omnipresent and undifferentiated. The light that shines in the sun and the moon, the energy that animates the gods, the intrinsic characteristic of the mind and the elements, the qualities and the faculties that exist in nature (like that in space which permits aircraft to move in it) and the infinite variety of manifestations of energy and intelligence are all the expansions and the functions of the one cosmic consciousness, which in itself is undivided and unmodified.

The infinite consciousness simultaneously pervades the three periods of time and experiences the infinite worlds. The consciousness experiences simultaneously what is sweet and what is bitter; it is tranquil and at peace. Because this consciousness is in itself free from all modifications (concepts and percepts), and because it is subtle and experiences all things at the same time, it is ever at peace and homogeneous, even while apparently experiencing the diversity of diverse phenomena.

When the apparently transformed becoming resorts to or rests on that being which has not undergone any modification, the former is freed from sorrow: and when what is is seen by what is not (or by the mind in which there is no movement of thought) that which is abandons its wickedness. When consciousness abandons the perception of the three modes of time, when it is freed from the bondage of objectivity or conceptualisation, it rests in utter tranquillity. It is as if it were unreal, because it is beyond description: hence some people declare that the self does not exist. Whether there is the self (Brahman) or not, that which is not subject to dissolution is the supreme liberation. On account of the modification (thought), this consciousness is apparently veiled and is not realised.

I salute the self! Salutations to myself — the undivided consciousness, the jewel of all the seen and the unseen worlds! You have indeed been reached very soon! You have been touched, you have been gained.

saṁbandhaḥ ko 'stu naḥ kāmair bhāvābhāvairathendriyaiḥ
kena saṁbadhyate vyoma kena saṁbādhyate manaḥ (32)

PRAHLĀDA continued to contemplate:

OM is the one non-dual consciousness devoid of all perversion. Whatever there is in the universe is the one self. In the past, present and in the future, here, there and everywhere, it is ever the same in all apparent modifications.

Utterly fearless and uninhibited, it is this consciousness that brings into manifestation and sustains the infinite variety of beings, from the Creator to the blade of grass. It is ever dynamic and active; yet it is more inactive than a rock and it is more unaffected by such activity than even the space.

It is this self or consciousness that activates the mind even as wind rustles the leaves; it makes the senses function as the rider guides the horse. Though the self is the lord of this body, it is ever engaged in diverse actions as if it is a slave.

This self alone is to be sought, adored and meditated upon. It is by resorting to it that one crosses this world-appearance with its cycle of birth and death and delusion. It is attained in one's own body, without even the need to call upon it: it manifests itself and reveals itself even if it is contemplated for an instant. Though it is the Lord of all and is endowed with all excellences, one who adores it is free from arrogance and pride.

It is not realised by all because not everyone enquires into the truth concerning the self. When it is seen, everything is seen; when it is heard, everything is heard; when it is touched, everything is touched — for the world is because IT is. It is awake even when one sleeps, it goads the unwise into wakefulness, it removes the distress of the suffering and bestows all desired objects. In this creation exists as if it were a jiva (living entity); it appears to enjoy the pleasures; and it seems to expand in the objects of this world.

This self is the emptiness in space. It is the motion in all things moving. It is the light in all things luminous. In all liquids it is taste. It is solidity in earth. It is heat in fire. It is coolness in the moon. It is the very existence of the worlds. Even as all these characteristic qualities exist in the corresponding substances, even so it exists as Lord in the body.

This self is the eternal existence. I, the self, alone am: in me there is no percept or concept. Let the body be subjected to happiness or unhappiness: how is the self affected by it? The self which exceeds or transcends all material existence is not bound by such materiality. **What relationship can exist between us (the self) and the cravings which spring from notions of existence and non-existence and from the senses? Who or what binds the space and by whom is the mind bound?**

stutyā praṇatyā vijñaptyā śamena niyamena ca
labdho 'yaṁ bhagavān ātmā dṛṣṭaścā 'dhigataḥ sphuṭaṁ (49)

PRAHLĀDA continued to contemplate:

Even if the body is cut into a hundred pieces, the self is not injured; even if the pot is pulverised, the space within it is not destroyed. Formerly, there was a mind which consisted of notions of happiness and unhappiness: but now that all such notions have ceased to be, where is my mind? In one who has attained liberation there is none of these. I neither entertain craving for pleasure, nor do I wish to get rid of it. Whatever comes, let it come; whatever goes, let it go. For so long I have been enslaved by the dreaded enemy known as ignorance who robbed me of my wealth of wisdom. But now, by the grace of lord Viṣṇu and through my own excellent self-effort, I have attained that wisdom.

The Lord who is the self has been seen by me by means of singing hymns, salutations, prayer, peace of mind and disciplined living.

The forest of ignorance has numerous anthills inhabited by deadly snakes in the form of sense-cravings, many blind holes known as death, and many forest-fires of sorrow; in it roam the thieves of violence and greed, as also the most deadly enemy of ego-sense. Now I am free of that by the grace of lord Viṣṇu as also by my own self-effort; and my intelligence has been fully awakened. In the light of that awakened intelligence I do not perceive an entity which can be called ego-sense.

Now that the goblin of ego-sense has been laid, I remain at peace within myself. Where is room for delusion, sorrows, hopes, desires and mental distress? Heaven and hell, as also delusions concerning liberation, exist only as long as the ego-sense exists: pictures are painted on canvas, not on empty sky! When the intelligence is free from the cloud of ego-sense and from the thunderstorm of cravings, it shines with the light of self-knowledge.

O self free from the mire of ego-sense, salutations to you. O self in whom the fearsome senses and all-consuming mind have attained quiescence, salutations to you. O self, the sun that dispels the darkness of ignorance in the heart, salutations to you. O self, the promoter of supreme love and the sustainer of all things in the universe, salutations to you.

Even as steel cuts the steel-beam which has been heated, I have subdued the mind with its own purified state. Egolessly, my body functions with its inherent energy. The past tendencies, mental conditioning and limitations have been completely destroyed. I begin to wonder: how was it that for such a long time I was caught up in the trap of the ego-sense! Freed from dependency, from habits of thought, from desires and cravings, from deluded belief in the existence of the ego, from the colouring of pleasure-seeking tendency and from revelry — my mind has reached a state of utter quiescence. With this, all sorrow has come to an end and the light of supreme bliss has dawned!

vācyavācakadṛṣṭyaiva bhedo yo 'yamihā ''vayoḥ
asatyā kalpanaiveṣā vicivicyambhasoriva (8)

PRAHLĀDA continued to contemplate:

At last, the self which is beyond all states or modes of consciousness has been realised. O self! I salute you, I embrace you: who but you is my friend and relative in the three worlds? You alone destroy, you alone protect, you give, you praise and you move; now, O self, you have been seen and attained — what will you do now and where will you go? From beginningless time the great wall of ignorance stood between us. Now that that wall has collapsed you are seen to be not distant at all. **O self, the distinction between you (the self) and me is verbal, like the distinction between the word and the substance it refers to; the distinction is unreal and imaginary, like the verbal distinction between the wave and the water in the wave.**

Salutations to the seer, the experiencer. Alas, on account of your identification with the embodiment, you O self had, as it were, forgotten your own nature. Hence, you had to undergo endless suffering in repeated births, experiencing external perceptions without self-knowledge. Now, Lord, you have been seen and reached. Hereafter you will not be deluded again: salutations to you. Lord, how is it that the self, which is the very light of the eyes and which fills the whole body as the innate intelligence, is not seen or experienced? How can that intelligence be distant from oneself — which as the intelligence in the sense of hearing, hears and produces goose-pimples? O self, now that you have been realised, the sense-pleasures that I revelled in before are no longer worthy of my attention!

Salutations to my self which is infinite and egoless: salutations to the formless self. You (self) dwell in 'me' in a state of equilibrium, as pure witness consciousness, without form and without the divisions of space and time. The mind gets agitated, the senses begin to stir and the energy begins to expand, setting in motion the twin-forces of prāṇa and apāna (two modifications of the life-force). Drawn by the power of desires, the driver (mind) carries away the body made up of flesh and blood, bone and skin. However, I am pure consciousness, not dependent upon the body or anything else: let this body rise or fall, in accordance with the desires that move it. In course of time the ego-sense arises and in course of time the ego-sense ceases to be, even as the universe dissolves at the end of the cosmic cycle. But, after a long time of such cyclic (birth and death) existence in this creation, I have attained the state of peace and rest, even as the whole cosmos comes to rest at the end of its own cyclic existence. Salutations to you, myself, who is transcendental and who is all: salutations to all of them that speak of us!

Being the light of the self, I open my eyes, as it were, and the universe comes into being: and I close my eyes and the universe ceases to be. You, O self, are the supreme atom in which the entire universe exists already. O self, you yourself appear in the cosmic space as the infinite variety of objects.

bhavānayamayaṁ cā 'haṁ tvaṁ śabdairevamādibhiḥ
svayamevātmanā ''tmānaṁ lilārthaṁ stauṣi vakṣi ca (56)

PRAHLĀDA continued to contemplate:

Abandon vanity, anger, impurity and violence, for great souls are not overcome by such base qualities. Remember past sorrows again and again, and with a cheerful attitude of mind enquire 'Who am I?' 'How could all this happen?' and be free from all that. O self, you are ever asleep, as it were: you are apparently awakened by your own energy for the purpose of becoming aware of the experiences being undergone. It is in fact that energy that comes into contact with the objects of such experiences: but on account of such awareness, you assume such experiences to yourself.

O self, you are the fragrance in the flower known as the body. Speech terminates in you, O self! It reappears somewhere else. Even as different ornaments are fashioned out of gold, all the countless objects of creation have been fashioned out of you: the distinction is verbal. **'This is you', 'This is I' — such expressions are used when you yourself adore yourself or describe yourself for your own delight.** Even as a huge forest fire momentarily assumes various forms though it is but a single flame, even so your non-dual being appears to be all these diverse objects in this universe. You are the string on which all these worlds are strung. The worlds are for ever potentially present in you: and by you they are made manifest, as the flavour of foodstuff is made manifest by cooking. However, though these worlds seem to exist, they will cease to be if you are not! Happiness and sorrow collapse when they approach you, even as darkness disappears when it approaches light.

Pleasure and pain, happiness and unhappiness owe their existence to you, O self: they are born of you and they lose their identity when their non-existence independent of you is realised. Even as an optical illusion comes into being and vanishes in the twinkling of an eye, the illusory experiences of pain and pleasure appear and disappear in the twinkling of an eye. They appear in the light of awareness and they disappear when they are perceived as non-different from that awareness; they are born the moment they die and they die the moment they are born — who is the perceiver of all this mystery? Everything is thus ever-changing all the time; how then can such momentary causes produce tangible and stable results? O self, you enjoy pleasure and pain as if they were real, while you perceive and receive them through the consciousness of a wise person, without ever abandoning the state of utter equanimity. But, what your experiences are when the same thing happens in the heart of an unwise or unawakened person, it is impossible for me to describe!

Hail, hail to you, O self who has manifested as the limitless universe. Hail to the self which is the supreme peace. Hail to you, O self who is beyond the reach of the scriptures. I am in a state of utter equilibrium and of supreme peace. I have reached self-knowledge. Salutations to myself; salutations to you.

daityodyogena vibudhāstato yajñatapaḥkriyāḥ
tena saṁsārasaṁsthānaṁ na saṁsārakramo 'nyathā (38/16)

VASIṢṬHA continued:

After thus contemplating, Prahlāda entered into the state in which there is no mental modification at all, but where there is supreme bliss, undisturbed by the movement of thought. He sat where he was, like a statue. A thousand years went by. The demons concluded that he was dead. Anarchy prevailed in the netherworld. There was utter disorder and the strong overpowered the weak.

In the meantime the protector of the universe, lord Viṣṇu, saw the state of the nether-world and that Prahlāda was deeply immersed in the transcendental state of consciousness.

LORD VIṢṆU thought:

Since Prahlāda is immersed in the transcendental state of consciousness, the leaderless demons have lost their power. In the absence of a threat from the demons, the gods in heaven have nothing to fear and hence nothing to hate. If they have nothing to fear or hate, they will soon rise to the transcendental state of consciousness and attain liberation! This universe, which ought to exist till the natural cosmic dissolution, will thus abruptly cease to be. I do not see any good in this: hence, I think that the demons should continue to live as demons. **If the demons function as the enemies of the gods, religious and righteous actions shall prevail in this creation: and thus will this creation continue to exist and flourish, not otherwise.**

Viṣṇu approached where Prahlāda was seated and roared aloud "Noble one, wake up!" and blew his conch. The life-force began to vibrate in the crown of Prahlāda's head. Prahlāda was fully awake to his surroundings and gazed upon the Lord.

LORD VIṢṆU said to Prahlāda:

Remember, O Prahlāda, your identity as the ruler of the netherworld. You have nothing whatsoever either to acquire or to reject: arise. You have to remain in this body till the end of this world-cycle: I know this as inevitable, as I know the law of this world-order. Hence, you have to rule this realm here and now, as a sage liberated from all delusion.

He is fit to die who is sunk in ignorance and sorrow. He who grieves, thinking 'I am weak, miserable, stupid' etc., is fit to die. He who is swayed by countless desires and hopes and he whose mind is restless is fit to die. Living is appropriate to one whose mind is well controlled by his self-knowledge and who is aware of the truth. He should live who does not entertain notions of egoism and who is unattached to anything, who is free from likes and dislikes and has a calm mind, whose mind has reached the state of no-mind. He, hearing of whom or listening to whom people experience great joy — life alone is appropriate to him, and not death.

dehasaṁstho 'pyadehatvād adeho 'si videhadṛk
vyomasaṁstho 'pyasakttatvād avyomeva hi mārutaḥ (4)

THE LORD continued:

The functioning or the existence of the body is known as the state of living, according to the people; and the abandonment of the body in order to get another body is known as death. You are free from these notions, O Prahlāda: to you what is death and what is life! I was only using the popular notions to explain myself to you: in truth, you neither live nor die. **Even though you are in the body, since you do not have the body you are bodiless. You are the observer, which is immaterial intelligence: just as, though air exists in space it is not attached to space, and hence it is free from spatial limitation.** Yet, in a manner of speaking, you are the body since you experience sensations through the body, even as, in a manner of speaking, space is responsible for the growth of a plant in as much as space does not arrest such growth.

You are enlightened. What is a body or embodiment to you? It is only in the eyes of the ignorant that even your form exists. At all times you are the all, you are the supreme inner light of consciousness. What is body or bodilessness to you, and what can you hold or abandon? Whether it is springtime or the day of cosmic dissolution, they are nothing to one who has transcended the notions of being and non-being. For in all conditions he is firmly established in self-knowledge. Whether all the beings in the universe live or perish, or they prosper, he remains firmly established in self-knowledge.

The supreme Lord dwells in the body, undying when the body dies and unchanging when the body changes. When you have given up the false notions 'I belong to the body' or 'The body belongs to me', there is no meaning in expressions like 'I shall give it up' or 'I shall not give it up', 'I have done this' and 'I shall do this now'.

Enlightened men, though they be constantly engaged in activity, do nothing. It is not by means of inaction that they reach the state of non-action! This very fact of non-action frees you from experiences, for there is no harvest where there is no sowing. When thus both the notions of 'I do' and 'I experience' have ceased, there remains only peace; when that peace is firmly grounded there is liberation.

To such an enlightened person, what is there to acquire or to renounce? For it is only when the notions of subject and object have ceased that there is liberation. Such enlightened persons (as you are) live in this world as if they are for ever in a state of deep sleep. Likewise, O Prahlāda, perceive this world as if you are half asleep! Enlightened beings do not exult in pleasure nor grieve in pain; they function non-volitionally, even as a crystal reflects the objects placed near it without intending to do so. They are fully awake in self-knowledge, but they are asleep, as it were, in relation to the world; they function in this world like children, without ego-sense and all the rest of its retinue. O Prahlāda, you have reached the plane of Viṣṇu; rule the netherworld for a world-cycle.

idaṁ sukhamidaṁ duḥkhamidaṁ nā 'stidamasti me
iti dolāyitaṁ ceto mūḍhameva na paṇḍitaṁ (12)

PRAHLĀDA said:

Lord, I was really overcome by fatigue and I took rest for a brief moment. By your grace, I have attained to the realisation in which there is no distinction between contemplation and non-contemplation. You were seen by me for a long time within myself: luckily, you are now seen in front of me. I have experienced the truth of the infinite consciousness within myself, in which there is no sorrow, no delusion, no concern with dispassion, no desire to abandon the body and no fear of this world-appearance. When the one single reality is known, where is sorrow, where is destruction, what is body, what is world appearance, what is fear or its absence? I was in that state of consciousness which spontaneously arose in me.

'Oh I am disgusted with this world and I shall abandon it' — such thoughts arise only in the ignorant. Only the ignorant think that there is sorrow when there is body and that there is no sorrow once the body is abandoned. **'This is pleasure', 'this is pain', 'this is', 'this is not' — only the mind of the ignorant swings like this, not of the wise.** Notions of 'I' and 'the other' exist only in the minds of the ignorant who have left wisdom far behind. 'This is to be acquired' and 'this is to be abandoned' — such thoughts arise only in the minds of the ignorant. When everything is pervaded by you, where is 'another' which can be acquired or abandoned? The entire universe is pervaded by consciousness. What is to be acquired and what abandoned?

I was naturally enquiring of myself in myself, and rested just for a moment without any notions of being or non-being, of acquisition or rejection. I have attained self-knowledge now and I shall do whatever pleases you. Pray, accept my worshipful adoration.

After receiving Prahlāda's worship, LORD VIṢṆU said to him:

Arise, O Prahlāda. I shall presently anoint you king of the netherworld while the gods and the sages who are here sing your glories. (After thus crowning him king of the netherworld, he continued:) Be thou ruler of the netherworld as long as the sun and the moon shine. Protect this realm without being swayed by desire, fear or hate, and looking upon all with equal vision. Enjoy the royal pleasures and may all prosperity attend you; but act in such a way that neither gods in heaven nor the humans on earth are unduly agitated or worried. Engage yourself in appropriate action, without being swayed by thoughts and motives. Thus will you not be bound by actions. O Prahlāda, you know everything already; what need have you to be instructed? From now the gods and demons will live in friendship; the goddesses and the demonesses will live in harmony. O king, keep ignorance at a great distance from you and live an enlightened life, ruling this world for a very long time to come.

ārādhayā ''tmanā ''tmānamātmanā ''tmānamarcaya
ātmanā ''tmānamālokya saṁtiṣṭhasvā ''tmanā ''tmani (43/19)

VASIṢṬHA continued:

Having said thus, lord Viṣṇu left the realm of the demons. By the grace and with the blessings of the Lord, the gods in heaven, the demons in the netherworld and the humans on earth lived happily, without distress.

RĀMA asked: How was it, O Lord, that Prahlāda, who was in the highest state of non-dual consciousness, was awakened by the conch-sound?

VASIṢṬHA replied: O Rāma, liberation is of two kinds: 'with body' and 'without body'. That state of liberation in which the mind is totally unattached to anything and in which there is no craving at all, is known as 'liberation with body'. That itself is known as 'liberation without body' when the body drops.

In the case of 'liberation with body', all the tendencies and mental conditioning are like fried seeds incapable of giving rise to future embodiment; but there still remains the conditioning of such purity, expansiveness and self-knowledge, though even this conditioning is unintentional and non-volitional (as in a sleeping person). As long as this trace remains, the sage who is 'liberated with body' can be awakened to world-consciousness even after a hundred years of inward contemplation. Such was the state of Prahlāda and hence he 'awoke' to the sound of the conch.

O Rāma, reach the vision which Prahlāda had and engage yourself in ceaseless enquiry: you will reach the supreme state.

RĀMA asked: Holy sir, you said that Prahlāda attained enlightenment by the grace of Lord Viṣṇu. If everything is achieved by self-effort, why was he not able to attain enlightenment without Viṣṇu's grace.

VASIṢṬHA replied: Surely, whatever Prahlāda attained was through self-effort, O Rāma, not otherwise. Viṣṇu is the self and the self is Viṣṇu: the distinction is verbal. At times one attains self-knowledge through self-enquiry undertaken through self-effort; at times this self-effort manifests as devotion to Viṣṇu who is also the self, and thus one attains enlightenment. Even if one worships Viṣṇu for a long time with great devotion, he does not bestow enlightenment on one who is not wise with self-knowledge. Thus, the foremost means for self-knowledge is self-enquiry; grace and such other factors are secondary means. If you think that lord Viṣṇu can be seen without self-effort, why do the birds and beasts not get uplifted by him? If it is true that the guru can spiritually uplift one without the need for self-effort, then why does a guru not so uplift a camel or a bull?

Hence, **adore the self by the self, worship the self by the self, behold the self by the self, and be firmly established by the self in the self.**

rāmā 'paryavasāneyaṁ māyā saṁsṛtināmikā
ātmacittajayenaiva kṣayamāyāti na 'nyathā (1)

VASIṢṬHA continued:

O Rāma, this cycle of birth and death is an interminable one; this Māyā ceases only by the mastery of one's own heart (mind), not otherwise. To illustrate this there is a legend which I shall presently narrate to you.

In this world there is a region known as Kosala. In it there was a brāhmaṇa known as Gādhi. He was very learned and the very embodiment of dharma. Right from his very childhood he was filled with the spirit of renunciation and dispassion. Once this brāhmaṇa went away to the forest in order to practise austerity. Desiring to behold Viṣṇu he entered the water of a river and there began to recite various mantrā, which soon completely purified his being.

After a period of eight months, LORD VIṢṆU appeared there and said to him: Ask of me the boon of your choice.

The BRĀHMAṆA said: Lord, I wish to behold your own illusory power (Māyā) which deludes all beings and keeps them in ignorance.

LORD VIṢṆU said: You will behold my Māyā and then you will at once abandon the illusory perception of objects.

After Lord Viṣṇu disappeared, Gādhi rose from the water. He was highly pleased. For several days thereafter Gādhi engaged himself in various holy activities, constantly immersed in the bliss which had resulted from his vision of Lord Viṣṇu.

One day he went to the river for his bath, still meditating upon the words of lord Viṣṇu. While he was immersed in the water he beheld himself dead and mourned by all. His body had fallen and his face had become pale and lifeless.

He saw himself surrounded by very many relatives who were all weeping and wailing aloud; they were inconsolably grief-stricken. His wife had caught hold of his feet and was shedding tears as if a dam had been breached. His mother, beside herself with grief, had caught hold of his face and was weeping bitter tears and crying aloud. He was surrounded by a number of grief-stricken relatives.

He saw himself lying silent, as if asleep or in deep meditation; he was taking a long rest, as it were. He listened to all the weeping and wailing of the relatives and wondered 'What does all this mean?'; he was curious about the nature of friendship and relationship.

Soon the relatives carried his body away to the crematorium. After the performance of the funeral rites they placed the body on the funeral pyre. They set the pyre alight and soon the body of Gādhi was consumed by the fire.

kiṁ me jīvitaduḥkhena maraṇaṁ me mahotsavaḥ
lokanindyasya durjantor jīvitānmaraṇaṁ varaṁ (46/43)

VASIṢṬHA continued:

O Rāma, Gādhi, who still remained immersed in the river, then saw that he was in the region known as Bhūtamaṇḍalaṁ in the womb of a tribal woman. In course of time he was born as her son. Soon he grew up into a robust young man. He was a good hunter. He got married to a tribeswoman. He became the father of a large family. His children were as violent and wicked as he was. He grew old. He did not die, but one by one he lost all his friends and relatives to death. Disgusted, he left his native realm and wandered away to foreign lands.

One day while thus wandering from one place to another, he entered the kingdom of Kīra which was obviously very rich and prosperous. He saw in front of him a huge royal elephant. The king who ruled over that kingdom had just died without an heir. In accordance with the custom, the royal elephant had been commissioned to find a suitable successor. The elephant picked up the hunter and placed him on its own back. At that very moment people exclaimed in great joy "Long live the king". The elephant had chosen the king. By and by, the very nature of his position taught him the art of ruling the kingdom: he became a well-known king named Gavala. He ruled the kingdom justly and wisely, with compassion and purity. Thus eight years passed. One day he roamed out of his inner apartments alone, and unadorned with regal dress and royal insignia. Outside the palace he saw a group of tribesmen who were singing familiar songs. Quietly he joined them and also began to sing with them. An aged tribesman recognised him and, rising from the crowd, addressed him: "O Kaṭanja! I am delighted to see you." Gavala ignored this, but the ladies of the royal household and the members of the court were shocked by the realisation that their king was an unworthy tribesman. They treated him as if he were a putrid corpse. Even the citizens avoided him and ran away at his very sight.

The leaders of the community held counsel among themselves and began to talk, "Alas, we have been polluted by the touch of this tribesman who lives on the flesh of dogs. There is no expiation for this pollution, other than death. Let us raise a huge pyre and throw our sullied bodies into it and thus purify our souls." Having decided this, they gathered firewood with which they built a huge funeral pyre. One by one they threw themselves into it.

The king Gavala reflected: "Alas, all this was brought about by me! **Why should I continue to live: death is preferable to life. For one who is dishonoured by the people death is better than life.**" Gavala calmly offered his body, too, into the fire. As fire began to consume the limbs of Gavala, Gādhi, who was reciting prayers immersed in the water of the river, regained his consciousness.

(At this stage, evening set in. Another day came to an end.)

manorājyamapi prājñā labhante vyavasāyinaḥ
gādhinā svapnasaṁdṛṣṭaṁ gatvā labdhamakhaṇḍitaṁ (47/37)

VASIṢṬHA continued:

Gādhi wondered "Who am I? What did I see? And how?" He concluded that because he was fatigued his mind had obviously played some tricks on him. He thought, "Surely, all that was illusory, for I do not perceive anything now!"

After some days another brāhmaṇa visited him: and Gādhi duly entertained the honoured guest. During the course of their conversation, Gādhi asked the guest: "Sir, why do you look so tired and worn out?" The guest answered: "Holy one, I shall tell you the truth! There is a kingdom in the north known as Kīra. I heard an extraordinary story there. They said, 'A tribesman ruled this kingdom for eight years. After that his identity became known. On account of him, very many brāhmaṇa of this place perished.' When I heard that, I too felt polluted and hence engaged myself in prolonged fasting. I am breaking this fast only today." The guest spent the night with Gādhi and left the following day.

GĀDHI contemplated further: "That which I saw in an hallucination, my guest saw as a factual event! Ah, I should verify the story for myself." Having thus resolved, Gādhi quickly proceeded first to the place known as Bhūtamaṇḍala. **Men of highly evolved consciousness can, by appropriate self-effort, attain even what they mentally visualise: Gādhi thus saw, after reaching the destination, whatever he had seen in his vision.**

There he saw a village which had been deeply impressed in his consciousness. He saw the very house of the tribesman (himself) and he saw the very objects which were used by him. The house was in a very bad shape. He saw there skeletons of animals whose flesh had been eaten by the family; for some time he saw that dreadful place which looked truly like a cemetery. He went to a nearby village and asked the villagers: "Do you know anything about that tribesman who lived in yonder house?" The villagers replied: "Holy sir, of course we know. There was a dreadful looking and fierce tribesman in that house who lived up to a ripe old age. When he had lost all his kinsmen he went away and become a king of Kīra and ruled for eight years. He was found out and as a result many people died and he too killed himself."

Hearing this, Gādhi was greatly puzzled. He travelled to the Kīra kingdom and enquired of the citizens: "Was this country ruled by a tribesman sometime ago?" They replied enthusiastically, "Oh yes: and he ruled for eight years, having been chosen by the royal elephant! When his identity was discovered, he committed suicide. It was twelve years ago."

Gādhi left the city at once and went to a mountain cave nearby and there performed intense austerity. Soon, lord Viṣṇu appeared before him and asked him to choose any boon he liked. GĀDHI asked the Lord: "The hallucination that I had as in a dream, how is it also seen in the wakeful state?"

tathāhi bahavaḥ svapnamekaṁ paśyanti mānavāḥ
svāpabhramada maireyamada manthara cittavat (49/11)

The LORD said:

O Gādhi! That which you see now is an illusion: it is truly naught but the self, but perceived by the mind which has not been purified and which has not realised the truth. It is the mind alone that is experienced as dream, illusion, illness, etc. In the mind are countless 'events' like flowers on a tree in full bloom. Is it any wonder that the mind which contains countless thought-forms should be able to manifest the idea 'I am a tribesman'? Even so, the same mind manifests other ideas like 'I have a brāhmaṇa-guest who told me the story, etc.' and 'I am going to Bhūtamaṇḍalaṁ' and 'I am in Kīra kingdom now'. All this was but hallucination! Thus, O Holy one, you have seen both forms of illusion: the one which you yourself thought was illusion and the other which you think is reality — both of which are hallucination in truth. You entertained no guest, and you did not go anywhere! All this, too, was but hallucination. You have really not been to Bhūtamaṇḍalaṁ or the Kīra kingdom — all these were also illusions.

O Gādhi, these incidents are reflected in your mind, though they took place unrelated to you, even as there appears to be a coincidental connection between the crow alighting upon a cocoanut tree and a cocoanut falling to the ground. Hence, they narrate the same story which you believe to be yours! Such coincidence is not uncommon: sometimes the same illusion is perceived by many. **Sometimes many people have the same dream: several people experience the same hallucination and many drunkards may all of them simultaneously experience that the world is revolving around them.** Several children play at the same game.

Whatever you saw in the Bhūtamaṇḍalaṁ and Kīra was possibly true. The tribesman known as Kaṭanja was indeed born sometime ago. He lost his kinsmen and became king of Kīra. All this was reflected in your consciousness. Even as the mind sometimes forgets what it actually experienced, it also thinks it has experienced what it has never seen. Just as one sees dreams and visions, one experiences hallucinations even during the wakeful state. Though Kaṭanja lived several years ago it appears to be in the present in your consciousness.

Because you are not fully enlightened your mind clings to the illusion of objective perception. Get up and meditate intensely for ten years.

(Gādhi engaged himself in intense meditation thereafter and attained self-realisation.)

vartamānamanāyāsaṁ bhajad bāhyadhiyā kṣaṇaṁ
bhūtaṁ bhaviṣyadabhajad yāti cittamacittatāṁ (16)

VASIṢṬHA continued:

This cosmic illusion (Māyā) creates great delusion and is of the nature of disequilibrium. It is extremely difficult to understand it. What comparison is there between a hallucination which lasts for the brief duration of an hour's dream, and a whole lifetime as a tribesman with all the varied experiences? Again, how can we relate what is seen in that hallucination and what is seen 'in front of our eyes'? Or, what is truly unreal and what has really undergone a factual transformation? Hence, I tell you, O Rāma, this cosmic illusion leads the unwary mind into endless difficulties.

RĀMA asked: But, O Holy sir, how can one restrain this wheel of cosmic illusion which revolves with such tremendous force?

VASIṢṬHA replied:

O Rāma, the mind is the hub around which this vicious cycle revolves, creating delusion in the minds of the deluded. It is by firmly restraining that hub through intense self-effort and keen intelligence that the whole wheel is brought to a standstill. When the hub's motion is stopped, the wheel does not revolve: when the mind is stilled, illusion ceases. One who does not know this trick and does not practise it, undergoes endless sorrow. The moment the truth is seen, behold! The sorrow comes to an end.

The disease of the perception of this world-illusion is not cured except through the mastery of the mind, which is its only remedy. Hence, O Rāma, abandon all other activities like pilgrimage, gifts and austerities, and bring the mind under your control for your ultimate good. This world-appearance abides in the mind, even as there is space within the pot; if the pot is broken, the illusory division of space vanishes; and if the mind ceases to be, the concept of a world within the mind also ceases to be. Even as an insect trapped within the pot attains freedom of movement when the pot is broken, you will also enjoy freedom when the mind ceases to be, along with the world-illusion contained in it.

Live in the present, with your consciousness externalised momentarily but without any effort: when the mind stops linking itself to the past and to the future it becomes no-mind. If from moment to moment your mind dwells on what is and drops it effortlessly at once, the mind becomes no-mind, full of purity. It is only as long as the mind continues to be agitated that it experiences the diversity of its own projection or expansion, even as rain falls only as long as there are clouds. And, it is only as long as the infinite consciousness limits itself into the finite mind, that such agitation and expansion take place. If consciousness ceases to be the finite mind, then know that the very roots of cyclic world-illusion (of birth and death) are burnt, and there is perfection.

cetanaṁ cittarikttaṁ hi pratyakcetanamucyate
nirmanaskasvabhāvaṁ tanna tatra kalanāmalaḥ (21)

VASIṢṬHA continued:

Consciousness free from the limitations of the mind is known as the inner intelligence: it is the essential nature of no-mind, and therefore it is not tainted by the impurities of concepts and percepts. That is the reality, that is supreme auspiciousness, that is the state known as the supreme self, that is omniscience — and that vision is not had when the wicked mind functions. Where there is mind, there flourish hopes and desires, and there arise the experiences of pain and pleasure. The consciousness which has been awakened to the truth does not fall into concepts and percepts: therefore, even though it seems to undergo various psychological experiences, it does not give rise to the world-illusion and the cycle of world-appearance.

In the case of those who have been awakened through the study of scriptures, company of holy men and unceasing and vigilant practice of truth, their consciousness has reached the pure state of non-objectiveness. Hence, one should forcefully uplift one's mind from the state of ignorance and vacillation and apply it to the study of scriptures and to the company of holy sages.

The self alone is the sole aid for the realisation of the supreme self or the infinite consciousness. It is one's own self that strives to abandon one's own sorrow; and for this the realisation of one's own self by oneself is the only course.

Hence, O Rāma, while yet remaining active in this world (talking, taking and leaving etc.) be without the mind and realise that you are pure consciousness. Abandon notions such as 'This is mine', 'That is he', 'This I am' and be established in the consciousness of undivided oneness. As long as the body lasts, consider the present and the future with an equanimous consciousness. Be forever established in the consciousness of the self in all states — youth, manhood and old age, pleasure and pain, in the waking, dream and sleep states. Abandon the impurity of objective perception, hopes and desires: remain established in self-knowledge. Give up notions of auspicious and inauspicious happenings, give up visions of the desirable and undesirable: know that you are the essence of consciousness. Realise that subject, object and actions do not touch you; remain as pure consciousness without any disturbance in it. Know 'I am the all' and live in the waking state as if in deep sleep. Be freed from conditions known as duality and non-duality, and remain in a state of equilibrium which is a state of pure consciousness and freedom. Realise that this cosmic consciousness is indivisible into 'I' and 'the other' and thus remain firm and unshakable.

bhogābhogatiraskāraiḥ kārśyaṁ neyaṁ śanairmanaḥ
rasāpahārais tajjñena kālenā 'jīrṇaparṇavat (56)

VASIṢṬHA continued:

Cut off all the fetters of desire and hope, solely with the intelligence that is unlimited and endowed with patience and perseverance, and go beyond dharma and adharma. When one is firmly rooted in self-knowledge even the worst of poisons turns into immortalising nectar. It is only when this self-knowledge is overpowered by ignorance that the delusion of world-appearance arises in the mind; but when one is firmly established in self-knowledge — which is infinite, unlimited and unconditioned — the delusion or ignorance that gave rise to world-appearance comes to an end. Then the light of your wisdom will radiate in the four directions, throughout the world.

To one who thus drinks the nectar of immortality in the shape of self-knowledge, the delights of sense-pleasures become painful. We resort to the company of only those who have attained self-knowledge; the others are donkeys in human garb. Even as elephants move with long strides, the sages who have reached the higher states of consciousness rise to the highest states of consciousness. They have no external help at all and no sun illumines their path. Self-knowledge alone is their light. In fact, the sun and the worlds become non-objects of perception to they who have gone beyond the realm of objective perception and knowledge, even as lamps lose their luminosity while the midday sun shines.

The sage of self-knowledge (the knower of truth) is supreme amongst those who are radiant, glorious, strong, great and endowed with other characteristics which are considered marks of excellence. These sages shine in this world like the sun, the fire, the moon and the stars put together. On the other hand, they who have not attained self-knowledge are worse than worms and insects.

The ghost of delusion afflicts one only as long as self-knowledge does not arise in him. The ignorant man is for ever sorrowful, though he roams everywhere to get rid of it. He is truly a walking corpse. Only the sage of self-knowledge is a living sentient being. Even as when dense clouds form in the sky the sun's light is veiled, when the mind becomes gross with impurities and ignorance the light of self-knowledge is veiled. **Therefore, one should abandon craving for pleasures (those that have been experienced in the past and others that have not yet been experienced but for which one craves) and thus gradually weaken the mind by the abandonment of a taste for them.** By the cultivation of a false relationship with what is not self (the body and those related to it such as wife, son, family, etc.) the mind becomes gross. The notions of 'I' and 'mine' make the mind dense and ignorant. This is further aggravated by old age, sorrow, ambitions, psychological distress, efforts to acquire and to abandon, attachments, greed, lust for wealth and sex and by the enjoyment of sense-pleasures, all of which are based on ignorance and delusion.

citena cetaḥ śamamāśu nītvā śuddhena ghorāstramivā 'strayukttyā
cirāya sādho tyaja cañcalatvaṁ vimarkaṭo vṛkṣa ivā 'kṣataśrīḥ (84)

VASIṢṬHA continued:

O Rāma, this mind is like a tree which is firmly rooted in the vicious field known as the body. Worries and anxieties are its blossoms; it is laden with the fruits of old age and disease and adorned with the flowers of desires and sense-enjoyments; hopes and longings are its branches and perversities are its leaves. Cut down this deadly poisonous tree, which looks as unshakable as the mountain, with the sharp axe known as enquiry.

O Rāma, this mind is like an elephant which roams the forest known as the body. Its vision is clouded by delusion, it has entered into the one (conditioned and ignorant) edge, it is incapable of resting in its own self-bliss and it is violent. Though it wishes to perceive the truth which it hears from wise men, it is caught up in the perception of diversity and conditioned by its own concepts of pleasure and pain and it is endowed with the fierce tusks of lust, etc. O Rāma, you are a lion among princes! Tear this elephant to pieces by your sharp intelligence.

O Rāma, this mind is like a crow which dwells in the nest of this body. It revels in filth; it waxes strong by consuming flesh; it pierces the hearts of others; it knows only its own point of view which it considers as the truth; it is dark on account of its ever-growing stupidity; it is full of evil tendencies and it indulges in violent expressions. It is a burden on earth, O Rāma. Drive it far, far away from yourself.

O Rāma, this mind is like a ghost. It is served by the female goblin known as craving, it rests in the forest of ignorance, it roams in countless bodies out of delusion. How can one attain self-knowledge if one does not lay this ghost with the help of wisdom and dispassion, the grace of the guru, self-effort, chanting of mantrā, etc.

O Rāma, this mind is like a venomous serpent which has killed countless beings; destroy this with the help of the eagle of the appropriate contemplative formula or instruction.

O Rāma, this mind is like a monkey. It roams from one place to another, seeking fruits (rewards, pleasures, etc.); bound to this world-cycle it dances and entertains people. Restrain it from all sides if you wish to attain perfection.

O Rāma, this mind is like a cloud of ignorance. Dispel it by the repeated renunciation of all concepts and percepts.

Even as a terrible weapon is encountered and destroyed by a more powerful weapon, tranquillise the mind with the help of the mind itself. Forever abandon every form of mental agitation. Remain at peace within yourself like a tree freed from the disturbance caused by monkeys.

kadopaśāntamanano dharaṇīdharakandare
sameṣyāmi śilāsāmyaṁ nirvikalpasamādhinā (33)

VASIṢṬHA continued:

O Rāma, do not take your stand on concepts and percepts of the mind, which are subtle and sharp; the mind has been put together by time and it has gained great strength in course of time. Bring it under control by wisdom, before time fells this creeper known as the body. By devoutly contemplating my words you will attain supreme bliss. I shall narrate to you, O Rāma, how the sage Uddālaka attained the supreme vision of truth.

In a corner of the earth there is a great mountain known as Gandhamādana. On one of its peaks there was a great tree. In that region there lived the sage Uddālaka. Even while he was a young boy he aspired to attain supreme wisdom through his own effort. Of course, then he was of little understanding and he had a restless mind, though he had a pure heart. He engaged himself in austerities, in the study of the scriptures and so on, and wisdom arose in him.

While sitting alone one day, the SAGE UDDĀLAKA reflected thus:

What is liberation, which is said to be the foremost among the objects to be attained, upon attaining which one does not experience sorrow and is not born again? When shall I rest permanently in that state? When will the mental agitations caused by desires and cravings cease? When will I be freed from thoughts like 'This I have done' and 'This I should do'? When will my mind cease to undergo perversities though living in relationship here, even as the lotus lying on water is not tainted by it? When will I, with the help of the boat of supreme wisdom, cross to the other shore of liberation? When will I be able to look upon the diverse activities of people with the playfulness of a child? When will the mind attain utter quiescence? When will the illusory division between the subjective and the objective experiences cease through the experience of the infinite consciousness? When will I be able to behold this concept known as time, without being involved in it? When will I, living in a cave with a mind in utter tranquillity, remain like a rock in a state in which there is no movement of thought at all?

Thus reflecting, Uddālaka continued his practice of meditation. But his mind continued to be agitated. Some days, however, his mind abandoned external objects and remained in a state of purity. At other times it was greatly disturbed. Greatly distressed by such changing moods, he roamed the forest. One day he reached a lonely spot in the forest which had not been visited by anyone else. There he saw a cave which appeared to be most conducive to the attainment of the state of utter tranquillity and peace. It was delightful in every way with beautiful creepers and flowers around it, with a moderate climate, and it shone as if it had been carved out of an emerald.

kurangālipatangebhamīnāstvekaikaśo hatāḥ
sarvair yukttair anarthais tu vyāptasyā 'jña kutaḥ sukhaṁ (21)

VASIṢṬHA continued:

Uddālaka entered that delightful cave and sat in a meditative posture. Intent on attaining the state of mind without the least movement of thought, he concentrated his attention on the latent tendencies in the mind, and

UDDĀLAKA reflected thus within himself:

O mind, what have you to do with this world-appearance? Wise men do not come into contact with what is called pleasure, which turns into pain later on. He who abandons the supreme peace that lies within and goes in search of sense-pleasure, abandons a delightful garden and goes into a bush of poison herbs. You may go where you like; you will never taste supreme peace except through perfect quiescence. Hence abandon all hopes and desires. For all these seemingly wondrous objects of the nature either of being or of non-being, are not meant for your happiness.

Do not perish like the deer which is trapped by the sound of music and bells, nor like the male elephant which is trapped with the help of the female elephant, nor like the fish whose sense of taste leads it to its death on the hook, nor like the moth which is attracted by the sight of a flame and perishes in it, nor like the bee whose sense of smell leads it to the flower, trapped in which it is destroyed when the flower folds up for the night.

O foolish mind, all these perish being subject to just one sense-craving (the deer by the sense of hearing, the bee by the sense of smell, the moth by the sense of sight, the elephant by the sense of touch and the fish by the sense of taste). But you are a victim to all the five temptations; how can you have happiness? Just as the silk-worm spins its cocoon and gets caught in it, you have woven the web of your own concepts and are caught in it. If you can get rid of all that, attain purity, overcome even the fear of life and death and thus attain to total equanimity, you have achieved the greatest victory. On the other hand, if you cling to this ever-changing phenomenon called the world, you will surely perish in sorrow.

Why do I instruct you thus, O mind? For if one investigates the truth he discovers that there is no such thing called mind! Mind is but a product of ignorance; when ignorance wears out, then the mind wears out, too. Hence you are in the process of being worn out. It is unwise and foolish to instruct one who is in the process of disintegrating! Since day by day you are becoming weaker and weaker, I renounce you; wise men do not teach one who is to be abandoned.

O mind, I am the egoless infinite and homogeneous consciousness; I have nothing to do with you who are the cause of the ego.

pādāṅguṣṭa chiro yāvat kaṇaśaḥ pravicāritam
na labdho 'sāvahaṁ nāma kaḥ syād ahamiti sthitaḥ (36)

UDDĀLAKA continued to contemplate thus:

The infinite self cannot possibly be squeezed into the mind any more than an elephant can be squeezed into a wood-apple fruit. The consciousness that, through the process of self limitation, is confined to finitude (and therefore to concepts and percepts) is known as the mind. This is the result of ignorance and hence I do not accept this. The ego-sense is only a child's ignorant concept and it is believed in by one who does not investigate the truth.

I have carefully investigated, I have observed everything from the tips of my toes to the top of my head, and I have not found anything of which I could say, 'This I am'. Who is 'I'? I am the all-pervading consciousness which is itself not an object of knowledge or knowing and is free from self-hood. I am that which is indivisible, which has no name, which does not undergo change, which is beyond all concepts of unity and diversity, which is beyond measure (small and big), and other than which naught else is. Hence, O mind, I abandon you who are the source of sorrow.

In this body in which there is flesh, blood, bone, etc., who says 'This I am'? Motion is the nature of energy, thinking is inherent in consciousness, old age and death are natural to the body — who says 'This I am'? This is the tongue, these are ears, this is nose, this is motion and these are eyes — who says, 'This I am'? I am none of these; nor am I you, O mind, nor these concepts. I am but the infinite consciousness, pure and independent. 'I am all this' or 'There is no I' are both expressions of the same truth; naught else is truth.

Alas, for so long I have been victimised by ignorance. But luckily, I have discovered that which robbed me of self-knowledge! I shall nevermore be the victim of ignorance. Even as the cloud sitting on top of a hill does not belong to the hill, though I seem to be associated with sorrow I am independent of it. In the absence of self-knowledge there arose ego-sense; but now I am free of ego-sense. Let the body, the senses and so on be, or perish — I have nothing to do with them. The senses (the eyes, etc.) exist in order to come into contact with their own objects for their own sake; who is the I that is deluded into thinking 'This is I', or 'I see' etc? These eyes etc. see or experience their objects naturally, without being impelled to do so by previous conditioning. Hence, if actions are performed spontaneously without mental conditioning, their experience will be pure and free from memories of past happiness or unhappiness. Hence, O senses, perform your functions without being hampered by memory. This memory or mental conditioning is not a fact, in truth. It is non-different from and not independent of the infinite consciousness. It can therefore be easily dispelled, by merely not reviving it in consciousness. Hence, O mind, abandon this perception of diversity and realise the unreality of your own independence from the infinite consciousness. That is liberation.

tenā 'haṁ nāma nehā 'sti bhāvābhāvopapattimān
anahaṅkārarūpasya saṁbandhaḥ kena me kathaṁ (15)

UDDĀLAKA continued to reflect thus:

In reality, consciousness cannot be conditioned. It is unlimited and subtler than the subtlest atom, hence beyond the influence of mental conditioning. The mind rests in the ego-sense and the reflected consciousness in the senses; and from this there arises the illusion of self-limitation of consciousness. When this is experienced and thought of again and again, the ego-sense and the illusion of self-limitation acquire a false validity. But, I am consciousness which is untouched by any of these.

Let the body continue to live in a world brought into being by its ignorant activities, or let it abandon it: I am consciousness unaffected by any of these. Consciousness, being infinite and all-pervading, has no birth nor death, nor is it possessed by anyone. It has nothing to gain by 'living' as a separate entity, since it is all-pervading. Birth and death are mental concepts, they have nothing to do with the self. Only that which entertains notions of the ego-sense can be grasped and bound. The self is free from the ego-sense and therefore beyond being and non-being.

The ego-sense is vain delusion, the mind is like a mirage and the objects of the world are inert substances. Who is it that says 'I am'? The body is an aggregate of flesh, blood, etc., the mind vanishes on enquiry into its nature, self-limitation of consciousness and such other concepts are insentient (non-sense) — what is the ego? The senses exist and are engaged in self-satisfying activity all the time, the substances of the world are the substances of the world — where is the ego? Nature is nature and its qualities interact on one another (like the sight and light, hearing and sound, etc.), and what is, rests in itself — where is the ego?

The self, which is consciousness, exists as the supreme self of all, everywhere in all bodies at all times. Whom am I, what am I made of, what is my form, made by whom? What shall I acquire and what shall I reject? **There is thus nothing which can be called 'I' and which undergoes being and non-being. When there is no ego-sense in truth, how can that ego-sense be related, and to whom?** When thus it is realised that there is no relationship at all, then the false notion of duality vanishes. Thus, whatever there is is the one cosmic being (Brahman or the self). I am that reality, why do I suffer in delusion? When one alone exists as the pure omnipresent being, how can there even arise something known as the ego-sense? There is no substantiality in any substance in truth, the self alone exists. Even if one assumes the substantiality to be real, there is no relationship between that and the self. The senses function as senses, the mind exists as mind, the consciousness is untouched by these — what is relationship and how does it come into being? Just because they exist side by side it is not right to assume a relationship: a stone and an iron rod may lie side by side, totally unrelated to each other.

ahaṅkārabhramasyā 'sya jātasyākāśavarṇavat
apunaḥ smaraṇaṁ manye nūnaṁ vismaraṇaṁ varaṁ (25)

UDDĀLAKA continued to reflect:

It is only when this false ego-sense has arisen that the perverse notions 'This is mine' and 'That is his' arise. And, when it is seen that all these are tricks of the false ego-sense, these unreal notions cease to be. There is in truth naught else but the self; hence I realise that all this is the one cosmic being or Brahman. **The delusion known as the ego-sense is like the blueness of the sky: it is better not to entertain that notion once again, but to abandon it.** After having abandoned the very root of the ego-sense, I rest in the self which is of the nature of peace.

The ego-sense is the source of endless sorrow, suffering and evil action. Life ends in death, death leads to birth, and what is is disrupted by its own end — such notions entertained by the ego-sense lead to great sorrow. The anxiety caused by thoughts like 'I have got this now', 'I shall get that too' burns the ignorant. Such notions as 'This is' and 'That is not' cause restlessness in the egotist. But if the ego-sense ceases to be, then the illusory world-appearance does not germinate again and all cravings come to an end.

This universe has surely come into being without any valid cause for its creation: how can one accept the truth of a creation which had no cause or purpose? From time immemorial all these bodies have been inherent in the cosmic being, even as pots are forever inherent in clay. Even as ocean exists in the past, present and future as ocean, and the same water temporarily assumes the form of a wave, all this is forever the cosmic being at all times. It is only a fool who entertains a feeling 'This I am' in relation to that temporary appearance known as the body, etc.

In the same way, the mind was consciousness in the beginning and will be consciousness again in the end (after its nature and function as mind have ceased). Why then is it called differently in the middle (now)?

All these phenomena seem to have a transient reality, like dream experiences, visions in a state of delirium, hallucinations of a drunkard, optical illusions, psychosomatic illness, emotional disturbances and psychotic states. But, O mind, you have conferred a permanent reality upon them, even as a lover suffers from the very imagination of his beloved's separation. But, of course, this is not your fault; it is my fault that I still cling to the notion that you, my mind, are a real entity. When I realise that all these are illusory appearances, then you will become no-mind and all the memories of sense-experiences, etc. will come to an end. When consciousness realises itself and abandons its self-limiting mental conditioning, the mind is freed from its colouring and rests in its essential nature, which is consciousness. When the mind, gathering to itself all its limbs, offers itself into the fire of pure consciousness, it is purified and attains immortality.

kṣīyate manasi kṣīṇe dehaḥ prakṣīṇavāsanaḥ
mano na kṣīyate kṣīṇe dehe tat kṣāpayen manaḥ (66)

UDDĀLAKA continued to contemplate:

When the mind perceives the body as distinct from it, abandons its own conditioning (the concepts) and recognises its own transient nature, it is victorious. Mind and body are each other's foes; hence, supreme happiness follows their destruction. For, when they come together there is a host of suffering on account of their mutual conflict.

The mind gives birth to the body through its own thought-force and throughout the body's lifetime the mind feeds it with its (the mind's) own sorrow. Thus tortured by sorrow the body wishes to destroy the mind, its own parent! There is no friend nor enemy in this world; that which gives us pleasure is considered our friend and that which causes pain is our enemy!

When thus the mind and the body are constantly engaged in mutual destruction, how can one have happiness? It is by the destruction of the mind that there can be happiness; hence the body tries every day (in deep sleep) to destroy the mind. However, until self-knowledge is attained, one unwittingly promotes the strength of the other and they seem to function together for a common purpose — even as water and fire, though opposed to each other, work together for a common cause (e.g. cooking).

If the mind ceases to be, the body ceases to be, too, on account of the cessation of thought-force and mental conditioning; but the mind does not cease to be when the body dies. Hence, one should strive to kill the mind. Mind is like a forest with thought-forms for its trees and cravings for its creepers. By destroying these, I attain bliss. When the mind is dead, whether the body (composed of flesh, blood, etc.) exists or not does not matter to me. That I am not the body is obvious, for the corpse does not function!

Where there is self-knowledge there is neither mind nor the senses, nor the tendencies and habits (the concepts and percepts). I have attained that supreme state. I have emerged victorious. I have attained liberation (nirvāṇa). I have risen above all relationships with the mind, body and the senses, even as the oil pressed out of the seeds has no relation to them. To me now the mind, body and the senses are playthings. Purity, total fulfilment of all desires (hence, their absence), friendliness to all, truthfulness, wisdom, tranquillity and blissfulness, sweetness of speech, supreme magnanimity, lustrousness, one-pointedness, realisation of cosmic unity, fearlessness, absence of divided consciousness, non-perversity — these are my constant companions. Since at all times everything everywhere happens in every manner, in me there is no desire or aversion towards anything, whether pleasant or unpleasant. Since all delusion has come to an end, since the mind has ceased to be and all evil thoughts have vanished, I rest peacefully in my own self.

antaḥ kuṇḍalinīṁ prāṇāḥ pūrayāmāsurādṛtāḥ
cakrānuvartaprasṛtāṁ payāṁsīva saridvarāṁ (26)

VASIṢṬHA continued:

The sage Uddālaka then sat down in the lotus posture, with his eyes half closed, in meditation. He uttered the holy word OṀ which bestows the highest state. He intoned OṀ in such a way that its vibrations filled his whole being right up to the crown of his head. As the first part of his practice, he exhaled his breath completely. It was as if his life-force had abandoned the body and was roaming in the space (dimension) of pure consciousness. The fire that arose from his heart burnt the whole of his body. (All this, Uddālaka practised without the violence involved in Haṭha Yoga; for Haṭha Yoga gives rise to pain.)

With the second utterance of the holy word OṀ, he reached the state of equilibrium and there happened in him a spontaneous retention of the breath (life-force) without agitation or vibration. The life-force stood still, as it were, neither outside, nor inside, neither below nor above. After reducing the body to ashes, the fire burnt itself out and vanished; only the pure ashes were visible. It was as if the very bones had turned into camphor which was being burnt in adoration. The ashes were blown by a powerful wind and dispersed in space. (All this happened without the violence of Haṭha Yoga; for Haṭha Yoga gives rise to pain.)

In the third stage, when the holy word OṀ reached its culmination or tranquillity, there arose the inhalation of breath (the drawing in of the life-force). During this stage the life-forces, which were in the very centre of the nectar of consciousness, spread out in space as a cool breeze. These forces reached the region of the moon. There they spread out as auspicious rays, which thereupon rained on the ashes that remained of the body.

Instantly, there arose from the ashes a radiant being with four arms like lord Viṣṇu. Uddālaka shone like a divinity, his whole being transmuted into a divinity. **The life-force filled the inner kuṇḍalinī which was spread out like a spiral.** Uddālaka's body had thus been completely purified. Then he, who was already seated in the lotus posture, made the posture firm, 'tied up' his senses and proceeded to make his consciousness absolutely free from the least movement of thought. With all his strength he restrained his mind from distraction. His half-closed eyes were still and motionless. With his mind established in inner silence, he equalised the movement of the twin life-forces, prāṇa and apāna. He withdrew his inner senses from contact with their objects, even as oil is separated from the seed. Thereupon he became directly aware of the mental conditioning created by past experiences, and unconditioned the awareness and made it pure. Then, he firmly closed his rectum and the other outlets to the body (the eyes, etc.). With his life-force and awareness thus prevented from externalisation by perfect discipline, he held his mind in his heart.

ānande pariṇāmitvādanānandapadaṁ gataḥ
nā ''nande na nirānande tatastatsaṁvidā babhau (68)

VASIṢṬHA continued:

Uddālaka's mind had attained absolute tranquillity and no distraction could afflict it. Directly he beheld in his heart the darkness of ignorance that veiled the light of self-knowledge. With the light of knowledge that arose in him, he dispelled even that darkness. He then beheld the light within. However, when that light dimmed, he experienced sleep. But, he dispelled the dullness of sleep, too. Once the drowsiness of sleep had been dispelled, his mind threw up diverse brilliant forms. He cleared his consciousness of these visions. Then he was overcome by a great inertia, like one intoxicated. He got over that inertia, too. After this, his mind rested in another state which was different from all these so far described. After resting for a while in this state, however, his mind awoke to the experience of the totality of existence. Immediately after this he experienced pure awareness. This awareness, which till then had been associated with other factors, had now regained its purity and independence, even as when the muddy water in an earthen pot has completely evaporated the mud becomes an integral part of the pot made of the same substance. Even as the wave merges in the ocean and becomes one and non-different from it, the consciousness abandoned its objectivity and regained its absolute purity. Uddālaka was enlightened. He enjoyed the supreme bliss that gods like Brahmā enjoy. His state was beyond description. He was one with the ocean of bliss.

Soon Uddālaka beheld great sages in that infinite consciousness. He ignored them. He continued with the experience of supreme bliss. He attained the state of 'liberated while living'. He beheld the gods and the sages, and he even beheld the members of the trinity. He went beyond even that state. **He was completely transmuted into bliss itself and hence he had gone beyond the realm of bliss. He experienced neither bliss nor non-bliss.** He became pure consciousness. He who experiences this even for a moment is disinterested even in the delights of heaven. This is the supreme state, this is the goal, this is the eternal abode. He who rests in this is not again deluded and is no longer caught in the subject-object relationship. He is fully awakened and never again entertains the notion of objectivity or conceptualisation. Of course this is not an 'attainment'.

Uddālaka remained for six months in this state, vigilantly avoiding the temptation of psychic powers. Even sages and gods adored him. He was invited to ascend to heaven; he declined the invitation. Totally freed from all desires, Uddālaka roamed as a sage liberated while living. Often he would spend days and months in meditation in the caves of mountains. Though at other times he engaged himself in the ordinary activities of living, he had reached the state of perfect equilibrium. He looked upon all with equal vision. His inner light shone at all times, never rising and never setting. With all notions of duality totally at rest, he lived devoid of body-consciousness, established in pure being.

**upaśaśāma śanair divasairasau katipayaiḥ svapade vimalātmani
taruraşaḥ śaradanta ivā 'male ravikaraujasi janmadaśātigaḥ (23)**

In answer to Rāma's question concerning pure being, VASIṢṬHA said:

When the mind has ceased to be because of the total absence of the notions of material existence, consciousness exists in its own nature as consciousness. That is known as pure being. When consciousness devoid of notions of objectivity merges in itself losing its separate identity, as it were, it is pure being. When all external (material) and internal (notional) objects merge in consciousness, there is pure being of consciousness. This is the supreme vision which happens to all liberated ones, whether they seem to have a body or they are without one. This vision is available to one who has been 'awakened', to one who is in a state of deep contemplation and to a man of self-knowledge; it is not experienced by the ignorant person. Sages and the members of the trinity are established in this consciousness, O Rāma. Having reached this state of consciousness Uddālaka lived for some time.

In course of time, in his mind there arose the wish, 'Let me drop this embodiment'. He went to a mountain-cave and seated himself in the lotus posture, with his eyes half closed. He closed off the nine apertures of the body, by pressing his heel against the rectum, etc. He withdrew the senses into his heart. He restrained his life-force (prāṇa). He held his body in a state of perfect equilibrium. He pressed the tip of the tongue against the root of his palate, his jaws were slightly parted from each other. His inner vision was directed neither inward nor outward, neither above nor below, neither in substantiality nor void. He was established in pure consciousness and he experienced pure bliss within himself. He had reached the consciousness of pure being, beyond the state of bliss. His whole being had become absolutely pure.

Uddālaka remained in this totally pure state for some time, like a painted picture. **Gradually, day by day, he attained perfect quiescence; he remained in his own pure being. He had risen above the cycle of birth and death.** All his doubts were set at rest, perverse thoughts had ceased, all impurities of the heart had been washed away. He had attained that state of bliss which is beyond description, in which one regards even the joy of the king of heaven as worthless. His body remained thus for a period of six months.

After that, one day several goddesses led by Pārvati arrived at that spot in response to the prayers of a devotee. Pārvati who was worshipped by the gods themselves, saw the body of Uddālaka which had been dried by the scorching rays of the sun, and quickly placed it on the crown of her head.

Such is the glorious story of the sage Uddālaka, O Rāma, which awakens the highest wisdom in the heart of one who takes shelter in its shade.

praśāntajagadāstho 'ntarvītaśokabhayaiṣaṇaḥ
svastho bhavati yenā "tmā sa samādhiriti smṛtaḥ (20)

VASIṢṬHA continued:

O Rāma, living like this, constantly enquiring into the nature of the self, attain peace. This state of consciousness can be attained by the cultivation of dispassion, the study of scriptures, the instructions of a guru and by the persistent practice of enquiry. But, if the awakened intelligence is keen and sharp, you will attain it even without the other aids.

RĀMA asked:

Holy sir, some there are who rest in self-knowledge, who are enlightened and yet engage themselves in activities; and there are others who isolate themselves and practise contemplation (samāḍhi). Of these who is the better?

VASIṢṬHA replied:

O Rāma, that is samāḍhi (contemplation or meditation) in which one realises the objects of the senses as not-self and thus enjoys inner calmness and tranquillity at all times. Having realised that the objects are related only to the mind, and therefore constantly resting in inner peace, some are engaged in activity while others live in isolation. Both of them enjoy the bliss of contemplation. If the mind of one who appears to be in samādhi is distracted, he is a mad man; on the other hand, if the mind of one who appears to be a mad man is free from all notions and distraction, he is enlightened and he is in unbroken samādhi. Whether he is engaged in activity or he lives in isolation in a forest, in enlightenment there is no distinction. The mind which is free from conditioning is not tainted even while it is engaged in activity. The non-action of the mind is known as quiescence (samādhāna); it is total freedom, it is blessedness.

The difference between contemplation and its absence is indicated by whether or not there is movement of thought in the mind. Hence make the mind unconditioned. The unconditioned mind is firm, and that in itself is meditation, freedom and peace eternal. The conditioned mind is the source of sorrow. The unconditioned mind is a non-actor and attains to the supreme state of enlightenment. Hence one should work to remove all mental conditioning. **That is known as contemplation or samāḍhi in which all the desires and hopes concerning the world have ceased, which is free from sorrow, fear and desire, and by which the self rests in itself.**

Mentally renounce all false identification of the self with objects here and then live where you like, either at home or in a mountain-cave. To the householder whose mind has attained utter quiescence, his house itself is the forest. If the mind is at peace and if there is no ego-sense, even cities are as void. On the other hand, forests are like cities to him whose heart is full of desires and other evils. The distractions of the mind subside in deep sleep; enlightenment attains enlightenment. Do as you please.

paramātmamaṇeścittvād yad antaḥ kacanaṁ svayaṁ
cetanātmapade cā 'ntar ahamityādi vettyasau (15)

VASIṢṬHA continued:

O Rāma, the infinite consciousness becomes aware of the pungency of the chilli; this gives rise to the ego-sense, with all its differentiation in time and space. The infinite consciousness becomes aware of the savour in salt and that gives rise to the ego-sense with all the differentiation which seems to exist in time and space. The infinite consciousness becomes aware of the sweetness in sugarcane and thereby arises the awareness of its particular characteristic. Similarly, the infinite consciousness being the indwelling omnipresence, becomes aware of the nature of rock, a mountain, a tree, water and space, and thus self-consciousness or individuality arises.

Thus the natural combination of atomic particles and molecules (which is indwelt by consciousness) apparently acts as a dividing wall, thus giving rise to the divisions of 'I', 'you', etc. and these then appear to be outside of consciousness as its object. In fact, all these are but reflections in the consciousness which, becoming aware of them within itself, bestows upon them their apparent individuality. Consciousness tastes itself, the awareness being non-different from consciousness; and that appears to give rise to the ego-sense, etc., naught else. **The crystal of this infinite consciousness reflects its own light of consciousness which is present in all these combinations of atomic particles; and they then gain an apparent self-consciousness and think 'I am' etc.**

In reality, because the inner awareness in all these combinations is non-different from the infinite consciousness, there is no subject-object relationship between them: hence one does not experience the other, gain the other, or change or modify the other. O Rāma, all that I have said above is but a play of words to help your comprehension: there is no such thing as 'I' or 'the world' (the combination of atomic particles etc.). There is neither mind, nor an object of knowledge, nor the world-illusion. Just as water acquires the appearance of a whirlpool with a personality of its own, consciousness seems to give the appearance of 'I' etc., within itself. But consciousness is consciousness only, whether it thinks of itself as lord Śiva or as a little jīva.

All this diversity of 'I', 'you', etc., and of the material substances, arises for the satisfaction of the ignorant. Whatever the ignorant person imagines in the infinite consciousness, that alone he sees. In the light of awareness, life is seen as consciousness; when it is regarded as life, life appears to be no more than life! There is in reality no essential distinction between life and consciousness. In the same way, there is no real and essential distinction between the individual (jīva) and the cosmic being (Śiva). Know all this to be undivided and indivisible infinite consciousness.

yāvatsarvaṁ na saṁtyakttaṁ tāvadātmā na labhyate
sarvāvasthāparityāge śeṣa ātmeti kathyate (58/44)

VASIṢṬHA continued:

In this connection, O Rāma, pray listen to an interesting legend.

In the Himālaya mountain range there is a mountain known as Kailāsa. At the foot of that mountain there lived a hill-tribe known as Hemajaṭa (yellow-haired). Suraghu was their king. He was just in his rule, blessing and punishing those who deserved to be thus blessed and punished. In all this activity, however, his spiritual vision became obscured.

One day, the sage Māṇḍavya came to visit the king. Suraghu welcomed the sage, bowed to him, worshipped him and asked: "Lord I am tormented by the anxieties that the blessing and punishment that I inflict upon my subjects will return to me. Please help me to gain equal vision and save me from prejudice and partiality".

MĀṆḌAVYA said:

All mental weaknesses come to an end by self-effort based on the wisdom which arises in one who is firmly rooted in self-knowledge. The distress of the mind is got rid of by enquiry into the nature of the self. When you have gained self-knowledge and when your consciousness has infinitely expanded, your mind no longer falls into the cesspool of this world. **Not till one renounces everything is self-knowledge gained: when all points of view are abandoned, what remains is the self.** This is true even of life in this world: one does not get what one desires unless the obstacle to it is removed. It is even more so in self-knowledge.

When the sage Māṇḍavya had departed after saying this, SURAGHU contemplated thus:

What is it that is known as 'I'? I am not the mountain, the mountain is not mine. I am not the hill-tribe, nor the hill-tribe mine. This is merely called my kingdom: I abandon that notion. Now, the capital city is left. I am not this city nor is it mine. That notion, too, is abandoned. Even so I abandon the notions of family relationships — wife, sons, etc.

Let me enquire into this body. I am not the inert substances like flesh and bones — nor am I the blood nor the organs of action. I am not the mind which is the root cause of this ignorant cycle of birth and death. I am not the faculty of discrimination nor am I the ego-sense.

Now, what is left? What remains is the sentient jīva. But, it is involved in subject-object relationship. That which is the object of knowledge or comprehension is not the self. Thus do I abandon that which is knowable — or the object. What now remains is the pure consciousness which is free from the shadow of doubt. I am the infinite self.

na nirghṛṇo dayāvān no na dvandvī nā 'tha matsarī
na sudhīr nā 'sudhīr nā 'rthī nā 'narthī sa babhūva ha (60/6)

VASIṢṬHA continued:

By such enquiry, Suraghu attained to the supreme state of consciousness. Never again did he grieve; but from that time onwards he performed his work, ever remaining in a balanced state of mind. **Compassionate, yet not uncontemptuous; not avoiding the pairs of opposites and not jealous; neither intelligent nor non-intelligent; neither motivated nor non-motivated — he lived** with equal vision and inner calmness. He had realised that all this is but the diverse manifestation of consciousness. He was therefore peaceful in both pain and pleasure, having attained to the fullness of understanding.

Thus he ruled in this world for a considerable time, and then of his own accord discarded his body. He attained oneness with the infinite consciousness. O Rāma, thus live and rule the world with an enlightened mind.

RĀMA asked: But, O Lord, the mind is so unsteady. How can one reach the state of perfect equanimity?

VASIṢṬHA replied:

O Rāma, a dialogue which is relevant to this problem took place between that very king Suraghu and the sage Parigha. Listen to it.

There was a king in Persia named Parigha who was a close friend of the king Suraghu. Once there was a great famine in the kingdom of Parigha. Sore distressed at heart at the very sight of his people's suffering, and seeing that all his attempts at bringing relief to them proved fruitless, Parigha, unbeknown to his people, went away to the forest to perform austerities. He lived on dried leaves, and earned the name Parnāda. After a thousand years of penance and contemplation he attained self-knowledge. Thereafter he roamed the three worlds freely.

One day he met the king Suraghu, whom he had known before. The two enlightened kings duly worshipped each other. After that, Parigha asked Suraghu: "Even as you attained self-knowledge through the instructions of the sage Māndavya, I reached it through the grace of the Lord earned by penance. Pray tell me: is your mind at perfect rest now? Are your subjects living in peace and prosperity? Are you firmly established in dispassion?"

SURAGHU replied:

Who can truly understand the course of the divine will? You and I had been separated by a great distance so far; but now we have been brought together. What is impossible for the divine? We have been truly blessed by your holy visit. By your very presence in our midst we have all been rid of all sins and defects and I feel that all prosperity stands in front of us in your form. Company of good and holy men is indeed equal to the supreme state of liberation.

tattvāvabodho bhagavan sarvāśātṛṇapāvakaḥ
prokttaḥ samādhiśabdena na tu tūṣṇīmavasthitiḥ (62/8)

PARIGHA asked:

O king, all actions that are performed by one who is firmly established in equanimity are productive of joy, not those done by others. Are you established in that state of supreme peace in which no thoughts or notions arise in your mind, and which is known as samādhi?

SURAGHU replied:

Holy sir, please tell me why only that state of mind which is free from thoughts and notions is called samādhi? If one is a knower of truth, whether he be engaged in constant action or in contemplation, does his mind ever lose the state of samādhi? No. The enlightened ones are forever in samādhi, even though they engage themselves in the affairs of the world. On the other hand, one whose mind is not at peace does not enjoy samādhi by merely sitting in the lotus posture.

Knowledge of truth, Lord, is the fire that burns up all hopes and desires as if they are dried blades of grass. That is what is known by the word samādhi — not simply remaining silent! That is known as the state of samādhi in which there is eternal satisfaction, clear perception of what is, egolessness, not being subject to the pairs of opposites, freedom from anxiety and from the wish to acquire or to reject. From the very moment of the dawn of self-knowledge, the state of samādhi becomes permanent in the sage. He neither loses it nor is it interrupted, even for a moment. Even as time does not forget to move on, the man of self-knowledge does not forget the self. Even as a material object is forever material, the sage of self-knowledge is forever a sage of self-knowledge.

Hence, I am always awakened, pure, at peace within myself and in a state of samādhi. How can it be otherwise? How can there be anything other than the self? When at all times and in all ways the self alone is all in all, how can there be a state other than samādhi? And what can be termed samādhi?

PARIGHA said: Surely, O king, you have attained total enlightenment. You shine, radiant with bliss, with peace, with sweetness and with purity. In you there is no ego-sense, desire or aversion.

SURAGHU continued: O sage, there is indeed nothing which is worth desiring or renouncing. For as long as these things are seen as objects, they are nothing but concepts, percepts and notions. When nothing is worth acquiring it follows that nothing is worth renouncing. Good and evil, great and small, worthy or unworthy, are all based on the notion of desirability. When desirability has no meaning, the others do not arise at all. There is truly no essence in all that is seen in this world — the mountains, the oceans, the forests, the men and women and all the objects — hence there is no desire for them. When there is no desire, there is supreme peace at heart.

tāni mitrāṇi śāstrāṇi tāni tāni dināni ca
virāgollāsavān yebhya ātmacittodayaḥ sphuṭaṁ (64/19)

VASIṢṬHA continued:

After thus considering the illusory nature of the world-appearance and after mutually worshipping each other, Suraghu and Parigha continued to engage themselves in their respective duties. O Rāma, be firmly established in this wisdom and discard the impure notion of ego-sense from your heart. Thereafter, even if you engage yourself in activity you are unattached to it and therefore not tainted by it, even as the eyes of fish are not affected by sea-water. **They alone are friends, scriptures and days that generate in one's heart true dispassion and also self-knowledge.**

There is a great mountain which is as high as the three worlds put together. On it there is the hermitage of the sage Atri. In it there dwelt two sages known as Bṛhaspati and Śukra, each of whom had a son, known as Vilāsa and Bhāsa respectively.

In course of time the two elder sages, Bṛhaspati and Śukra, left this world. Grief stricken, the two young men performed the appropriate funeral rites. On account of the loss of their fathers they felt disinterested in property, wealth, etc., and both of them thereupon went away to the forest, each in a different direction, to lead a nomadic life. After a considerable time, once again they met each other.

VILĀSA said to his friend Bhāsa:

What a delight to meet you again, O my dearest friend. Tell me what you have been doing since we parted. Did your austerities bear fruit? Has your mind rid itself of the burning fever of worldliness? Have you attained self-knowledge? Tell me: are you well and happy?

BHĀSA replied:

I consider myself extremely fortunate to see you again, my very dear friend and brother. However, how can we who are wandering in this world-appearance ever be well and happy unless and until we attain the highest wisdom, until the psychological perversions cease? Until we cross this ocean of world-cycle, how can we be well and happy? Until the hopes and desires born of the mind have been completely destroyed, how can we be well and happy?

Until we attain self-knowledge we shall return to this plane of birth and death, to undergo childhood, youth, manhood, old age and death; again and again we shall engage ourselves in the same essenceless actions and experiences. Cravings destroy wisdom. Lost in satisfying sensual appetites, life ebbs away fast. The mind falls into the blind well of sense pleasure. It is a wonder how and why this body, which is an excellent vehicle to take us to the other shore of self-knowledge, falls into the mire of worldliness! In the twinkling of an eye this little ripple known as the mind assumes terrible proportions. Man foolishly ascribes to the self the sorrow and sufferings that do not touch it in the least, and becomes miserable.

Thus conversing with each other and enquiring into the nature of the world, they soon attained the supreme wisdom.

antaḥsakttaṁ mano baddhaṁ mukttaṁ sakttivivarjitaṁ
antaḥsaṁsakttirevaikaṁ kāraṇaṁ bandhamokṣayoḥ (34)

VASIṢṬHA continued:

O Rāma, I tell you that there is no way other than self-knowledge for the cutting asunder of bondage and for crossing this ocean of illusion. To the enlightened person this ocean of sorrow is like a little puddle. He views the body as a spectator looks at a distant crowd. Hence he is not affected by the pains that the body is subjected to. The existence of the body does not diminish the omnipresence of the self any more than waves diminish the fullness of the ocean.

What is the relationship of a swan, a rock or a piece of wood to the water which surrounds them? Even so, the supreme self has no relationship with this world-appearance. A falling tree seems to raise waves on the water: similar is the experience by the self of the pleasure and pain that appear on the body. Even as by its proximity to water wood is reflected in the water, the body is reflected in the self. But even as a rock falling in the water does not injure the water nor is injured by it, even so when the body comes into contact with other material substances (such as wife, children, or material objects) there is no injury or pain to anyone.

The reflection of an object in the mirror can be said to be neither real nor unreal. It is indescribable. Even so, the body which is reflected in the self is neither real nor unreal, but is indescribable. The ignorant person accepts as real whatever he sees in this world; not so the wise one. Even as a piece of wood and water in which it is reflected has no real relationship, the body and the self have no real relationship. Moreover, there is in fact no duality where such relationship could exist. One infinite consciousness alone exists without subject-object division. In this, diversity is imagined, and that which is untouched by sorrow believes itself to be miserable, even as one who thinks he sees a ghost, sees a ghost! On account of the power of thought this imaginary relationship assumes the force of reality. The self is ever untouched by pain and pleasure; but thinking itself to be the body, it undergoes the experiences of the body. The abandonment of this ignorant belief is liberation.

They who are not thus overcome by false identification or attachment are freed at once from sorrow. It is this conditioning that is the seed of old age, death and delusion; when it ceases one goes beyond the ocean of delusion. The conditioned mind creates bondage even in ascetics; the unconditioned mind is pure even in a householder. **The mind that is thus conditioned is bondage; liberation is freedom from conditioning (inner contact, attachment or identification). This inner contact (which presupposes fictitious division) alone is the cause for bondage and liberation.** Actions performed by the unconditioned are non-action; the conditioned mind acts even while outwardly refraining from it. Action or non-action is in the mind; the body does nothing. Hence, one should resolutely abandon this false inner division.

saṁsakttir dvividhā proktā vandyā vandhyā cā rāghava
vandhyā sarvatra mūḍhānāṁ vandyā tattvavidāṁ nijā (21)

RĀMA asked:

What is conditioning, O Lord, and how does it cause bondage; and what is liberation and how is it attained?

VASIṢTHA continued:

Conviction in the reality of the body in one who has abandoned the distinction between the body and the self is known as conditioning. He who believes that the infinite self is limited and therefore seeks pleasure, thus gets bound. He who enquires, "All this is indeed the self, what do I desire and what should I renounce?" is established in the unconditioned state of liberation. He who knows "I am not, nor is there another" or, "Let these be or not be" and does not seek pleasure, is liberated. He is neither addicted to inaction nor does he get lost in the results of action; he is not given to exultation or to depression. He renounces the fruits of actions by his mind (not by action!). It is by the rejection of the conditioning that bondage is got rid of and the highest good gained. Conditioning is the cause of all sorrow.

Conditioning can be illustrated by the following examples: (1) the donkey is led by the master's rope and, afraid, it carries a heavy burden; (2) the tree rooted to the ground bears heat, cold, wind and rain; (3) the worm lies in a hole in earth, biding its time; (4) the hungry bird rests on the branch of a tree, fearful of predators; (5) the tame deer peacefully goes about grazing and falls a prey to the hunter's shot; (6) numerous people are born again and again as worms and insects; (7) the countless creatures that arise and fall in this creation like waves on the surface of the ocean; (8) the weak human beings who, unable even to move about, die again and again; (9) those shrubs and creepers which derive their nourishment from the earth and grow on earth; and (10) this very world-illusion which is like a river that carries in its stream the countless sorrows and sufferings. All these are the expansions of conditioning.

Conditioning (or inner contact, attachment or self-limitation) is of two kinds: the adorable and the sterile or barren. The sterile or barren conditioning is seen everywhere in fools; the adorable conditioning is seen among those who know the truth. That conditioning which exists in the minds of those who are ignorant of self-knowledge, which arises from things like the body and which is conducive to repeated birth and death, is barren and sterile. The other form of conditioning which is found in adorable beings who have self-knowledge arises from the realisation of true wisdom; this enables one to avoid birth and death.

Note: The adorable conditioning recognises 'natural' limitations, e.g., the eyes and ears etc. are limited in their perception. The fool's is self-imposed conditioning and he regards the infinite self to be identical with the physical body. The word used in the text, viz. saṁsaktti is usually translated 'attachment'. However, attachment implies division and duality which is limitation of the infinite and conditioning of the unconditioned.

antaḥ saṁsaṅgamaṅgānāṁ aṅgāraṁ viddhi rāghava
anantaḥ saṅgamaṅgānām viddhi rāma rasāyanaṁ (50)

VASIṢṬHA continued:

The god who holds in his hands the conch, the discus, etc., protects the three worlds on account of the 'adorable conditioning'. It is thanks to the same type of conditioning that the sun shines and the cosmic body of the Creator continues to direct this vast creation. And lord Śiva, too, shines as a divinity on account of this type of conditioning. The gods that sustain this world and function in various ways are endowed with their faculties by this adorable conditioning or self-limitation.

On the other hand, under the influence of the sterile or barren conditioning, the mind falls a prey to the desire for pleasure in the deluded belief that such experience is delightful.

Even the functioning of the cosmic elements is due to conditioning. And it is because of it that the gods in heaven, the humans on earth and the demons in the netherworld arise and fall, like waves on the ocean. Even as in the ocean the big fish eat the small ones, all these countless beings feed upon one another and are helplessly blown around in space on account of their conditioning. And the stars in space move in their own orbits because of conditioning. Now rising, now setting, now bright, now dark (and said to have several spots or defects), the moon continues to revolve around the earth and is not abandoned, because of conditioning.

Oh Rāma, behold this mysterious creation brought into being by who-knows-who in response to the mental concepts of beings. This universe has been conjured up in empty space merely by mental conditioning. It is not a reality. And in this universe, craving for pleasure gnaws at the very vitals of all beings who are attached to the world, the body etc. No one can count their number any more than the number of particles of sand along the ocean beaches. The Creator of this universe has brought this universe into being, as it were, only in response to the mental conditioning of these countless beings. These beings are indeed excellent dry fuel for the flaming fire of hell here. Whatever suffering is found in this world, know that it is meant only for those beings. Even as rivers flow rapidly towards the ocean, suffering flows towards those who are mentally conditioned. This whole creation is thus pervaded by ignorance. However, if one cuts asunder this craving for pleasure, the limitation of mental conditioning yields to a great expansion. **Mental conditioning (or attachment to the finite and the perishable) is burning pain to the limbs, O Rama; but infinite expansion (or devotion to the infinite) is the magic cure for the burning pain.** That mind which is unattached to anything, which is established in the peace of infinite expansion, is conducive to delight. He who stands rooted in self-knowledge is liberated here and now.

Note: In this chapter the real significance of 'conditioning' is brought out, though the word used again is saṁsaṅgaṁ which may also be translated as 'contact' or 'attachment'. It is 'identification' or 'conditioning' that is really implied.

eṣaiva rāma sauṣupti sthitir abhyāsayogataḥ
praudhā satī turyamiti kathitā tattvakovidaiḥ (70/26)

VASIṢṬHA continued:

O Rāma, doing what is appropriate, at all times, the mind should not be attached to the action, the thoughts or the object. Neither should it be attached to the heavens above, nor what is below nor in the other directions. It should not be bound to external relations, to the natural movement of the inner senses, nor to the life-force. The mind should not rest in the head, inside the palate, between the eyebrows, at the tip of the nose or in the mouth or eyes. It should not repose either in the darkness or in the light or even in the cave of the heart. The states of wakefulness, dream and sleep should not hold it, and even the wide, pure space should not be its home. Unattached to the spectrum of colours, to movement and steadiness, to the beginning, the middle, the end and elsewhere, the mind should not rest either at a distance or nearby, in front, in objects or in the self. Sense experiences, the deluded state of happiness, concepts and percepts should have no hold over the mind.

The mind should rest in pure consciousness as pure consciousness, with just a little externalised movement of thought, as if aware of the utter vanity of the objects of this world. When thus all attachments have been snapped, the jīva becomes no-jīva.

That state in which the mind is freed from its characteristic movement of thought and in which there is only the experience of peace, is known as 'deep sleep in wakefulness.' When this same state of 'deep sleep in wakefulness' matures, it is known as turīya or the fourth state. Firmly established in that, the sage perceives the universe as if it is a cosmic playground and life in it is a cosmic dance. The state beyond that (which is the state of those who have transcended body-consciousness) is not for words to describe. This is the 'state beyond the turīya'. O Rāma, strive to reach that.

Truly, the cause for this world-appearance is ignorance or the non-investigation into the nature of reality. Even as a lamp instantly removes darkness, the light of self-knowledge dispels the darkness of ignorance instantly. Hence, one should enquire into what is known as jīva or mind or the inner psychological factor. The supreme self, which alone is the truth, is right in the middle between the inert and the intelligent: that alone creates diversity and is known by all these diverse names. Just as a nanny takes the baby from one place to another in order to distract it, this mental conditioning (or the psychological habit or tendency) takes the jīva here and there. Thus, tied to the rope of mental conditioning, the jīva goes through repeated births in various species, enduring interminable suffering.

(As the sage Vasiṣṭha said this, another day came to an end and the assembly dispersed for their evening prayers.)

dṛśyadarśanasaṁbandha vistāraistad vijṛmbhate
dṛśyadarśanasaṁbandhe yatsukhaṁ pāramātmikaṁ
anubhūtimayaṁ tasmāt sāraṁ brahmeti kathyate (72/33)

VASIṢṬHA continued:

The self, on account of its ignorant self-limitation as the mind, becomes as if tainted by the objects of the world; but the same self, when it is awakened to its true nature, abandons its ignorant delusion and regains self-knowledge. Then the mind sees the body as if from a great height. Recognising the body as an aggregate of the elements, it transcends body consciousness and becomes enlightened.

All that is, is but the expansion of the relationship between pure experiencing and its experience. That experience is truly the delight of self-bliss. It is pure experiencing itself. Hence it is known as Brahman the absolute. That delight which arises in the contact of this pure experiencing with experience, is the highest: to the ignorant it is worldliness, and to the wise it is liberation. This pure experiencing is in itself the infinite self; when it is bent towards objects it is bondage, but when it is free it is liberation. When such experiencing is free from decay or curiosity, it is liberation. When such experiencing is freed from even this contact (the subject-object relationship), then the world-appearance ceases entirely. Then arises the turiya consciousness or 'deep sleep in wakefulness'.

O Rāma, by the following attitude you will also gain divine insight and remain firmly established in self-knowledge: 'I am the space. I am the sun. I am the directions, above and below. I am the gods. I am the demons. I am all beings. I am darkness. I am the earth, the oceans, etc. I am the dust, the wind, the fire and all this world. I am omnipresent. How can there be anything other than me?' By adopting this attitude you will rise beyond joy and sorrow.

Both the following attitudes are conducive to liberation: one is 'I am the extremely subtle and transcendent self' and the other is 'I am all and everything'. There is another attitude with regard to the 'I', and that is the attitude of 'I am this body'; this attitude is the source of endless sorrow. Abandon all these three attitudes, O Rāma, and remain as pure consciousness.

Abandon these two false concepts of bondage and liberation, and live an enlightened life here. There is no liberation in the sky or on earth or in the nether world; liberation is but a synonym for pure mind, correct self-knowledge and a truly awakened state.

Of the mind and the ego-sense — if one ceases the other ceases to be. Hence, instead of entertaining the notion of bondage and that of liberation, abandon all cravings, and through wisdom and dispassion bring about the cessation of the mind. If even the wish 'May I be liberated' arises within you, the mind is revived; and the mind entertaining other notions, creates a body. Then there arise other concepts like 'I do this', 'I enjoy this' and 'I know this'. All these concepts are unreal, like a mirage in the desert.

tiryagyoniṣvapi sadā vidyante kṛtabuddhayaḥ
devayoniṣvapi prājñā vidyante mūrkhabuddhayaḥ (75/32)
sarvaṁ sarvena sarvatra sarvathā sarvadaiva hi
saṁbhavatyeva sarvātmanyātmanyātatarūpiṇī (75/33)

VASIṢṬHA continued:

He who is endowed with desirelessness (hope-lessness) treats the whole world as if it were the footprint of a calf, the highest mountain as the stump of a felled tree, space as a small box and the three worlds as a blade of grass. The knower of truth regards even the most beautiful woman as a painted image; that is the truth, for both of them are made of the same substance (earth, water, etc.).

When thus the truth is seen, desire to possess does not arise in the heart. Even as a woman who has a lover goes about doing her housework with her heart absorbed in contemplation of that lover, the enlightened sage functions in this world while his consciousness is firmly established in the truth. In both these cases it is impossible for anyone to prevent such behaviour — i.e. make the woman forget her lover or make the sage forget the truth.

Very many such liberated beings exist in the universe, O Rāma. Some of them are sages, others are kings, others shine as stars and planets, others are divinities and others are demons. **O Rāma, there are liberated beings even among worms and insects; and there are stupid fools among the gods. The self is in all; it exists as the all everywhere at all times and in all ways.** The self alone is the Lord and all the divinities. There is void (space) in substances and substantiality in the void or space. What is inappropriate appears appropriate on enquiry. People are righteous because they are afraid of the consequences of sin. Even what is not, leads to what is — the contemplation of space or void leads to the attainment of the supreme truth! What is not comes into being, guided by time and space. On the other hand, what appears to be strong and powerful reaches its own destruction. Thus perceiving the truth, O Rāma, abandon joy and sorrow, grief and attachment. The unreal appears to be real and the real appears to be unreal: hence give up hope and hopelessness and attain equanimity.

In this world, O Rāma, liberation is at hand at all times everywhere. There have been countless beings in this world who have attained self-knowledge and liberation while yet living, like the emperor Janaka. Therefore, do thou become liberated here and now. The attainment of inner peace by utter non-attachment to anything here is known as liberation; this is possible whether the body exists or not. He who is freed from all attachment is liberated.

One should wisely and intelligently exert oneself to attain this liberation; one who does not exert cannot even jump over the footprint of a calf. Hence, O Rāma, resort to spiritual heroism, to right exertion, and by the right self-enquiry strive to reach the perfection of self-knowledge. For one who thus strives, the entire universe is like the footprint of a calf.

cidātmana imā ittham prasphurantiha śakttayaḥ
ityasyā ''ścaryajāleṣu nā 'bhyudeti kutūhalam (77/30)

VASIṢṬHA continued:

All these worlds, O Rāma, appear in Brahman the absolute but they are apprehended as an independent substantial reality on account of ignorance or non-wisdom. Such an erroneous notion ceases on the arising of wisdom. Erroneous perception makes all this appear as 'the world'; right perception brings about the cessation of this error. O Rāma, this error is not dispelled except by right exertion with the right attitude and wisdom. Fie on that person, O Rāma, who, though such possibility of overcoming this illusion exists, remains sunk in the mire of world-illusion. Blessed are you, Rāma, that the right spirit of enquiry has already manifested in your heart. When the truth is realised through such enquiry, strength, intelligence and radiance increase.

The sage who has realised the truth and who is liberated from error here and now beholds this world as he would in deep sleep, without the least craving. He does not apprehend with his inner intelligence even those objects and experiences which seek him unsought, for his own heart is withdrawn into itself. He has no hopes for the future, he does not recall the past nor does he even live in the present; and yet he does all. Asleep, he is awake; awake, he sleeps. He does all, yet he does nothing. Inwardly having renounced everything, though outwardly he appears to be busy, he is ever in a state of equilibrium. His actions are entirely non-volitional.

The sage is unattached to anything or anybody. Hence, his behaviour appears to be devout to the devout and harsh to the harsh. He is a child among children, old man among old men, hero among heroes, youth among youth and sorrowing among the sorrowful. His soft and sweet words are full of wisdom. He has nothing to gain from noble deeds, yet he is noble; he has no longing for pleasure and hence is not tempted by it. He is not attracted to bondage or even to liberation. The net of ignorance and error having been burnt by the fire of wisdom, the bird of his consciousness flies away to liberation.

He is not elated when his efforts bear fruit, nor is he worried if they do not. He appears to take and to abandon with the playfulness of a child. He is not surprised if the moon shines hot and the sun shines cool. Knowing that **the self which is the infinite consciousness can bring all these about, he is not surprised even by such wondrous phenomena.** He is not timid and he is not given to outbursts of anger.

Knowing that beings are constantly born and that they die constantly, he does not give way to joy or grief. He knows that the world arises in his own vision even as the dream-objects arise when one dreams, and hence all these objects are of momentary existence. Therefore, he does not feel any justification for either pity or joy. When all such concepts as pleasure and pain, desirable and undesirable cease, all notions in the mind cease. Error does not arise again, even as oil is not obtained from burnt seed.

prāṇaspandāccitaḥ spandas tatspandādeva saṁvidaḥ
cakrāvartavidhāyinyo jalaspandādivormayaḥ (14)

VASIṢṬHA continued:

O Rāma, just as when a firebrand is swung around, an illusory circle of fire is formed, there is an illusory appearance of the world due to the vibration that arises in consciousness. Vibration and consciousness are inseparably one like the whiteness of snow, the oil in the sesame seed, the fragrance of the flower and the heat of fire. Their description as distinct categories is an error. Mind and movement of thought are inseparable; and the cessation of one is the cessation of both.

O Rāma, there are two ways in which this cessation can be achieved: one is the way of yoga which involves the restraint of the movement of thought, and the other is the way of knowledge which involves the right knowledge of truth.

In this body, that energy (lit. air) which circulates in the energy-channels (nādi lit. means 'channel of motion', not necessarily a nerve though for convenience it may be called so) is known as prāṇa. In accordance with its diverse functions in the body, it is also known by the names apāna, etc. This prāṇa is indistinguishably united with the mind. In fact, the consciousness that tends towards thinking on account of the movement of prāṇa, is known as the mind.. **Movement of thought in the mind arises from the movement of prāṇa; and movement of prāṇa arises because of the movement of thought in consciousness. They thus form a cycle of mutal dependence, like waves and movement of currents in water.**

The wise ones declare that the mind is caused by the movement of prāṇa; and hence by the restraint of the prāṇa, the mind becomes quiescent. When the mind abandons the movement of thought, the appearance of the world-illusion ceases. The movement of prāṇa is arrested at the moment when all hopes and desires come to an end in one's heart through the earnest practice of the precepts of the scriptures and sages, and by the cultivation of dispassion in previous life-spans or through endeavouring to practise contemplation or meditation and reaching a stage of devotion to a single truth in a single-minded way.

The movement of prāṇa is also arrested by the effortless practice of breathing, without strain, in seclusion, or the repetition of the sacred OṀ with the experience of its meaning, when the consciousness reaches the deep sleep state. The practice of exhalation, when the prāṇa roams in space without touching the limbs of the body, of inhalation, leading to the peaceful movement of prāṇa, and of retention, bringing it to a standstill for a long time, all lead to the arrest of the movement of prāṇa. Likewise the closure of the posterior nares by the tip of the tongue as the prāṇa moves towards the crown of the head, the practice of meditation where there is no movement of thought, the holding of the consciousness steadily at a point twelve inches from the tip of the nose, the entering of the prāṇa into the forehead through the palate and upper aperture, the fixing of the prāṇa at the eyebrow centre, the sudden cessation of the movement of thought, or cessation of all mental conditioning through meditation on the space in the heart-centre over a long period of time, all these lead to this arrest of the movement of prāṇa.

saṁvinmātraṁ tu hṛdayamupādeyaṁ sthitaṁ smṛtaṁ
tadantare ca bāhye ca na ca bāhye na cā ''ntare (78/35)

RĀMA asked:

Lord, what is the heart that is spoken of by you?

VASIṢṬHA continued:

O Rāma, two aspects of the 'heart' are spoken of here: one is acceptable and the other is to be ignored. The heart that is part of this physical body and is located in one part of the body may be ignored! **The heart which is acceptable is of the nature of pure consciousness. It is both inside and outside, and it is neither inside nor outside.** That is the principal heart. In it is reflected everything which is in the universe and it is the treasure-house of all wealth. Consciousness alone is the heart of all beings, not the piece of flesh which people call the heart! Hence, if the mind, freed of all conditioning, is gathered into pure consciousness, the movement of prāṇa is restrained.

By any one of these methods, propounded by the various teachers, the movement of prāṇa can be restrained. These yoga methods bring about the desired results if they are practised without violence or force. When one is firmly established in such practice with simultaneous growth in dispassion, and when the mental conditioning comes under perfect restraint, there is fruition of the restraint of the movement of prāṇa.

During the practice one may use as a focus of attention the eyebrow centre, the palate, the tip of the nose or the top of the head (twelve inches from the nose); thus the prāṇa will be restrained. Again, if by steady and persistent practice the tip of the tongue can touch the uvula, the movement of prāṇa will be restricted. Surely, all these practices appear to be distractions; but by their steady practice one reaches the absence of distractions. It is only by such steady practice that one is freed from sorrow, and experiences the bliss of the self. Hence, practice yoga. When through practice the movement of prāṇa is restrained, then nirvāna or liberation alone remains. In it is all; from it is all; it is all; it is everywhere. In it this world-appearance is not, nor is this from it, nor is the world-appearance like it! He who is firmly established in it is liberated while living.

He whose mind is firmly established in peace through the practice of yoga has the right vision of the truth. To see that the supreme self is without beginning and without end and that these countless objects are in fact the self and no other, is the right vision. Erroneous vision leads to rebirth; right vision ends rebirth. In it there is no subject-object (knower-knowable) relationship; for the self (consciousness) is the knower, knowledge and the knowable, too, and the division is ignorance. When this is directly seen there is neither bondage nor liberation. When the sage rests in his own self, with his intelligence firmly established in the inner self, what pleasures can bind him in this world?

mṛtaṁ mano mṛtā cintā mṛto 'haṅkārarākṣasaḥ
vicāramantreṇa samaḥ svasthastiṣṭhāmi kevalaṁ (80/38)

VASIṢṬHA continued:

One who engages himself in enquiry is not tempted by distractions. The eyes but see: the notions pleasant, unpleasant, etc. arise, not in the eyes, but elsewhere. It is even so with the other senses. Hence, the sense functions are not evil. If egoistic thought is linked to these sense functions (which arise and cease in a moment) there is mental agitation.

O eyes! The objects of your experience arise and fall, and they are but appearances. Do not let your gaze linger on them, lest the eternal indwelling consciousness suffer mortality. Be an onlooker that you truly are. O mind! Countless scenes are seen by the eyes in accordance with their natural function; why do you get involved in them?

Indeed, it is through repeated thinking, that this ignorant relationship is strengthened; but I shall now destroy it through right enquiry. When ignorance is destroyed, such illusory relationship between scene, sight and mind will never again arise. The mind alone provides the senses with their intelligence; hence this mind should be destroyed. For a very long time this ghost of a mind generated countless evil notions like lust, anger, etc. Now that the ghost has been laid, I laugh at my own past foolishness. **The mind is dead; all my worries and anxieties are dead; the demon known as ego-sense is dead, too: all this has been brought about through the mantra of enquiry. I am free and happy now.**

All my doubts have ceased. I am without the fever of agitation. Whatever I am, I am — but without craving. When the mind ceases to be, the craving ceases to be, too. When the mind is dead and the craving is dead, delusion has vanished and egolessness is born. Hence I am awakened in this state of wakefulness. When there is only one truth and diversity has no reality at all, what shall I investigate?

I am the eternal self that is omnipresent and subtle. I have reached that state of reality which is unreflected in anything, which is beginningless and endless and which is utterly pure. Whatever is and whatever is not, the mind and the inner reality are all the one infinite consciousness, which is supreme peace beyond comprehension and by which all this is pervaded. Let the mind continue to be or let it die. What is the sense in enquiring into all this, when the self is established in utter equanimity? I remained in a conditioned state as long as I was foolishly engaged in this enquiry. Now that through this enquiry I have reached the unconditioned being, who is the enquirer?

Such thoughts are utterly useless, now that the mind is dead; they may revive this ghost known as the mind. Hence I abandon all these thoughts and notions; contemplating the OM, I shall remain in the self, in total inner silence.

The above line of enquiry was adopted by the sage Saṁvarta who himself described it to me.

tyajadevā 'nugṛhṇāti vṛttīrindriyavardhitāḥ
yasmānnivāryate tasminpronmatta iva dhāvati (14)

VASIṢṬHA continued:

There is another mode of enquiry which was adopted by the sage Vītahavya. This sage used to roam the forests in the mountain ranges known as Vindhyā. At one stage he became totally disenchanted with the affairs of the world which create delusion, and through the contemplation which is free from all perverse notions and thoughts he abandoned the world as a worn-out illusion. He entered his hermitage, seated himself in the lotus posture and remained firm like a mountain peak. Having withdrawn the senses and having turned the attention of the mind upon itself, he began to contemplate as follows:

How fickle is the mind! Even if it is introverted it does not remain steady, but gets agitated in a moment like the surface of the ocean. Tied to the senses (like the sight) it bounces again and again like a ball. **Having been nourished by the senses, the mind grasps the very objects that it has given up; and like a demented person it runs after the very things from which it had been restrained.** It jumps from one object to the other like a monkey.

I shall now consider the character of the five senses through which the mind thus gets distracted. O senses, has the time not yet arrived for you all to attain self-knowledge? Do you not remember the sorrow that followed your pursuit of pleasure? Then, give up this vain excitement. Truly, you are inert and insentient; you are the avenue through which the mind flows out to reach objective experience. I am your Lord, I am consciousness and I alone do all these as the pure intelligence. You, O senses, are false. There is no connection whatsoever between you and the consciousness which is the self. In the very light of the consciousness which is non-volitional, you function even as people perform various actions in the light of the sun. But do not entertain the false notion, O senses, that 'I am intelligent', for you are not. Even the notion 'I am alive', that you entertain falsely, is conducive only to sorrow.

There is nothing but consciousness, which is beginningless and endless. O wicked mind, what then are you? The notions that arise in you, viz., 'I am the doer' and 'I am the enjoyer', which appear to be great rejuvenators, are in fact deadly poisons. Do not be so deluded, O mind; in truth you are neither the doer of anything nor are you the experiencer. You are inert and your intelligence is derived from some other source. How are pleasures related to you? You yourself do not exist; how do you have relations? If you realise 'I am but pure consciousness', then you are indeed the self. Then how does sorrow arise in you, when you are the unlimited and unconditioned consciousness?

kriyate yattu yacchakttyā tattenaiva kṛtaṁ bhavet
lūṇāti dātraṁ puṁśakttyā lāvakaḥ procyate pumān (39)

VĪTAHAVYA continued to contemplate:

O mind, I shall gently bring home to you the truth that you are indeed neither the doer nor the experiencer. You are indeed inert; how can a statue made of stone dance? If your intelligence is entirely dependent upon the infinite consciousness, then may you live long in that realisation. However, **what is done with the intelligence or the energy of another, is considered to be done by the latter. The sickle harvests with the energy of the farmer; and hence the farmer is said to be the harvester.** Similarly, though it is the sword that cuts, the man who wields the sword is the killer. You are inert, O mind; your intelligence is derived from the infinite consciousness. That self or the infinite consciousness knows itself by itself, experiences itself in itself by itself. The Lord endeavours to enlighten you continuously, for the wise should thus instruct the ignorant in a hundred ways. The light of the self alone exists as consciousness or intelligence; that itself has come to be known as the mind. If you realise this truth you will instantly be dissolved.

O fool, when you are in truth the infinite consciousness, why do you grieve? That is omnipresent, that is the all: when you realise it, you become the all. You are not, the body is not: the one infinite consciousness alone exists and in that homogeneous being the diverse concepts of 'I' and 'you' appear to exist. If you are the self, then the self alone exists, not you! If you are inert, but different from the self, then you do not exist either! For the self or the infinite consciousness alone is all; there is naught else. There is no possibility of the existence of a third thing, apart from the consciousness and the inert substance.

Hence, O mind, you are neither the doer nor the experiencer. You have been used as a channel of instruction by the wise ones in their communication with the ignorant. But, in fact, that channel is unreal and inert; the self alone is the reality. If the farmer does not use the sickle, can it harvest? The sword has no power to kill either. O mind, you are neither the doer nor the experiencer. Hence, grieve not. The Lord (consciousness) is not like you; hence do not grieve for him! He does not gain anything by either doing or not-doing. He alone pervades all; there is naught else. Then, what shall he do and what shall he desire?

You have no relationship to the self, except as fragrance to a flower. Relationship exists only between two independent beings of similar nature when they strive to become one. You, O mind, are ever agitated; the self is ever at peace. There can thus be no relationship between you two. If, however, you enter into the state of samādhi, or utter equanimity, you will remain firmly established in consciousness without the distraction of diversity or the notions of either many or one, and realise that there is but one self, the infinite consciousness which shines as these countless beings.

svātmabhāvastava sukhaṁ manye mānavatāṁ vara
tameva bhāvayā 'bhāvaṁ sukhatyāgo hi mūḍhatā (28)

VĪTAHAVYA continued to contemplate:

O senses, I feel that you have all been dispelled by the light of my admonitions, for you are born of darkness of ignorance. O mind, surely your emergence as an appearance is for your own grief! See how, when you exist, countless beings get deluded and enter into this ocean of sorrow with all its prosperity and adversity, illness, old age and death; how greed gnaws at all the good qualities and destroys them; how lust or desire distracts and dissipates their energy.

O mind, when you cease to be, all the good and noble qualities blossom. There is peace and purity of heart. People do not fall into doubt and error. There is friendship, which promotes the happiness of all. Worries and anxieties dry up. When the darkness of ignorance is dispelled, the inner light shines brightly. Mental distraction and distress cease, just as the ocean becomes calm when the wind ceases to agitate its surface. There arises self-knowledge within, and the realisation of truth puts an end to the perception of the world-illusion. Infinite consciousness alone shines. There is an experience of bliss not granted to the ignorant who are full of desires. Even as new shoots may arise from burnt leaves, a new life may emerge from this. However, he who would avoid entanglement in delusion once again, rests in self-knowledge constantly. Such are the fruits of your absence, O mind, and there are countless others. O mind, you are the support of all our hopes and desires; when you cease to be, all these hopes and desires cease. You can now choose either to be one with the reality or to cease to be an independent entity.

Your existence as identical with the self and non-different from it, is conducive to happiness, O mind. Hence, be firmly rooted in the realisation of your non-existence. Surely, it is foolish to neglect happiness. If you exist as the inner being or consciousness, who will wish for your non-existence? But, you are not a real entity; hence your happiness is delusion. You were not real, you came into being through ignorance and delusion, but now through enquiry into your nature and that of the senses and self, you have once again ceased to be. You exist as long as one does not undertake this enquiry. When the spirit of enquiry arises there is total equanimity or homogeneity. You were born of the ignorance which is the absence of wisdom and discrimination. When this wisdom arises, you cease to be. Hence, I salute wisdom! O mind, you were awakened by many means. Now that you have lost the false characteristic of a mind, you exist as the supreme being or the infinite consciousness, freed from all limitation and conditioning. That which arose in ignorance perishes in wisdom. In spite of yourself, O good mind, this enquiry has arisen in you; this is surely for the attainment of bliss. There is indeed no mind, O mind: the self alone exists, it alone is, there is naught else. I am that self, hence there is naught other than me in the universe. I am the infinite consciousness whose kinetic state alone appears as the universe.

yathāsthitamidaṁ viśvam śāntamākāśanirmalaṁ
brahmaiva jīvanmukttānāṁ bandhamokṣadṛśaḥ kutaḥ (84/30)

VASIṢṬHA continued:

After this enquiry, the sage Vītahavya remained in a state of total quiescence (samādhi) and even his prāṇa did not move. Thus he spent three hundred years as if it were an hour. The body which was reflected in the consciousness was protected by it. After this period, his mind began to move in his heart and there arose in it notions of a creation. Then he spent a hundred years as a sage in mount Kailāsa. For a hundred years he was a demi-god. Then he ruled as Indra, the king of heaven, for a period of five world-cycles.

Whatever, wherever and however the infinite consciousness conceives the order, so does it become. Thus he saw all this in his own heart, which was free from all conditioning. On account of his attainment of the infinite consciousness, therefore, these notions apparently arose in it non-volitionally.

After this he served as an attendant of lord Śiva for a whole epoch. All this the liberated sage, Vītahavya, experienced. O Rāma, **for the liberated sages this world exists in all its purity, peace and perfection, as Brahman the infinite: how can there be bondage and liberation for them?** Since Vītahavya had become one with the infinite consciousness he experienced the experiences of all, and he does so even now!

RĀMA asked: If the creation of the sage was fictitious and imaginary, how were the embodied beings in it conscious and sentient?

VASIṢṬHA replied: If the creation of Vītahavya was fictitious, O Rāma, so is this! That and this are both pure infinite consciousness, their appearances being the result of the delusion of the mind.

RĀMA asked: Lord, please tell me how Vītahavya revived his body in the cave.

VASIṢṬHA replied:

The sage had realised the infinite consciousness; and he knew that the mind, called Vītahavya, was but a trick of the infinite consciousness. He thought of seeing that body of Vītahavya. In his own consciousness he saw all the other embodiments that he had had — some of them had come to an end and others were still functioning. And, he saw the body known as Vītahavya sunk like a worm in mud.

Seeing it thus, he reflected: "Surely, this body of mine is devoid of life-force and is therefore unable to function. I shall now enter into the solar orbit and with the help of the solar power known as piṅgala I shall enter that body. Or, shall I abandon it, for what have I to do with the body of Vītahavya?" The sage's subtle body then entered into the orbit of the sun. The sun ordained his own energy to execute the task. The energy of the sun led the way. It descended right where the body of the sage was lying covered in mud, in order to raise it. Following it, the subtle body of Vītahavya also entered that body. The body was instantly revived. Piṅgala returned to the solar orbit and the sage proceeded towards the lake for his bath and ablution.

vismṛtir vismṛtā dūraṁ smṛtiḥ sphuṭamanusmṛtā
satsajjātam asaccā 'sat kṣataṁ kṣiṇaṁ sthitaṁ sthitaṁ (22)

VASIṢṬHA continued:

In the evening the sage once again entered the forest with which he was familiar, for the practice of intense meditation. He thought: "I have already realised the falsity of the senses; any further enquiry concerning them will be a contradiction." Having abandoned all vain imagination ('This is' and 'This is not'), he sat in the lotus posture again and in him arose the knowledge 'I am established in the consciousness of total equanimity. Awake, I remain as if in sleep. Established in the transcendental state of consciousness I shall continue to be till the body drops away.'

Thus resolved, he meditated for six days, which passed as if in a moment. After that he lived a long time as a liberated sage. He was free from exultation and sorrow. At times, he would address his mind thus: "O mind, look how blissful you are, now that you are in a balanced state! Remain like that all the time."

He would address his senses as follows: "O senses! The self does not belong to you, nor do you belong to the self. May you all perish! Your cravings have ceased. You will no longer be able to rule me. The error of your existence arose from ignorance of the self, even as the non-perception of the rope gives rise to the erroneous perception of a snake. All these errors exist in the darkness of non-wisdom, and in the light of wisdom they vanish."

"O senses! You are different from the self, the doer of actions is different from all these, the experiencer of experiences is again different and the infinite consciousness is again different from all these — what is whose error and how does it arise? It is like this: trees grow in the forest, ropes are made of other fibres with which the timber is bound together, the blacksmith fashions an axe, etc. and with all these the carpenter builds a house for his own livelihood, not because he wants to build a house! Thus in this world all things happen independently of one another and their coincidence is accidental — like the ripe cocoanut falling coincidentally when a crow alights on it, making ignorant people feel that the crow dislodged the cocoanut. Who is to blame for all these? When this truth is known, **error remains error, knowledge becomes clear knowledge, the real is real, the unreal is unreal, what has been destroyed is destroyed and what remains, remains."**

Thus reflecting and established in this knowledge, the sage lived in this world for a very long time. He was established in that state which is totally free from ignorance and error, and which ensures that he is not born again. Whenever there was contact with the objects of the senses he resorted to the peace of contemplation, and enjoyed the bliss of the self. His heart was free from attraction and aversion even when all manner of experiences came to him unsought.

mitrakāya mayā yattvaṁ tyajyase cirabāndhavaḥ
tvayaivā ''tmanyupānitā sātmajñānavaśāt kṣatiḥ (36)

VASIṢṬHA continued:

Once the sage Vītahavya felt inclined to abandon his body and to ensure that he would never again return to embodiment. He resorted to a cave on the Sahya mountain, sat in the lotus posture and

VĪTAHAVYA said this within himself:

O attraction, abandon your force of attraction. O hate, abandon hatred. You have played long enough with me. O pleasures, salutations to you; you have indeed sustained me all these years and even made me forget the self. O sorrow, salutations to you; you spurred me on my quest for self-knowledge, and it is by your grace that I have attained this self-knowledge; hence you are indeed the bestower of delight.

O body, my friend, permit me to go to my eternal abode of self-knowledge. Such indeed is the course of nature; everyone has to abandon the body at some time or the other. **O body, my friend, you have been my relation for a long time. I abandon you now. You yourself have brought on this separation by nobly leading me to the realisation of the self.** How wonderful! In order to enable me to attain self-knowledge, you have destroyed yourself.

O mother craving! Give me leave to go; you are now left alone to wither away, because I have reached the state of supreme peace. O lust! In order to conquer you, I befriended your enemy dispassion; forgive me. I proceed to freedom. Bless me. O merit! Salutations to you, for you rescued me from hell and led me to heaven. Salutations to demerit, the source of all pain and punishment. Salutations to delusion, under which I laboured for a long time, and which is not seen by me even now.

O cave, the companion of samādhi (meditation), salutations to you. You have given me shelter when I was tormented by the pains of worldly existence. O staff, you have been my friend too, protecting me from snakes and saving me from falling. Salutations to you.

O body, return to the elements of which you are composed. Salutations to activities like bathing, and salutations to all the activities in this world. Salutations to the life-forces (prāṇa) that have been my companions. Whatever I did in this world was done only with you, through you and because of your energy. Pray, return to your own source, for now I shall merge in the infinite consciousness (Brahman). All things that come together in this world have to part one day or the other. O senses, return to your own sources, the cosmic elements.

I shall now enter into the self by the self indicated by the culmination of the OṀ-sound — as a lamp without fuel. I am free from all the activities of this world and from all notions of perceptions and experiences. My heart is established in the peace indicated by the resonance of the OṀ. Gone are delusion and error.

acinmayaṁ cinmayaṁ ca neti neti yaducyate
tatastat saṁbabhūvā 'sau yadgirāmapyagocaraḥ (87/16)

VASIṢṬHA continued:

With all the desires in the mind utterly silenced and having well grounded himself in the plane of non-dual consciousness, sage Vītahavya uttered the holy word OṀ. Contemplating the esoteric significance of the OṀ he perceived the error of confusing the reality with the appearance. By the total abandonment of all concepts and percepts he renounced the three worlds. He became utterly quiescent, as when the potter's wheel comes to rest. By the utterance of the OṀ he dispelled the web of sense-organs and their objects, even as wind disperses scent. After this, he pierced the darkness of ignorance. He beheld the inner light for just a split second, but renounced that too immediately. He transcended both light and darkness. There remained just a trace of thought-form; this, too, the sage cut asunder in the twinkling of an eye, through the mind. Now the sage remained in the pure infinite consciousness, not modified in the least; it was like the state of consciousness of the just-born infant. He abandoned all objectivity of consciousness and even the slightest movement of consciousness. He crossed the state known as 'paśyantī' and reached the deep-sleep consciousness. He continued beyond that, too, and reached the transcendental or turīya consciousness. It is a state of bliss that is not its description, which is both the 'is' and the 'is not', both something and not-something, light and darkness. **It is full of non-consciousness and (objectless) consciousness, it can only be indicated by negation (not this, not this). He became that which is beyond description.**

That state is the void, Brahman, consciousness, the Puruṣa of the Sāṅkhya, Īśvara of the yogi, Śiva, time, Ātman or self, non-self and the middle etc. of the mystics holding different views. It is that state which is established as the truth by all these scriptural viewpoints, that which is all — in that the sage remained firmly established.

When the sage had thus become one with the infinite consciousness, the body decomposed and the elements returned to their respective source.

Thus have I told you, O Rāma, the auspicious story of the sage Vītahavya. Reflect over it. Whatever I have said to you and whatever I shall say to you now is born of direct perception, direct experience and deep contemplation.

Meditate upon this, O Rāma, and attain wisdom. Liberation is attained only by wisdom or self-knowledge. Only through such wisdom does one go beyond sorrow; destroy ignorance and attain perfection.

What has been described as Vītahavya is only a notion in our mind; so am I and so are you. All these senses and the whole world are nothing but the mind. What else can the world be, O Rāma?

avidyāmapi ye yukttyā sādhayanti sukhātmikām
te hyavidyāmayā eva na tvātmajñāstathākramāḥ (15)

RĀMA asked:

Lord, why do we not see many of these liberated sages traversing the sky now?

VASIṢṬHA replied:

Flying in the sky and other powers are natural to some beings, O Rāma. The extraordinary qualities and faculties which are observed in this world are natural to those beings — not to the sages of self-knowledge. Supernatural faculties (like flying in the air) are developed by even those who are devoid of self-knowledge or liberation, by the utilisation of certain substances or by certain practices. All this does not interest the man of self-knowledge who is utterly content in himself. **They who, in pursuit of pleasures, acquire these powers tainted by ignorance, are surely full of ignorance; the sages of self-knowledge do not adopt such a course.**

Whether one is a knower of truth or ignorant of it, powers like flying in the air accrue to one who engages himself in some practices. But the sage of self-knowledge has no desire to acquire these. These practices bestow their fruit on anyone, for such is their nature. Poison kills all, wine intoxicates all, even so these practices bring about the ability to fly, etc., but they who have attained the supreme self-knowledge are not interested in these, O Rāma. They are gained only by those who are full of desires; but the sage is free from the least desire for anything. Self-knowledge is the greatest gain; how does the sage of self-knowledge entertain any desire for anything else? In the case of Vītahavya, however, he did not desire these powers: they sought him unsought.

RĀMA asked: How is it that worms and vermin did not destroy Vītahavya's body when it lay abandoned in the cave? And how was it that Vītahavya did not attain disembodied liberation in the first place?

VASIṢṬHA replied: O Rāma, the ignorant man's body is composed and decomposed on account of the states of his mental conditioning; in the case of one who has no such conditioning, there is no momentum for decomposition. Again, the mind of all beings responds to the qualities of the object with which it comes into contact. When a violent creature comes into contact with one who has reached utter equanimity, it also becomes temporarily equanimous and tranquil, though it may return to its violence when this contact is lost. Hence, too, Vītahavya's body remained unharmed. This applies even to material substances like earth, wood, etc. for consciousness pervades all. Since Vītahavya's consciousness did not undergo any change, no change happened to his body. Since there was no movement of prāṇa in it, even decomposition could not take place. The sage is independent and free to live or to abandon the body. That he did not abandon the body at one time and did so later is purely coincidental; it may be related to his karma etc., but in truth he is beyond karma, beyond fate and devoid of mental conditioning. Again, it is like the crow dislodging the ripe cocoanut — purely coincidental.

manastāṁ mūḍhatāṁ viddhi yadā naśyati sā 'nagha
cittanāśābhidhānaṁ hi tadā sattvamudetyalaṁ (16)

VASIṢṬHA continued:

When the mind of Vītahavya had become unattached and totally free through the practice of enquiry, there arose in him noble qualities like friendliness, etc.

RĀMA asked:

When the mind has been dissolved in Brahman the absolute, in whom do qualities like friendliness arise?

VASIṢṬHA answered:

O Rāma, there are two types of 'death of the mind'. One is where the form of the mind remains and the other is where even the form ceases to be. The former happens when the sage is still alive and the latter happens when he is disembodied. The existence of the mind causes misery and its cessation brings joy. The mind that is heavily conditioned and caught in its own conditioning brings about repeated births. Such a mind brings unhappiness. That which regards as 'my own' the qualities that are beginningless is the jiva. It arises in the mind which has no self-knowledge and which is therefore unhappy.

As long as there is mind, there is no cessation of sorrow. When the mind ceases the world-appearance also ceases to be. The mind is the seed for misery.

I shall now describe how the mind ceases to be. When both happiness and unhappiness do not divert a man from his utter equanimity, then know that his mind is dead. He in whom the notions 'this I am' and 'this I am not' do not arise, thus limiting his consciousness — his mind is dead. He in whom the very notions of calamity, poverty, elation, pride, dullness and excitement do not arise — his mind is dead, and he is liberated while living.

The very nature of the mind is stupidity. Hence when it dies, purity and noble qualities arise. Some wise men refer to 'the pure mind' as that state of utter purity that prevails in a liberated sage in whom the mind is dead. Such a mind of the liberated sage is, therefore, full of noble qualities like friendliness, etc. The existence (sattā) of such natural goodness in a liberated sage is known as satva, purity, etc. Hence, this is also called 'death of the mind where form remains'.

The death of the mind where even the form vanishes pertains to the disembodied sage. In the case of such a mind, no trace is left. It is impossible to describe it in a positive way. In it there are neither qualities nor their absence, neither virtues nor their absence, neither light nor darkness, no conditioning and no notions at all, neither existence nor non-existence. It is a state of supreme quiescence and equilibrium. They who have risen beyond the mind and the intelligence reach that supreme state of peace.

dve bije cittavṛkṣasya vṛttivratatidhāriṇaḥ
ekaṁ prāṇaparispando dvitiyaṁ dṛḍhabhāvanā (14)

RĀMA asked:

Lord, what is the seed of this fearful tree known as the mind, and what is the seed of that seed, and so on?

VASIṢṬHA replied:

Rāma, the seed for this world-appearance is the body within, with all its notions and concepts of good and evil. That body also has a seed which is the mind, which flows constantly in the direction of hopes and desires and which is also the repository of notions of being and non-being and the consequent sorrow. The world-appearance arises only in the mind, and this is illustrated by the dream state. Whatever is seen here as the world is but the expansion of the mind, even as pots are transformations of clay.

The two seeds for the tree known as the mind, which carries within it innumerable notions and ideas, are movement of prāṇa (life-force) and obstinate fancy. When there is movement of prāṇa in the appropriate channels, then there is movement in consciousness and mind arises. Again, it is the movement of prāṇa alone (when it is seen or apprehended by the mind) that is seen as this world-appearance, which is as real as the blueness of the sky. The cessation of the movement of prāṇa is the cessation of the world-appearance too. The omnipresent consciousness is 'awakened', as it were, by the movement of prāṇa. If this does not happen, then there is supreme good.

When consciousness is 'awakened' thus, it begins to apprehend objects, ideas arise and thence sorrow. On the other hand, if this consciousness rests in itself, as if fast asleep, then one attains what is most desirable, and that is the supreme state. Therefore, you will realise the unborn state of consciousness if you either restrain the movement of prāṇa in your own psychological ground (of concepts and notions), or refrain from disturbing the homogeneity in consciousness. It is when this homogeneity is disturbed and the consciousness experiences diversity that the mind arises, and the countless psychological conditions spring up into activity.

In order to bring about quiescence of the mind, the yogi practises prāṇāyāma (restraint of the movement of the life-force), meditation and such other proper and appropriate methods. Great yogī regard this prāṇāyāma itself as the most appropriate method for the achievement of tranquillity of the mind, peace, etc.

I shall now describe to you the other viewpoint, that of the men of wisdom, born of their direct experience: they declare that the mind is born of one's obstinate clinging to a fancy or deluded imagination.

hṛdi saṁvedyamāpyayva prāṇaspando 'tha vāsanā
udeti tasmāt saṁvedyaṁ kathitaṁ bījametayoḥ (64)

VASIṢṬHA continued:

When obstinately clinging to a fancy and therefore abandoning a thorough enquiry into the nature of truth, one apprehends an object with that fancy — such apprehension is described as conditioning or limitation. When such fancy is persistently and intensely indulged in, this world-appearance arises in consciousness.

When the psychological conditioning or limitation is not dense, when it has become transparent, one becomes a liberated sage who apparently lives and functions by past momentum (even as a potter's wheel rotates after the initial impulse has been withdrawn), but he will not be born again. In his case the seed has been fried, as it were, and will not germinate into world-illusion. When the body falls he is absorbed into the infinite.

Of the two seeds for this world-illusion (viz., movement of prāṇa and clinging to fancy), if one is got rid of, the other also goes away; for the two are interdependent. The mind creates the world-illusion and the mind is created by the movement of prāṇa in one's own conditioning. Again, this movement of prāṇa also takes place because of the mental conditioning or fancy. Thus this vicious circle is completed; one feeds the other, one spurs the other into action. Motion is natural to prāṇa and when it moves in consciousness, mind arises; then the conditioning keeps the prāṇa in motion. When one is arrested, both fall.

Rāma, the notion of an object (of knowledge, of experience) is the seed for both movement of prāṇa and for the clinging to a fancy, for it is only when such desire for experience arises in the heart that such movement of prāṇa and mental conditioning take place. When such desire for experience is abandoned, both these cease instantly.

Of course, the indwelling consciousness is the seed for this desire for experiencing: for without that consciousness the desire for such experience will not arise at all. However, it has no object of experience either outside or inside. When this truth is realised, the illusion ceases to be. Hence, O Rāma, strive to eradicate the desire for experience. Get rid of idleness. Free yourself from all experiences.

RĀMA asked:

Lord, how can these two be reconciled? Can I seek freedom from all experiences and freedom from inactivity at the same time?

VASIṢṬHA replied:

He who has no desire or hope for anything here, nor entertains a wish to rest in inactivity, such a one does not exist as a jiva; he is neither inactive nor does he seek to experience. He who does not lean towards experience or perception of objects, though he is engaged in ceaseless activity, is neither inactive nor does he do anything or experience anything. The objective experiences do not touch the heart at all: hence, he whose consciousness is not inactive is a liberated sage here and now.

adhyātmavidyādhigamaḥ sādhusaṅgama eva ca
vāsanāsaṁparityāgaḥ prāṇaspandanirodhanam (35)

RĀMA asked: Holy sir, kindly tell me how one may quickly destroy all these seeds of distraction and reach the supreme state.

VASIṢṬHA said:

These seeds of sorrow, O Rāma, can each be destroyed by destruction of the previous one. But, if you can at one stroke cut off all mental conditioning and by great self-effort rest in the state of pure existence (if you rest in that state even for a second) in no time you will be established in it. If however you wish merely to find your foot-hold in pure existence, you can achieve it by even greater effort. Similarly, by contemplating the infinite consciousness, too, you can rest in the supreme state: but that demands greater effort.

Meditation is not possible on objects of experience: for they exist only in consciousness or the self. But if you strive to destroy the conditioning (the concepts, notions, habits, etc.), then in a moment all your errors and illnesses will vanish. However, this is more difficult that the ones described earlier. For, until the mind is free from the movement of thought, cessation of conditioning is difficult, and vice versa; and unless the truth is realised, the mind does not cease to function, and vice versa. Yet, again, until the conditioning ceases, the unconditioned truth is not realised, and vice versa. Since realisation of truth, cessation of the mind and the ending of conditioning are interwoven, it is extremely difficult to deal with them individually and separately.

Hence, O Rāma, by every means in your power renounce the pursuit of pleasure and resort to all three simultaneously. If all these are simultaneously practised for a considerable time, they become fruitful, not otherwise. O Rāma, this world-appearance has been experienced as truth for a very long time and it needs persistent practice of all these three simultaneously to overcome it.

Wise ones declare that the abandonment of conditioning and the restraint of prāṇa are of equal effect: hence, one should practise them simultaneously. Prāṇa is restrained by the practice of prāṇāyāma and the yoga āsanā, as taught by the guru, or by other means. When desires, aversions and cravings do not arise in the mind even though their objects are seen in front, then it is to be inferred that mental conditioning has weakened; thence wisdom arises, further weakening the conditioning. Then the mind ceases.

It is not possible to 'kill the mind' without proper methods. **Knowledge of the self, company of holy men, the abandonment of conditioning and the restraint of prāṇa** are the means to overcome the mind. Ignoring these and resorting to violent practices like Haṭha Yoga, austerities, pilgrimage, rites and rituals, is a waste of time. Self-knowledge alone bestows delight on you. A man of self-knowledge alone lives. Hence, gain self-knowledge, O Rāma.

bhāvābhāve padārthānāṁ harṣāmarṣavikāradā
malinā vāsanā yaiṣā sā saṅga iti kathyate (84)

VASIṢṬHA continued:

He who acts without attachment, merely with the organs of action, is not affected by anything, neither by joy nor by sorrow. His actions are non-volitional. He sees not, though eyes see; he hears not, though ears hear; he touches not, though the body touches. Surely, attachment (contact, association) is the cause for this world-illusion; it alone creates objects. Attachment causes bondage and endless sorrow. Therefore, holy ones declare that the abandonment of attachment is itself liberation. Abandon attachment, O Rāma, and be a liberated sage.

Attachment is that, O Rāma, which makes the conditioning of the mind more and more dense, by repeatedly causing the experiences of pleasure and pain in relation to the existence and the non-existence of the objects of pleasure, thus confirming such association as inevitable and bringing about an intense attachment to the objects of pleasure. In the case of the liberated sage, however, this conditioning is freed from the experiences of joy and sorrow: hence it is purified, i.e., the conditioning is weakened if not destroyed. Even if it exists in an extremely weakened state till the death of the body, the actions that spring from such a weakened and so pure conditioning do not result in rebirth.

On the other hand, the dense conditioning which exists in the unwise is itself known as attachment. If you abandon this attachment which causes perverse notions in you, the actions that you may spontaneously perform here will not affect you. If you rise beyond joy and sorrow and therefore treat them alike, and if you are free from attraction, aversion and fear, you are unattached. If you do not grieve in sorrow, if you do not exult in happiness and if you are independent of your own desires and hopes, you are unattached. Even while carrying on your activities here, if you do not abandon your awareness of the homogeneity of the truth, you are unattached. If you have gained self-knowledge and if, endowed with equal vision, you engage yourself in spontaneous and appropriate action in the here and now, you are unattached.

By effortlessly remaining established in non-attachment, live here as a liberated sage without being attracted by anything. The liberated sage lives in the inner silence, without pride or vanity, without jealousy and with his senses fully under his control. Even when all the objects of the world are spread out in front of him, the liberated sage, who is free from cravings, is not tempted by them, but engages himself in mere natural actions. Whatever is inevitable and appropriate, he does; his joy and delight, however, he derives from within; thus he is freed from this world-appearance. Even as milk does not abandon its colour when it is boiled, he does not abandon his wisdom even when it is severely tested by terrible calamities. Whether he is subjected to great pain or he is appointed the ruler of heaven, he remains in a balanced state of mind.

anayaiva dhiyā rāma viharannaiva badhyase
anyathā 'dhaḥ patasyāśu vindhyakhāte yathā gajaḥ (1/26)

VASIṢṬHA said:

I have thus provided you with a net woven with words which are indicative of the highest truth: tie down the bird of your mind with this net and let the mind then rest in your heart. Thus shall you attain self-knowledge. O Rāma, have you absorbed this truth imparted by me, although it is mixed with various expressions and illustrations, even as the proverbial swan is able to separate milk from water when these are mixed together, and to drink the milk alone?

You should contemplate this truth again and again, and reflect upon it from beginning to end. You should march along this path now, O noble one. **Though engaged in diverse activities, you will not be bound if your intelligence is saturated with this truth; otherwise, you will fall, even as an elephant falls from the cliff.** Again, if you conceptualise this teaching for your intellectual entertainment and do not let it act in your life, you will stumble and fall like a blind man.

In order to reach the state of perfection or liberation taught by me you should live a life of non-attachment, doing what is appropriate in every situation as it reaches you. Rest assured that this is the vital factor in the teachings of all scriptures.

VĀLMĪKI said:

Given leave to depart, all the kings and the sages of the assembly left for their abode. They contemplated Vasiṣṭha's teachings and discussed it among themselves, spending only a couple of hours in pleasant and deep sleep.

Next morning, Rāma, Lakṣmaṇa and all the others proceeded swiftly to the hermitage of the sage Vasiṣṭha. All of them took their allotted seats as on the previous days.

VASIṢṬHA said:

O Rāma, do you remember what I have so far said to you, the words which are capable of awakening a knowledge of truth or self-knowledge?

By resorting to dispassion (the unconditioned mind) and a clear understanding of the truth, this ocean of saṁsāra (bondage to life and death) can be crossed. The one infinite absolute existence or cosmic consciousness alone is. Knowing this, be free of the ego-sense and rejoice in the self. There is no mind, no ignorance, no individual soul: these are all concepts that arose in the Creator. As long as one considers the body as the 'I' and as long as the self is related to what is seen, as long as there is hope in objects with the feeling 'this is mine', so long will there be delusion concerning mind, etc.

jīvanmuktā mahātmāno ye parāvaradarśinaḥ
teṣāṁ yā cittapadavī sā sattvamiti kathyate (42)

VASIṢṬHA continued:

The illusory notion of the existence of the mind, etc. persists only as long as the sublime realisation of the truth is not experienced through the company of the wise who are totally unattached, and as long as wickedness has not been weakened. As long as the experience of this world as a reality has not been shaken by the energy derived from the clear perception of the truth, so long the existence of the mind etc., seems to be self-evident. Such a notion continues as long as there is blind dependence, on account of craving for objective experience, and as long as there are wickedness and delusion as a consequence.

But in the case of one who is not attracted by pleasure, whose heart is cool because of its purity and who has shattered the cage of desires, cravings and hopes, the deluded notion of the existence of the mind ceases to be. When he sees even his body as the deluded experience of a non-entity, how can a mind arise in him? He who has the vision of the infinite and into whose heart the world-appearance has merged, does not entertain the deluded notion of a jīva, etc.

When incorrect perception has come to an end and when the sun of self-knowledge arises in the heart, know that the mind is reduced to naught. It is not seen again, even as burnt dry leaves are not seen. **The state of mind of the liberated ones who are still living and who see both the supreme truth and the relative appearance, is known as satva (transparency).** It is improper to call it the mind: it is really satva. These knowers of truth are mindless and are in a state of perfect equilibrium; they live their life here playfully. They behold the inner light all the time, even though they seem to be engaged in diverse actions. Concepts of duality, unity or such others do not arise in them, for there are no tendencies in their heart. The very seed of ignorance is burnt in the state of satva and it does not again give rise to delusion.

O Rāma, you have reached that state of satva and your mind has been burnt in the fire of wisdom. What is that wisdom? It is that the infinite Brahman is indeed the infinite Brahman, the world-appearance is but an appearance whose reality is Brahman. The appearance (for instance, your body as 'Rāma') is insentient, is unreal; its reality is the reality of its substratum which is consciousness. Why then do you grieve? However, if you feel that all this is consciousness, there need not arise in you the notions of diversity. Recollect your essential nature as the infinite consciousness. Abandon the notions of diversity. You are what you are: nay, not even that as a concept, but beyond it you are the self-luminous being. Salutations to you, O cosmic being that is infinite consciousness.

mahātaraṅga gambhīra bhāsurātma cidarṇavāḥ
rāmābhidhormistamitaḥ samaḥ saumyo 'si vyomavat (3/4)

VASIṢṬHA continued:

That which is known as Rāma is in truth the magnificent and infinite ocean of consciousness in which numerous universes appear and disappear like ripples and waves. Remain in a state of total equanimity. You are like infinite space. Fire is inseparable from heat, fragrance from lotus, blackness from collyrium, whiteness from snow, sweetness from sugarcane and light from a luminary. Even so, experiencing is inseparable from consciousness. Even as waves are inseparable from the ocean, the universes are inseparable from consciousness.

Experiencing is non-different from consciousness, the ego-sense is non-different from experiencing, the jīva is non-different from ego-sense and the mind is non-different from the jīva (non-different or inseparable). The senses are non-different from the mind, the body is non-different from the senses, the world is non-different from the body and there is nothing but this world. This catalogue of dependent categories has existed for a very long time; yet this has neither been set in motion by anyone, nor can we say whether it has existed for a very long or a very short time. The truth is, O Rāma, that all this is naught else but the self-experiencing of the infinite.

There is an emptiness in the empty, Brahman pervades Brahman, the truth shines in the truth and fullness fills fullness. The wise man, though functioning in this world, does nothing, for he seeks nothing. Even so, O Rāma, remain pure at heart like space, but outwardly engage yourself in appropriate action; in situations which could provoke exultation or depression, remain unaffected by them like a log of wood. He who is friendly even to one who is about to murder him, is a seer of truth. Adoration of one who has not thus risen above likes and dislikes (rāga and dveṣa) is futile effort. Only he who is free from egoistic or volitional activity and who is utterly non-attached to anything here, is liberated: even if he should destroy the world, he does nothing.

He in whom all concepts and habitual tendencies have ceased has overcome all mental conditioning and bondage. He is like a lamp which is not fed with oil.

You have listened intently to my words: and on account of that the veil of ignorance has been lifted in you. Even ordinary human beings are profoundly influenced by the words of their family preceptor: how can it be different in one who possesses an expanded vision, as you do?

RĀMA said:

All my doubts have been dispelled. I am free from attraction and resistance. I am established in nature. I am well (svasthah: I rest in the self) and I am happy. I am Rāma in whom the worlds find their refuge. Salutations to me, salutations to you.

bhedamabhyupagamyā 'pi śṛṇu buddhi vivṛddhaye
bhavedalpaprabuddhānām api no duḥkhitā yathā (2)

VASIṢṬHA continued:

O Rāma, you are dear to me: hence I declare the truth to you once again. Listen attentively. **Listen, though for doing so, you have to assume the existence of diversity. Your consciousness will expand. And the truth that I shall expound will save from sorrow even they who are not fully awakened.**

When one is ignorant, one entertains the wrong notion that the body is the self; his own senses prove to be his worst enemies. On the other hand, he who is endowed with self-knowledge and knows the truth enjoys the friendship of his senses, which are pleased and contented; they do not destroy him. The self is not affected by the body, nor is the body in any way related to the self. They are like light and darkness.

Correct understanding of the body and the intelligence that dwells in the body enables one to understand the entire creation in its material and its spiritual aspects, as easily as one sees objects illumined by a lamp. It is only when there is not this right understanding that deluded and wrong notions rise and flourish within one's heart — notions which are utterly devoid of substance. Befuddled by these wrong notions which arise in the absence of the light of true knowledge, one is constantly and restlessly carried hither and thither like a blade of grass in wind.

In the absence of the 'taste' (direct knowledge) of cosmic intelligence, the senses endeavour to apprehend their objects and vainly imagine that such contact gives rise to meaningful experience! Surely, the infinite and inexhaustible intelligence (consciousness) dwells in all these; however on account of the absence of self-knowledge, it appears to be ignorant of itself and therefore limited and finite.

The life-force and its retinue function here merely to provide energy for the movements inherent in living, not with any other motive. In the absence of self-knowledge, all the talking and roaring which people indulge in are like the sound produced by a gun! They inevitably proceed towards destruction and do not lead to salutory results. Fools enjoy the fruits of their labour, not knowing that they are resting and sleeping on a rock that is burning hot.

Keeping company with such fools is like sitting in a forest on a tree which is about to be felled. Whatever you do for the sake of such people is like beating the air with a rod. What is given to them is thrown into mud, and to converse with them is as meaningful as a dog barking at the sky.

Ignorance of the self is the source of all troubles and calamities. Is there a single trouble that does not spring from ignorance of the self? This entire creation is pervaded by ignorance which sustains it. One who is ignorant is visited again and again by terrible sorrow and rarely by pleasure.

janma bālyam vrajatyetad yauvanam yuvatā jarām
jarā maraṇamabhyeti mūḍhasyaiva punaḥ punaḥ (6/45)

VASIṢṬHA continued:

Only in the heart of the wicked man grows the dreadful tree of infatuation. In the forest of his vicious heart rages the fire of hate. His mind is flooded with jealousy, giving rise to the growth of the weeds of destructive criticism of others; the only lotus his heart knows is envy, which is sought by the bees of endless worry. Death is meant only for such vicious fools. **Birth and childhood lead to youth, youth leads to old age, and old age ends in death — and all these are repeatedly experienced by the ignorant.**

With a small piece of flesh (the eyes) the foolish man sees a little particle of earth which he regards as mountains, lakes, forests and cities. They whom one regards as radiant women decked with pearls and other jewels are but the creation of one's own delusion: they are the ripples that arise in the ocean of lust. It is on account of delusion that one seeks wealth and prosperity — which are sweet in the beginning to the dull-witted, which are the cause of the pairs of opposites (happiness and unhappiness, pleasure and pain, success and failure) in the middle, and which come to an end very soon. From the pursuit of prosperity arise countless branches of pleasure and numberless branches of unhappiness.

This delusion flows like a river from beginningless time and it is muddied and darkened by useless actions and their reactions. Such actions are like an ill-wind that raises a cloud of dust whose particles are physical and mental illness, old age and the various relationships. All these lead to death (or the passage of time) which has an insatiable and voracious appetite and which consumes all the worlds when they are ripe, as it were.

Youth is haunted by the goblins of worries and anxieties which dance when the wisdom-moon does not shine; and youth proceeds towards denser darkness of delusion. One's tongue (the faculty of speech) is overworked in the service of the common and uncultured folk here and it grows debilitated. In the meantime, poverty spreads its thousands of branches yielding the fruits of unhappiness and hard labour. Yet greed which is empty and insubstantial and destructive of one's own spiritual elevation, continues to proclaim victory in the darkness of delusion. Stealthily the cat of senility catches the mouse of youth.

This creation is essenceless; yet, it gains a false reality. It even grows the fruits of dharma (righteous living) and artha (pursuit of prosperity). This world, enveloped by the sky and endowed with the eyes of the sun and the moon, is upheld by the delusion of its substantiality. In the lake of this world-appearance lilies known as bodies blossom and they are resorted to by the bees known as life-forces.

ajñānād vṛddhim āyāti tadeva syāt phalaṁ sphuṭaṁ
jñānenā ''yāti saṁvittis tāmevā 'nte prayacchati (8/6)

VASIṢṬHA continued:

The decadent concept of the world-existence lies imprisoned in the senses, bound by self-limitation and conditioning and by the powerful thread of hopes and desires. This world-appearance is like a delicate creeper which constantly trembles in the wind of the movement of prāṇa or life-force and which constantly sheds all kinds of beings, abandoning them to their destruction.

There are many noble people who have risen above the quagmire of this hell known as world-existence and, devoid of all doubt, rejoice for a little while. There are the divine beings who dwell like lotuses in the blue expanse of the firmament. In this creation, actions are like the lily which is polluted by vain desire for the fruits of such actions. This world-appearance is like a little fish which comes into being in this infinite space and which is soon swallowed by the obstinate and invincible old vulture known as kṛtānta (the end or conclusion of action). Yet, diverse scenes arise and cease day after day, as ripples and waves appear and disappear on the surface of the ocean. Such is the state of this creation. But since the ignorant are bound fast to their own false notions, neither the transiency of the world nor the hard blow they suffer in their life is able to awaken them.

Whereas the immobile creatures stand contemplating the mystery of time, as it were, the mobile creatures swayed by the twin-forces of attraction and repulsion, love and hate, and afflicted by the terrible illness known as pleasure and pain, old age and death, become debilitated and decadent. Among the latter, the worms and vermin silently and patiently endure the fruits of their own past evil actions, contemplating them, as it were, all the time. But the imperceptible time (or death), which is beyond even contemplation, devours all and everything.

All prosperity and all adversity, childhood, youth, old age and death, as also suffering, what is known as being immersed in happiness and unhappiness and all the rest of it: all these are the extensions of the dense darkness of ignorance.

That ignorance expands by means of ignorance, and yields greater ignorance; when it seeks wisdom, it feeds on wisdom and grows into wisdom in the end. This creeper of ignorance is made manifest in its various pastimes and psychological states or modes. Somewhere at some time it falls on (comes into contact with) wisdom, and is purified; but it gets attached again. It is the source of all emotions and sense-experiences. Its sap is the memory of past experiences. Vicāra or enquiry into the nature of the self is the termite that eats it away. This creeper itself is manifest as all these: the stars and planets, the living beings, the plants, the elements, heaven and earth, the gods as well as the worms and vermin. Whatever there is in this universe is pervaded by this ignorance. When it is transcended you will attain self-knowledge.

udetyavidyā vidyāyāḥ salilādiva budbudaḥ
vidyāyāṁ līyate 'vidyā payasīva hi budbudaḥ (16)

RĀMA asked:

Lord, I am puzzled by your statement that even the gods like Viṣṇu and Śiva are part of this ignorance or avidyā. Pray explain that statement further.

VASIṢṬHA replied:

The truth or existence-consciousness-bliss absolute is beyond thought and understanding, it is supreme peace and omnipresent, it transcends imagination and description. There arises naturally in it the faculty of conceptualisation. This self-understanding is considered to be threefold: subtle, middling and gross. The intellect that comprehends these three regards them as satva, rajas and tamas. The three together constitute what is known as prakṛti or nature. Avidyā or ignorance is prakṛti or nature, and it is threefold. This is the source of all beings; beyond it is the supreme.

These three qualities of nature (satva, rajas and tamas) are subdivided again into three each, i.e. the subtle, middling and gross of each of these. Thus you have nine categories. These nine qualities constitute the entire universe.

The sages, the ascetics, the perfected ones, the dwellers of the netherworld, the celestials and the gods are the sātvika part of ignorance. Among these, the celestials and the dwellers of the netherworld form the gross (tāmasa), the sages form the middling (rājasa) and the gods Viṣṇu, Śiva, etc. form the sātvika part. They who come under the category of satva are not born again: hence they are considered liberated. They exist as long as this world lasts. The others (like the sages), who are liberated while living (jīvanmukta), shed their body in course of time, reach the abode of the gods, dwell there during the period of existence of the world and then are liberated. Thus this part of avidyā or ignorance has become vidyā or self-knowledge. **Avidyā arises in vidyā just as ripples arise in the ocean; and avidyā dissolves in vidyā just as ripples dissolve in the water.**

The distinction between the ripples and the water is unreal and verbal. Even so, the distinction between ignorance and knowledge is unreal and verbal. There is neither ignorance here nor even knowledge! When you cease to see knowledge and ignorance as two distinct entities, what exists alone exists. The reflection of vidyā in itself is considered avidyā. When these two notions are abandoned, what remains is the truth: it may be something or it may be nothing! It is omnipotent, it is more empty than space and yet it is not empty because it is full of consciousness. Like the space within a pot, it is indestructible and everywhere. It is the reality in all things. Just as a magnet makes iron filings move by its very presence, it causes cosmic motion without intending to do so. Hence, it is said that it does nothing at all.

parijñāya parityāgo vāsanānāṁ ya uttamaḥ
sattāsāmānyarūpatvaṁ tat kaivalyapadaṁ viduḥ (14)

VASIṢṬHA continued:

Thus, all this world-appearance with all the mobile and immobile beings in it is naught whatsoever. Nothing has really become physical or material. If conceptualisation (which gives rise to notions of being and non-being) is eliminated, then it is realised that all these jīvā (the individual souls), etc. are empty expressions. All the relationships that arise in one's heart on account of ignorance are seen to be non-existent. Even when the rope is mistaken for a snake, no one can be bitten by that snake!

It is absence of self-knowledge that is known as ignorance or delusion. When the self is known one reaches the shores of limitless intelligence. When consciousness objectifies itself and regards itself as its own object of observation, there is avidyā or ignorance. When this subject-object notion is transcended, all the veils that envelop the reality are removed. The individual is nothing more than the personalised mind. Individuality ceases when that mind ceases; it remains as long as the notion of a personality remains. So long as there is a pot there is also the notion of a space enclosed within or confined to that pot; when it is broken, the infinite space alone is, even where the pot-space was imagined before.

RĀMA asked:

Lord, please tell me how this cosmic intelligence becomes things like insentient rocks.

VASIṢṬHA replied:

In these substances like rocks, consciousness remains immobile, having abandoned the thinking faculty but not having been able to reach the state of no-mind. It is like the state of deep sleep, far away from the state of liberation.

RĀMA asked again:

But, if they exist as in a state of deep sleep without any concepts or percepts, I think they are close to liberation!

VASIṢṬHA replied:

Mokṣa, liberation or the realisation of the infinite is not existence as an immobile creature! Liberation is attained when one arrives at the state of supreme peace after intelligent enquiry into the nature of the self and after this has brought about an inner awakening. **Kaivalya or total freedom is the attainment of pure being after all mental conditioning is transcended consciously and after a thorough investigation.** The wise ones say that one is established in pure being or Brahman only after one has investigated the nature of the truth as expounded in the scriptures, in the company of and with the help of enlightened sages.

yatrā 'sti vāsanābījaṁ tat suṣuptaṁ na siddhaye
nirbīja vāsanā yatra tatturyaṁ siddhidaṁ smṛtaṁ (20)

VASIṢṬHA continued:

As long as psychological limitation and conditioning remain in the heart, even in their subtle 'seed' state, it should be regarded as the deep sleep state; it gives rise to rebirth, even if a state of tranquillity is experienced and even when the mind appears to be self-absorbed. It is an inert state and is the source of unhappiness. Such is the state of the insentient and immobile objects like rocks, etc. They are not free of self-limitation (vāsanā) but self-limitation is hidden and latent in them even as flowers are latent in seeds (which sprout, grow and yield flowers) and pots in clay. **Where the seed of vāsanā (self-limitation, conditioning or tendency) exists, that state is like deep sleep; it is not perfection. When all vāsanā are destroyed and even the potentiality of the vāsanā does not exist, that state is known as the fourth (beyond waking, dream and deep sleep) and transcendental state. It brings about perfection.** Vāsanā, fire, debt, disease, enemy, friendship (or glue), hate and poison— all these are bothersome even if a little residue is left after their removal.

On the other hand, if all the vāsanā have been completely removed, then one is established in the state of pure being; whether such a one is alive or not, he is not again afflicted by sorrow. The cit-śakti (energy-consciousness) lies in immobile creatures, etc., as latent vāsanā. It is this cit-śakti that determines the nature of each object; it is the fundamental characteristic of the very molecules of each object.

If this is not realised as ātma-śakti (the energy of the self or infinite consciousness) it creates the delusion of world-appearance; if it is realised as the truth, which is infinite consciousness, that realisation destroys all sorrow. The non-seeing of this truth is known as avidyā or ignorance; such ignorance is the cause of the world-appearance which is the source of all the other phenomena. Even as the arising of the first thought disturbs sleep and ends it, the slightest awakening of inner intelligence destroys ignorance. When one approaches darkness with light in hand, wishing to behold it, the darkness vanishes; when the light of enquiry is turned on ignorance, ignorance disappears. When one begins to enquire: "What is 'I' in this body composed of blood, flesh, bone, etc.?" at once ignorance ceases to be. That which has a beginning has an end. When all things that have a beginning are ruled out, what remains is the truth which is the cessation of avidyā or ignorance. You may regard it as something or as no-thing: that is to be sought which IS when ignorance has been dispelled. The sweetness one tastes is not experienced by another: listening to someone's description of the cessation of avidyā does not give rise to your enlightenment. Each one has to realise it. In short, avidyā is the belief that 'There exists a reality which is not Brahman or cosmic consciousness'; when there is the certain knowledge that 'This is indeed Brahman', avidyā ceases.

punaḥ punar idaṁ rāma prabodhārthaṁ mayocyate
abhyāsena vinā sādho nā 'bhyudety ātmabhāvanā (1)

VASIṢṬHA continued:

Again and again I repeat all this, O Rāma, for the sake of your spiritual awakening; the realisation of the self does not happen without such repetition (or spiritual practice). This ignorance, known as avidyā or ajñāna, has become dense by having been expressed and experienced by the senses in thousands of incarnations, within and outside this body. But, self-knowledge is not within the reach of the senses. It arises when the senses and the mind, which is the sixth sense, cease.

O Rāma, live in this world firmly established in self-knowledge, even as king Janaka lives having known what there is to be known. In his case the truth is realised all the time whether he is active or not, whether he is awake or not. Lord Viṣṇu incarnates in this world and takes on embodiment fully established in this self-knowledge. Even so, lord Śiva remains established in self-knowledge, and lord Brahmā too is established in self-knowledge. Be established in self-knowledge, O Rāma, as they are.

RĀMA asked:

Lord, pray tell me: What is the nature of the self-knowledge in which all these great ones are established?

VASIṢṬHA replied:

Rāma, you know this already, yet in order to make it abundantly clear you are asking about it again.

Whatever there is and whatever appears to be the world-jugglery, is but the pure Brahman or the absolute consciousness and naught else. Consciousness is Brahman, the world is Brahman, all the elements are Brahman, I am Brahman, my enemy is Brahman, my friends and relatives are Brahman, Brahman is the three periods of time, for all these are rooted in Brahman. Even as the ocean appears to be expanded on account of the waves, Brahman seems to be expanded on account of the infinite variety of substances. Brahman apprehends Brahman, Brahman experiences or enjoys Brahman, Brahman is made manifest in Brahman by the power of Brahman himself. Brahman is the form of my enemy who displeases me who am Brahman: when such is the case, who does what to another?

The modes of the mind like attraction and repulsion and likes and dislikes have been conjured up in imagination. They have been destroyed by the absence of thoughts. How then can they be magnified? When Brahman alone moves in all which is Brahman, and Brahman alone unfolds as Brahman in all, what is joy and what is sorrow? Brahman is satisfied with Brahman, Brahman is established in Brahman. There is neither 'I' nor another!

mano buddhirahaṅkāras tanmātrāṇimdriyāṇi ca
brahmaiva sarvaṁ nānātmā sukhaṁ duḥkhaṁ na vidyate (43)

VASIṢṬHA continued:

All the objects in this world are Brahman. 'I' am Brahman. Such being the case, both passion and dispassion, craving and aversion are but notions. Body is Brahman, death is Brahman, too: when they come together, as the real rope and the unreal imaginary snake come together, where is the cause for sorrow? Similarly, body is Brahman and pleasure is Brahman; where is the cause of rejoicing when body experiences pleasure? When, on the surface of the calm ocean, waves appear to be agitated, the waves do not cease to be water! Even when Brahman appears to be agitated (in the world-appearance), its essence is unchanged and there is neither 'I'-ness nor 'you'-ness. When the whirlpool dies in the water, nothing is dead! When the death-Brahman overtakes the body-Brahman, nothing is lost.

Water is capable of being calm and of being agitated: even so Brahman can be quiescent and restless. Such is its nature. It is ignorance or delusion that divides the one into 'This is sentient jiva', and 'This is insentient matter'; the wise ones do not hold such erroneous views. Hence, to the ignorant the world is full of sorrow; to the wise the same world is full of bliss, even as to a blind man the world is dark and to one who has good eyesight the world is full of light.

When the one Brahman alone pervades all, there is neither death nor is there a living person. The ripples play on the surface of the ocean, they are neither born nor do they die! Even so do the elements in this creation. 'This is' and 'This is not' — such deluded notions arise in the self. These notions are not really caused nor do they have a motivation, even as a crystal reflects different coloured objects without a motivation.

The self remains itself even when the energies of the world throw up endless diversities on the surface of the ocean of consciousness. There are no independent entities in this world known as 'body' etc. What is seen as the body and what are seen as notions, the objects of perception, the perishable and the imperishable, the thoughts and feelings and their meaning — all these are Brahman in Brahman the infinite consciousness. There is duality only in the eyes of the deluded and ignorant. **The mind, the intellect, the ego-sense, the cosmic root-elements, the senses and all such diverse phenomena are Brahman only; pleasure and pain are illusions** (they are words without substance). Even as a single sound produced amongst hills echoes and re-echoes into diversity, the one cosmic consciousness experiences multiplicity within itself, with the notions 'This is I' and 'This is mine' etc. The one cosmic consciousness sees diversity within itself even as a dreamer dreams of diverse objects within himself.

svayaṁ prabhur mahātmaiva brahma bramavido viduḥ
aparijñātam ajñānam ajñānām iti kathyate (47)

VASIṢṬHA continued:

When gold is not recognised as such it gets mixed up with the earth: when Brahman is not thus recognised, the impurity of ignorance arises. **The knower of Brahman declares that such a great one is himself the Lord and Brahman; in the case of the ignorant the non-recognition of the truth is known as ignorance.** (Or, it is the opinion of the knowers of Brahman that the very same Lord or supreme being is regarded as ignorance in the ignorant.) When gold is recognised as such it 'becomes' gold instantly; when Brahman is recognised as such it 'becomes' Brahman instantly.

Being omnipotent, Brahman becomes whatever it considers itself to be without any motivation for doing so. The knowers of Brahman declare that Brahman is the Lord, the great being which is devoid of action, the doer and the instrument, devoid of causal motivation and of transformation or change.

When this truth is not realised it arises as ignorance in the ignorant, but when it is realised, the ignorance is dispelled. When a relative is not recognised as such, he is known as a stranger; when the relative is recognised, the notion of stranger is instantly dispelled.

When one knows that duality is illusory appearance, there is realisation of Brahman the absolute. When one knows 'This is not I', the unreality of the ego-sense is realised. From this arises true dispassion. 'I am verily Brahman' — when this truth is realised the awareness of the truth arises in one, and all things are then merged in that awareness. When such notions as 'I' and 'you' are dispelled, the realisation of the truth arises and one realises that all this, whatever there is, is indeed Brahman.

What is the truth? 'I have nothing to do with sorrow, with actions, with delusion or desire. I am at peace, free from sorrow. I am Brahman' — such is the truth. 'I am free from all defects, I am the all, I do not seek anything nor do I abandon anything, I am Brahman' — such is the truth. 'I am blood, I am flesh, I am bone, I am body, I am consciousness, I am the mind also, I am Brahman' — such is the truth. 'I am the firmament, I am space, I am the sun and the entire space, I am all things here, I am Brahman' — such is the truth. 'I am a blade of grass, I am the earth, I am a tree-stump, I am the forest, I am the mountain and the oceans, I am the non-dual Brahman' — such is the truth. 'I am the consciousness in which all things are strung and through whose power all beings engage themselves in all their activities; I am the essence of all things' — such is the truth.

This is certain: all things exist in Brahman, all things flow from it, all things are Brahman; it is omnipresent, it is the one self, it is the truth.

cid ātmā brahma sat satyam ṛtaṁ jña iti nāmabhiḥ
procyate sarvagaṁ tattvaṁ cinmātraṁ cetyavarjitaṁ (66)

VASIṢṬHA continued:

The truth which is omnipresent and which is pure consciousness devoid of objectivity, is referred to variously as consciousness, self, Brahman, existence, truth, order and also as pure knowledge. It is pure and in its light all beings know their own self. I am the Brahman which is pure consciousness after its own appearance as the mind, the intellect, the senses and all other such notions have been negated. I am imperishable consciousness or Brahman in whose light alone all the elements and the entire universe shine. I am the consciousness of Brahman, sparks from whom arise continually radiating reflected consciousness throughout the universe. Even when seen by a pure mind it is expressed in silence. Though it appears to be in contact with the ceaseless experiences of the ego-sense of countless beings who thus derive the delight that is of Brahman, yet it is beyond the reach of these and untouched by them. For, though it is truly the ultimate source of all happiness and delight, it is of the nature of deep sleep (devoid of diversity), peaceful and pure. In subject-object relationship and the consequent experience of pleasure the bliss of Brahman is infinitesimally experienced.

I am the eternal Brahman free from the wrong notions of pleasure and pain, etc., and therefore pure; I am the consciousness in which there is true and pure experiencing. I am that pure consciousness in which the pure intelligence functions without thought interference. I am Brahman which is the intelligent energy that functions in all the elements (earth, water, fire, etc.). I am the pure consciousness which manifests as the characteristic taste, etc. of the different fruits.

I am the changeless Brahman which is realised when both elation at having gained what one desires and depression at not having gained it, are transcended. When the sun shines and the objects of the world are seen in that light, I am the pure consciousness that is in the middle between these two, and which is the very self of the light and of the illumined object. I am that pure consciousness or Brahman which exists unbroken in the waking, dream and deep sleep states, and which is therefore the fourth or the transcendental truth.

Even as the taste of the juice of sugarcane cultivated in a hundred different fields is uniform and same, even so the consciousness indwelling all beings is the same — that consciousness I am. I am that conscious energy (cit-śakti) which is larger than the universe and yet subtler than the minutest atomic particle and therefore invisible. I am the consciousness that exists everywhere like butter in milk, and whose very nature is experiencing.

akhilamidamahaṁ mamaiva sarvaṁ
tvahamapi nā 'hamathetaracca nā 'ham
iti viditavato jagatkṛtaṁ me
sthiramathavā 'stu gatajvaro bhavāmi (112)

VASIṢṬHA continued:

Even as ornaments made of gold are only gold, I am the pure consciousness in the body. I am the self that pervades all things within and without. I am that consciousness which reflects all experiences without itself undergoing any change, and which is untouched by impurity.

I salute that consciousness which is the bestower of the fruits of all thoughts, the light that shines in all luminaries, the supreme gain; that consciousness pervades all the limbs, ever awake and alert, vibrates constantly in all substances, and is ever homogeneous and undisturbed as if it were in deep sleep though wide awake. That consciousness is the reality that bestows the individual characteristic on each and every substance in the universe, and though within all and so nearest to all, is far on account of its inaccessability to the mind and the senses. Continuous and homogeneous in waking, dreaming, deep sleep and in the fourth (transcendental) state of consciousness, it shines when all thoughts have ceased, when all excitements have ceased and when all hate has ceased. That consciousness is devoid of desire and ego-sense and cannot be divided into parts.

I have attained that consciousness which is the indweller of all; and yet though all, is beyond diversity. It is the cosmic net in which the infinite number of beings are caughts like birds; in it all these worlds manifest, though in fact nothing has ever happened. That consciousness is of the nature of being and non-being and the resting place of all that is good and divine. It plays the roles of all beings and it is the source of all affection and peace, though it is forever united and liberated. It is the life of all living beings, the uncreated nectar that cannot be stolen by any-one, the ever existent reality. That consciousness which is reflected in sense-experiences is yet devoid of them and cannot be experienced by them. In it all beings rejoice, though it itself is pure bliss beyond all joy — like the space but beyond space, glorious yet devoid of all expansions and glory. Though seemingly it does all, it does nothing.

All this is 'I' and all this is 'mine'. But I am not and I am not 'other than I'. I have realised this. Let this world be an illusion or substantial, I am free from the fever of distress.

The verses in the text that constitute the second paragraph above are inspiring.

saṁsārottaraṇe yukttir yogaśabdena kathyate
tāṁ viddhi dviprakārāṁ tvam cittopaśamadharmiṇīṁ (13/3)

VASIṢṬHA continued:

Established in this realisation of the truth, the great sages lived forever in peace and equanimity. They were free from psychological predisposition and hence they did not seek nor reject either life or death. They remained unshaken in their direct experience like another Meru-mountain. Yet, they roamed the forests, islands and cities, they travelled to the heavens as if they were angels or gods, they conquered their enemies and they ruled as emperors and they engaged themselves in diverse activities in accordance with scriptural injunctions, as they realised that such was appropriate conduct. They enjoyed the pleasures of life: they visited pleasure gardens and were entertained by celestial damsels. They duly fulfilled the duties of the household life, they even engaged themselves in great wars and they retained their equanimity even in those disastrous situations where others would have lost their peace and balanced state of mind.

Their mind had fully entered the state of satva or divinity and was therefore utterly free from delusion, from egoistic notion ('I do this') and from the desire for achievement — though they did not reject such achievement or the rewards for their actions. They did not indulge in vain exultation when they defeated their enemies, nor did they give way to despair and grief when they were defeated. They were engaged in natural activities, allowing all actions to proceed from them non-volitionally.

Follow their example, O Rāma. Let your personality (ego-sense) be egoless and let appropriate actions spontaneously proceed from you. For the infinite indivisible consciousness alone is the truth; and it is that which has put on this appearance of diversity which is neither real nor unreal. Hence live completely unattached to anything here. Why do you grieve as if you are an ignoramus?

RĀMA said:

Lord, by your grace I am fully awakened to the reality. My delusion has vanished. I shall do as you bid me to do. Surely, I rest peacefully in the state of one who is liberated even while living. Pray, Lord, tell me how one reaches the state of liberation by the restraint of the life-force (prāṇa) and by the annihilation of all self-limitations or psychological conditioning.

VASIṢṬHA continued:

They call it yoga, which is the method by which this cycle of birth and death ceases. It is the utter transcendence of the mind and is of two types. Self-knowledge is one type and restraint of the life-force is another. However, yoga has come to mean only the latter, yet both the methods lead to the same result. To some, self-knowledge through enquiry is difficult; to others yoga is difficult. But my conviction is that the path of enquiry is easy for all, because self-knowledge is the ever-present truth. I shall now describe to you the method of yoga.

sa yathā jīvati khagas tatheha yadi jīvyate
tadbhavej jīvitaṁ puṇyaṁ dīrghaṁ codayameva ca (14/11)

VASIṢṬHA continued:

In the infinite and indivisible consciousness there is a mirage-like world-appearance in one corner, as it were. The Creator who is the apparent cause for this world-appearance, dwells there. I am his mind-born son. Once when I was in heaven, I heard from sages the stories of long-lived beings. In the course of this discussion, the great sage Śātātapa said:

"In one corner of the mount Meru there is a wish-fulfilling tree. On that tree there dwells a crow known as Bhuśuṇḍa, who is utterly free from all attraction and aversion. There is none on earth or in heaven who has lived longer than he has. **If any of you can live as he lives, that shall be regarded as a highly laudable and meritorious life.**"

I heard these words. I was greatly inspired. Soon I set out to meet this Bhuśuṇḍa. Instantly I reached that peak of the mount Meru and the tree where Bhuśuṇḍa lived. Perfected sages who could assume any form they liked also dwelt on it. It was an enormous tree of immeasurable dimensions.

I saw the different types of birds that dwelt on that tree. At a great distance on that tree I saw crows. Among them I saw the great Bhuśuṇḍa, the long-lived. He had lived through several world-cycles. He remembered even those who lived aeons ago. He remained silent. He was free from I-ness and mine-ness. He was the friend and relative of all.

I descended right in front of Bhuśuṇḍa. He knew that I was Vasiṣṭha and welcomed me appropriately. He then said to me: "I consider it a great blessing that after a long time you have given us your darśan (visit). You are the greatest among those who are worthy of adoration and you have come here only as a result of my accumulated merit. Pray tell me the immediate reason for this visit."

I replied as follows: "You are truly blessed in that you enjoy the supreme peace all around you, in that you are endowed with the highest wisdom (self-knowledge) and in that you are not caught in the net of illusion known as world-appearance. Pray enlighten me in regard to a few facts concerning yourself. In what clan were you born? How did you acquire the knowledge of that which alone deserves to be known? What is your age now? Do you remember anything concerning the past? Who is it that ordained that you shall be long-lived and that you shall live on this tree?"

BHUŚUṆḌA replied:

Since you ask these questions concerning me, O sage, I shall duly answer them. Pray listen attentively. The story I am about to narrate is so inspiring that it will destroy the sins of those who relate it and those who listen to it.

tāta. jñātamalaṁ jñeyaṁ brāhmyā devyāḥ prasādataḥ
kintv ekāntasthiteḥ sthānam abhivāñchāma uttamaṁ (19/25)

BHUŚUṆḌA said:

In this universe there is a great divinity known as Hara, who is the god of gods and who is adored by all the gods in heaven. His consort occupies one half of his body. His lieutenants are goblins that have heads and hands like razors and that have faces like a bear, a camel, a mouse etc. And female deities who feed on the beings in the fourteen worlds dance in front of him. Of these, Alaṁbusā is the most famous. Her vehicle is the crow Caṇḍa which is extremely powerful and which is blue in colour.

Once upon a time all these female deities assembled in space. They duly worshipped the divinity known as Tumburu (which is one of the aspects of Rudra) and engaged themselves in left-handed ritual which reveals the supreme truth. They began to perform various rites intoxicated, as they were, by wine. Soon they began to discuss an important question: how is it that the Lord of Umā (Hara) treats us contemptuously? They made up their mind thus: "We shall demonstrate our prowess in such a way that he does not do so hereafter." They overwhelmed Umā by their magic powers, and separated her from her lord Hara. All the female deities sang and danced in ecstasy. Some drank, some sang, some laughed, some roared, some ran, some fell, and some ate flesh.

The female swans (which were the vehicles of goddess Brāhmi) danced along with the crow Caṇḍa which was Alaṁbusā's vehicle. One by one, all the swans mated with the crow (Caṇḍa), as they were all drunk. Soon they became pregnant. The swans informed Brāhmi of everything that happened.

The goddess Brāhmi said to them: "Since you are all big with child, you will not be able to perform your duties. Hence, for sometime go where you please." Having said this, the goddess sat in deep contemplation.

The swans laid twenty-one eggs at the proper time and they were soon hatched. Thus twenty-one of us were born in the family of Caṇḍa the crow. Along with our mothers, we adored the goddess Brāhmi. By her grace we attained self-knowledge and liberation. We then approached our father who fondly embraced us all. All of us then worshipped the goddess Alaṁbusā.

Caṇḍa said: "Children, have you gone beyond the dragnet known as the world-appearance after having cut the shackles of vāsanā or mental conditioning? If you have not, come let us adore the goddess by whose grace you will attain the highest wisdom." We replied: "**Father we have gained the knowledge that is worth gaining, by the grace of the goddess Brāhmi. We seek a secluded and excellent place to dwell.**"

In accordance with our father's instructions all of us came here and took up our abode in this nest.

tatastataśca paryastaṁ luṭhitaṁ na ca vṛttiṣu
nā 'parāmṛṣṭa tattvārthaṁ asmākaṁ bhagavan manaḥ (35)

BHUŚUṆḌA continued:

There was a world in days of yore which is not far beyond our memory, for we witnessed it ourselves.

VASIṢṬHA asked: What happened to your brothers, for I see only you here?

BHUŚUṆḌA continued:

A very long time has passed, O sage, and in course of time my brothers abandoned their physical existence and ascended to the heaven of lord Śiva. Indeed, even long-lived persons who may be holy and saintly and strong are consumed in course of time by Time (or death).

VASIṢṬHA asked again: How is it that you have remained unaffected by the heat and the cold and the wind and the fire?

BHUŚUṆḌA continued:

Truly, to be embodied as a crow held in contempt by the people is not a happy state, though the Creator has amply provided for the survival of even the humble crow. But, we have remained immersed in the self, happy and contented, hence we have survived in spite of ever so many calamities. We have remained firmly established in the self, having abandoned vain activities that are but torment of the body and the mind. To this physical body there is misery neither in life nor in death; hence we remain as we are, not seeking anything other than what is.

We have seen the fate of the worlds. We have mentally abandoned identification with the body. Established in self-knowledge and remaining on this tree I see the passage of time. Through the practice of prāṇāyāma I have risen above the division of time. Hence, I am at peace within my heart and I am not affected by the events of the world. Let all beings vanish or let them come into existence; we have no fear at all. Let all these beings enter into the ocean known as Time (or death), but we are seated on the shores of that ocean and are therefore unaffected. We neither accept nor reject; we appear to be, but we are not what appears to be. Thus do we remain on this tree.

Though we engage ourselves in diverse activities we do not get drowned in mental modifications and we never lose contact with the reality.

Lord, that nectar for which the gods churned the ocean is inferior to the nectarine blessing that flows from the very presence of sages like you. I consider nothing more praiseworthy than the company of sages who are free from all cravings and desires. Holy one, even though I have already attained self-knowledge I consider that my birth has been truly fulfilled, in that today I have seen you and have enjoyed your company.

brahmanniyatireṣā hi durlaṅghyā pārameśvarī
mayedṛśena vai bhāvyaṁ bhāvyam anyais tu tādṛśaiḥ (23)

BHUŚUṆḌA continued:

This wish-fulfilling tree is not shaken by the various natural calamities nor by the cataclysms caused by living beings. There have been several of the latter when demons have tried to destroy or overwhelm the earth, as also when the Lord has intervened and rescued the earth from the grip of the demons. During all these this tree has remained unaffected. Even the flood and the scorching heat of the sun attendant upon cosmic dissolution have not succeeded in shaking this tree. On account of this, we who dwell on this tree have also escaped harm. Evil overtakes one who lives in an unholy place.

VASIṢṬHA asked:

But at the end of the life of the cosmos, when everything is dissolved, how have you managed to survive?

BHUŚUṆḌA replied:

During that period, O sage, I abandon this nest, even as an ungrateful man abandons his friend. Then I remain united with cosmic space, totally free from all thoughts and mental modifications. When the twelve cosmic suns pour unbearable heat upon this creation, I practise the vāruṇi-dhāraṇā and remain unaffected. (Varuṇa is the lord of waters: vāruṇī-dhāraṇā is contemplation of Varuṇa.) When the wind blows with such force as to uproot even mountains, I practise the pārvatī-dhāraṇā and remain unaffected. (Parvata is mountain and pārvatī-dhāraṇā is contemplation of the mountain.) When the whole universe is flooded with the waters of cosmic dissolution, I practise vāyū-dhāraṇā and remain unaffected. (Vāyu is wind and vāyu-dhāraṇā is contemplation of the wind.) Then I remain as if in deep sleep till the beginning of the next cosmic cycle. When the new Creator begins to create a new cosmos, I resume my abode in this nest.

VASIṢṬHA asked:

Why is it that others are not able to do what you have done?

BHUŚUṆḌA replied:

O sage, the will of the supreme being cannot be transgressed: it is his will that I should be like this and that the others should be as they are. One cannot fathom nor measure what has to be. In accordance with the nature of each being, that which is to be comes to be. Therefore, in accordance with my thought-force or conception, this tree is found in every world-cycle at this place in this manner.

drṣṭānekavidhānalpa sargasaṅgagamāgamaḥ
kiṁ kiṁ smarasi kalyāṇa citramasmin jagatkrame (21/27)

VASIṢṬHA asked:

You enjoy such longevity as would suggest that you have attained final liberation! And you are wise, brave and a great yogi. **Pray, tell me what extra-ordinary events you remember, relating to this and the previous world-cycles.**

BHUŚUṆḌA said:

I remember that once upon a time there was nothing on this earth, neither trees and plants, nor even mountains. For a period of eleven thousand years the earth was covered by lava. In those days there was neither day nor night below the polar region: for in the rest of the earth neither the sun nor the moon shone. Only one half of the polar region was illumined.

Then demons ruled the earth. They were deluded, powerful and prosperous, and the earth was their playground.

Apart from the polar region the rest of the earth was covered with water. And then for a very long time the whole earth was covered with forests, except the polar region. Then there arose great mountains, but without any human inhabitants. For a period of ten thousand years the earth was covered with the corpses of the demons.

At one time the gods who used to roam the skies had vanished from sight on account of fear. And the earth had become more like a single mountain! I remember many such events — but let me narrate to you what is important.

During my lifetime I have seen the appearance and disappearance of countless Manū (the progenitor of the human race). At one time the world was devoid of the gods and the demons, but was one radiant cosmic egg. At another time the earth was populated by Brāhmaṇā (members of the priest class) who were addicted to alcohol, śūdrā (servant class) who ridiculed the gods, and polyandrous women. I also remember another epoch when the earth was covered with forests, when the ocean could not even be imagined and when human beings were spontaneously created. At another time there was neither mountain nor earth; the gods and the sages dwelt in space. At another time there were neither the gods nor the sages, etc.; darkness prevailed everywhere.

First there arose the notion of creation. Then light and the division of the universe arose. Then one after the other the diverse beings were created, as also the stars and the planets.

I saw that during one epoch it was lord Viṣṇu (generally considered the protector) who created the universe, during another it was Brahmā who created the universe and in another it was Śiva who became the creator.

Whatever is happening in the present creation has happened exactly in the same manner during three previous creations. But I remember the events of ten such creations.

andhīkṛtahṛdākāśāḥ kāmakopavikārajāḥ
cintā na parihiṁsanti cittaṁ yasya samāhitam (16)

VASIṢṬHA asked:

O Bhuśuṇḍa, how is it that your body has not been consumed by death?

BHUŚUṆḌA replied:

Death does not wish to kill one who does not have rāga-dveṣa (attraction and aversion) or false notions and mental habits. Death does not wish to kill one who does not suffer from mental illness, who does not entertain desires and hopes which give rise to anxieties and worry, who is not poisoned by greed, whose body and mind are not burnt by the fire of anger and hate, who is not churned and ground by the mill of lust, who is firmly established in the pure awareness of Brahman the absolute and whose mind is not distracted like a monkey. **He whose mind and heart are established in supreme peace is not touched by the blinding evils born of lust and hate.**

Even the contemplation of the self which is infinite consciousness banishes sorrow, terminates the long-dream vision of the world-appearance, purifies the mind and the heart, and dispels worries and misfortunes. But this contemplation of the self has comrades, as it were, that closely resemble such contemplation: among them is the contemplation of the life-force or prāṇa, which enables one to overcome sorrow and to promote auspiciousness. It is that contemplation of prāṇa that has bestowed longevity and also self-knowledge on me.

Lord, look at this enchanting body which is supported by three pillars (the three bodies or the three nāḍi?) and endowed with nine gates, and which is protected by the ego-sense which has eight consorts (the puryaṣṭaka) and several relatives (the root elements). Enclosed right in the middle of this body are the subtle idā and piṅgalā. There are three lotus-like wheels. These wheels are composed of bones and flesh. When the vital air wets the wheels, the petals or the radii of these lotus-like wheels begin to vibrate. The vital airs expand on account of their expansion. These nāḍī thereupon radiate above and below. Sages call these vital airs by different names — prāṇa, apāna, samāna, etc., on account of their diverse functions. These functions derive their energy from the central psychic centre which is the heart lotus.

That energy which thus vibrates in the heart-lotus is known as prāṇa: it enables the eyes to see, the skin to feel, the mouth to speak, the food to be digested, and it performs all the functions in the body. It has two different roles, one above and one below, and it is then known as prāṇa and apāna respectively. I am devoted to them; they are free from fatigue, shine like the sun and the moon in the heart, are like the cart-wheels of the mind which is the guardian of the city known as the body, and are the favourite horses of the king known as ego-sense. Being devoted to them I live as if in deep sleep, forever in homogeneous consciousness.

He who adores the prāṇa and the apāna thus is not reborn in this world again and he is freed from all bondage.

yatkaroti yad aśnāti buddhyaivā 'lam anusmaran
kuṁbhakādīn naraḥ svāntas tatra kartā na kiñcana (22)

BHUŚUṆḌA continued:

Prāṇa is constantly in motion inside and outside the body: prāṇa is that vital air which is established in the upper part. Apāna is similarly and constantly in motion inside and outside the body, but it dwells in the lower part. Pray, listen to the practice of the extension or the control of this life-force, which is conducive to the welfare of one who is awake or asleep.

The efflux of the vital force centred in the heart-lotus, of its own accord and without effort, is known as recaka or exhalation. The contact with the source of the pranic force which is located downward to the length of twelve 'fingers', in the heart-lotus, is known as pūraka or inhalation.

When the apāna has ceased to move and when the prāṇa does not arise and move out of the heart (and till these begin to happen) it is known as kumbhaka (retention as of a filled pot). There are said to be three points for the recaka, kumbhaka and pūraka: (1) outside (the nose); (2) from below the place known as dvādaśānta (above or in front of the forehead at a distance of twelve fingers); (3) the source of prāṇa (heart-lotus).

Pray listen to the natural and effortless movement of the life-force at all times. The movement of the vital air up to the extent of twelve fingers from oneself constitutes recaka. That state in which the apāna-force remains in the dvādaśānta, like the unfashioned pot in the potter's clay, should be known as external-kumbhaka.

When the outgoing air moves up to the tip of the nose, it is known as recaka. When it moves up to the extent of the dvādaśānta it is known as external-recaka. When the movement of prāṇa has ceased outside itself and as long as the apāna does not rise, they call it external-kumbhaka. When, however, the apāna flows inwards, without the prāṇa rising within, they call it internal-kumbhaka. When the apāna rises in the dvādaśānta and attains internal expansion, it is known as internal pūraka. He who knows these kumbhakā is not born again.

Whether one is going or standing, awake or asleep, these vital airs — which are naturally restless — are restrained by these practices. **Then whatever he does or eats, he who knows these kumbhakā is not the doer of those actions.** In a very few days he attains the supreme state. He who practises these kumbhakā is not attracted by external objects. They who are endowed with this vision — whether they are stationary or moving (active or inactive) — are not bound: they have attained that which is worthy of being attained.

Note: Dvādaśāntam suggests a magnetic field around the body twelve finger-widths all round. This magnetic field is also composed of prāṇa-apāna.

bāhye tamasi saṁkṣiṇe lokālokaḥ prajāyate
hārde tu tamasi kṣiṇe svāloko jāyate mune (44)

BHUŚUṆḌA continued:

When the impurity of one's heart and mind have been destroyed by thus being devoted to prāṇa and apāna, one is freed from delusion, attains inner awakening and rests in one's own self even while doing whatever has to be done.

Lord, prāṇa arises in the lotus of the heart and terminates at a distance of twelve finger-breadths outside the body. Apāna arises in the dvādaśānta (twelve finger-breadths from the body) and terminates in the lotus of the heart. Thus apāna arises where prāṇa terminates. Prāṇa is like a flame and it goes up and out; apāna is like water and it goes down towards the heart-lotus.

Apāna is the moon which protects the body from outside; prāṇa is like the sun or the fire and promotes the body's internal welfare. Prāṇa generates heat in the heart-space every moment, and after producing this heat it generates heat in the space in front of the face. Apāna, which is the moon, nourishes the space in front of the face and then it nourishes the space in the heart.

If one is able to reach that space where the apāna unites with the prāṇa, he does not grieve any more, nor is he born again.

In fact, it is only prāṇa that undergoes a modification and appears as apāna, after abandoning its burning heat. And then, the same prāṇa, having abandoned the coolness of the moon, gains its nature as the purifying fire of the sun. The wise ones enquire into the nature of prāṇa as long as it does not abandon its solar nature to become lunar. One who knows the truth concerning the rising and the setting of the sun and the moon in one's own heart, is not born again. He who sees the Lord, the sun, in one's heart, sees the truth.

In order to attain perfection one does not prevent nor protect external darkness, but one strives to destroy the darkness of ignorance in the heart. **When the external darkness goes, one is able to see the world; but when the darkness of ignorance in the heart is dispelled, there arises self-knowledge.** Hence one should strive to behold the prāṇa and the apāna, whose knowledge bestows liberation.

Apāna terminates in the heart where prāṇa arises. Where prāṇa is born, there apāna perishes; where apāna takes birth, there prāṇa ceases. When prāṇa has ceased to move and when apāna takes birth, there prāṇa ceases. When prāṇa has ceased to move and when apāna is about to rise one experiences external kumbhaka; rooted in this one does not grieve any more. When apāna has ceased to move and when prāṇa has arisen just a little, one experiences internal kumbhaka; rooted in this one does not grieve any more.

yatra prāṇo hy apānena prāṇenā 'pāna eva ca
nigīrṇau bahirantaś ca deśakālau ca paśya tau (57)

BHUŚUṆḌA continued:

If one practises kumbhaka (suspension of breath) after exhaling the prāṇa to a distance farther from where the apāna rises (the twelve finger-breadth distance), he is not subject to sorrow any more. Or, if one is able to see the space within oneself where the inhaled breath turns into the impulse for exhalation, he is not born again. By seeing where the prāṇa and the apāna terminate their motions, and by holding fast to that state of peace, one is not subject to sorrow again.

If one keenly observes the place and the exact moment at which the prāṇa is consumed by the apāna, he does not grieve. Or, if one keenly observes the place and the exact moment at which the apāna is consumed by prāṇa, his mind does not arise again. Therefore, **behold that place and that moment at which prāṇa is consumed by apāna and apāna is consumed by prāṇa inside and outside the body.** For that precise moment at which the prāṇa has ceased to move and the apāna has not begun to move, there arises a kumbhaka which is effortless: the wise regard that as an important state. When there is effortless suspension of breath, it is the supreme state. This is the self, it is pure infinite consciousness. He who reaches this does not grieve.

I contemplate that infinite consciousness which is the indwelling presence in the prāṇa, but which is neither with prāṇa nor other than prāṇa. I contemplate that infinite consciousness which is the indwelling presence in the apāna, but which is neither with apāna nor other than apāna. That which IS after the prāṇa and the apāna have ceased to be and which is in the middle between prāṇa and apāna — I contemplate that infinite consciousness. I contemplate that consciousness which is the prāṇa of prāṇa, which is the life of life, which alone is responsible for the preservation of the body; which is the mind of the mind, the intelligence in the intellect, the reality in the egosense. I salute that consciousness in which all things abide, from which they emerge, which is all and everywhere, and which is all in all and eternal; which is the purifier of all and whose vision is most meritorious. I salute that consciousness in which prāṇa ceases to move but apāna does not arise, and which dwells in the space in front (or, at the root) of the nose. I salute the consciousness which is the source for both prāṇa and apāna, which is the energy in both prāṇa and apāna, and which enables the senses to function. I salute that consciousness which is in fact the essence of the internal and the external kumbhaka, which is the only goal of the contemplation of prāṇa, which enables the prāṇa to function and which is the cause of all causes. I take refuge in that supreme being.

na bhūtaṁ na bhaviṣyaṁ ca cintayāmi kadācana
dṛṣṭim ālambya tiṣṭhāmi vartamānāmihā ''tmanā (8)

BHUŚUṆḌA continued:

By the regular and systematic practice of prāṇāyāma as described by me, I have gained the state of purity and I am not disturbed even when the mount Meru (or the north pole) is shaken. This state of samādhi or total equanimity is not lost whether I am walking or standing, whether I am awake, asleep or dreaming. In all conditions of life I rest in the self and with the self, with my vision turned upon itself, whatever changes may take place in the world or in the environment. Thus have I lived right from the time of the previous cosmic dissolution.

I do not contemplate either the past or the future: my attention is constantly directed to the present. I do what has to be done in the present, without thinking of the results. Without considerations of being or non-being, desirable or undesirable, I remain in the self: hence I am happy, healthy and free from illness.

My state is the fruit of contemplation of the moment of union of the prāṇa and the apāna (when the self is revealed). I do not entertain vain notions like, 'I have obtained this and I shall gain that, too'. I neither praise nor censure anyone (neither myself nor others) nor anything at any time; my mind does not exult on gaining what is considered good, nor does it become depressed on obtaining what is considered evil; hence my state of happiness and health. I embrace the supreme renunciation, having renounced even the desire to live; thus my mind does not entertain cravings, but is peaceful and balanced. I behold the one common substratum in all things (a piece of wood, a beautiful woman, a mountain, a blade of grass, ice, fire and space) and I am not worried by thoughts like, 'What shall I do now?' or 'What shall I get tomorrow morning?' I am not bothered by thoughts of old age and death, or by longing for happiness, nor do I regard some as 'mine' and others as 'not-mine'. I know that everything at all times, everywhere, is but the one cosmic consciousness. These are the secrets of my state of happiness and health.

I do not think, 'I am the body', even while engaged in physical activity, as I know this world-appearance to be illusory, and live in it as if fast asleep. I am disturbed neither by prosperity nor by adversity when they are granted to me, as I regard them with equal vision (even as I look upon both my arms as arms). Whatever I do is untainted by desire or the mud of ego-sense; thus I do not lose my head when I am powerful, or go begging when I am poor; I do not let hopes and expectations touch me, and even when a thing is old and worn out I look upon it with fresh eyes as if it were new. I rejoice with the happy ones and share the grief of the grief-stricken, for I am the friend of all, knowing I belong to none and none belongs to me. I know that I am the world, its intelligence, and all the activities in it. This is the secret of my longevity.

dīrghasvapnaṁ imaṁ viddhi dīrghaṁ vā cittavibhramaṁ
dīrghaṁ vā 'pi manorājyaṁ saṁsāraṁ raghunandana (28/28)

VASIṢṬHA said:

Thereupon I said to Bhuśuṇḍa, "Marvellous indeed is this, your autobiography, O Lord. Blessed indeed are they who can behold you. You are like a second Creator. Rare indeed are people like you. I have earned great merit by seeing you. May you continue to be blessed. Give me leave to depart."

O Rāma, on hearing this Bhuśuṇḍa worshipped me and, in spite of my remonstrances, accompanied me for some distance holding my hand tightly in a gesture of friendship. Then we parted, and parting of friends is indeed a difficult event. All this was in the previous (Kṛta) age and now it is the Treta-age. Such is the story of Bhuśuṇḍa. O Rāma: you too, practise the prāṇāyāma described by Bhuśuṇḍa and endeavour to live like him.

O Rāma, this house known as the body has not been made by anyone in fact! Dreams are real during the dream-state; even so the body is real when it is experienced as a real substance. The notion of 'I am this body' arises in relation to what is truly a piece of flesh with bones etc. because of a mental predisposition; it is an illusion. Abandon this illusion. There are thousands of such bodies which have been brought into being by your thought-force. When you are asleep and dreaming, you experience a body in the dream. Where does that body arise or exist?

'This is wealth', 'This is body' and 'This is a nation' — all these are notions, O Rāma. **Know this to be a long dream, or a long-standing hallucination, or day-dreaming, or wishful thinking.** When, by the grace of God or the self you attain awakening, you will then see all this clearly. I remarked that I was born of the mind of the Creator: even so the world arises in the mind as a notion. In fact, even the Creator is but a notion in the cosmic mind; the world-appearance, too, is a notion in the mind.

If a man resolutely seeks the source of the notions, he realises consciousness; otherwise he experiences the illusory world-appearance again and again. For by continually entertaining notions such as 'This is it', 'This is mine' and 'This is my world', they assume the appearance of substantiality. The permanency of the world is also an illusion: in the dream-state what is really a brief moment is experienced by the dreamer as a life-time. In a mirage only the illusory 'water' is seen and not the substratum: even so, in a state of ignorance one sees only the illusory world-appearance but not the substratum. However, when one has shed that ignorance, the illusory appearance vanishes. Even the man who is normally subject to fear is not afraid of an imaginary tiger; the wise man who knows that this world is naught but a notion or imagination is unafraid of anything. When one knows that the world is nothing but the appearance of one's self, of whom need one be afraid? When one's vision is purified by enquiry, one's deluded understanding concerning the world vanishes.

yatkiñcid uditaṁ loke yannabhaspatha vā divi
tat sarvaṁ prāpyate rāma rāgadveṣaparikṣayāt (28/74)

VASIṢṬHA continued:

When one realises that death is inevitable to all, why will he grieve over the death of relatives or the approach of one's own end? When one realises that everyone is sometimes prosperous and otherwise at other times, why will he be elated or depressed? When one sees that living beings appear and disappear like ripples on the surface of consciousness, where is the cause for sorrow? What is true is always true (what exists always exists) and what is unreal is ever unreal; where is the cause for sorrow?

Hence, one should not pin one's faith, hope and aspiration on that which is unreal; for such hope is bondage. O Rāma, do thou live in this world without entertaining any hope. What has to be done has to be done and what is inappropriate should be given up. Live happily and playfully in this world without considerations of desirable and undesirable. The infinite consciousness alone exists everywhere at all times. What appears to be is but an appearance. When the appearance is realised as appearance, that which is, is realised. Either realise that 'I am not and these experiences are not mine' or know that 'I am everything': you will be free from the lure of world-appearance. Both these attitudes are good. You will be freed from attraction and aversion (rāga-dveṣa).

Whatever there is in the world, in the firmament and in heaven is attained by one who has destroyed the twin forces of attraction and aversion. Whatever the ignorant man does, prompted by these forces, leads him to instant sorrow. One who has not overcome these forces, even if he is learned in the scriptures, is indeed pitiable and despicable.

O Rāma, for your spiritual awakening I declare again and again that this world-appearance is like a long dream. Wake up, wake up. Behold the self which shines like a sun.

(VASIṢṬHA, who suddenly became silent when he found that Rāma was completely absorbed in the self, resumed his discourse after an interval and after Rāma had returned to normal consciousness:)

O Rāma, you are thoroughly awakened and you have gained self-knowledge. Remain forever in this exalted state; do not get involved in this world-appearance.

The ignorant man who thinks he is suffering and whose face is streaming constantly with tears, is worse than a painting or a statue, for the latter is free from experience of sorrow! Nor is the statue subject to illness and death. The statue is destroyed only when someone destroys it, but the human body is certainly doomed to die. Even as when a statue is broken, no life is lost, when the body born of thoughts and notions is dead, nothing is lost. It is like the loss of the second moon when one is cured of diplopia. The self which is infinite consciousness does not die nor does it undergo any change whatsoever.

nirīho hi jaḍo deho nā "tmano 'syā 'bhivañchitaṁ
kartā na kaścidevā 'to draṣṭā kevalamasya saḥ (35)

VASIṢṬHA continued:

O Rāma, a man riding the merry-go-round sees the world whirling in the opposite direction: even so, a man whirling on the wheel of ignorance thinks that the world and the body are revolving. The spiritual hero, however, should reject this: this body is the product of thoughts and notions entertained by an ignorant mind. The creation of ignorance is false. Hence, even if the body seems to be active and doing all kinds of actions it is still unreal, even as the imaginary snake in the rope is forever unreal. What is done by an inert object is not done by it; though appearing to do, the body does nothing.

The inert body does not entertain any desire (to motivate its actions) and the self (which is the infinite consciousness) has no such desire either; hence there is in truth no doer of action but only the witnessing intelligence. Once the deluded notion that this false body is a reality has arisen, then like a ghost imagined by a little boy, there arises the goblin of ego-sense or the mind. This false mind or ego-sense then roars aloud in such a way that even great men, frightened by it, withdraw themselves in deep meditation. He who, however, lays the ghost known as the mind (or ego-sense) in the body, dwells without fear in the void known as the world. When the ego-sense is stripped of its coverings, ignored and abandoned by the awakened intelligence, it is incapable of doing you any harm. The self is infinite consciousness. Even if the ego-sense dwells in this body, how is the self affected?

Whatever a man does with the body is really done by the ego-sense with the help of the reins known as inhalation and exhalation. The self is indirectly regarded as the cause of all this, even as space is indirectly responsible for the growth of plants inasmuch as it (the space) does not prevent the plant from extending into space. Even as a lamp is considered responsible for the vision of an object, the self is regarded as responsible for the actions of the body and mind, which function in the light of the self.

You are the self, O Rāma, not the mind. What have you to do with the mind? Abandon this delusion. The goblin-mind residing in the body has nothing to do with the self, yet it quietly assumes 'I am the self'. This is the cause of birth and death. This assumption robs you of courage. Give up this ghost, O Rāma, and remain firm. Neither scriptures nor relatives nor even the guru or preceptors can protect the man who is utterly overpowered by the ghost known as the mind. On the other hand, if one has laid this ghost, the guru, the scriptures and relatives can easily aid him, even as one can easily rescue an animal from a mud-puddle. They who have laid this ghost are the good people who render some service to this world. Hence, one should uplift oneself from this ignorance, by laying this ghost known as ego-sense. O Rāma, do not wander in this forest of worldly existence like an animal in human garb. Do not wallow in this mud known as family-relationship for the sake of this impermanent body. The body was born of someone, it is protected by the ego-sense and in it happiness and sorrow are experienced by someone else: this indeed is a great mystery.

ākārādi paricchinne mite vastuni tatkutaḥ
akṛtrimam anādyantaṁ devanaṁ cicchivaṁ viduḥ (122)

VASIṢṬHA continued:

I lived in the abode of Lord Śiva, known as Kailāsa, for sometime, worshipping Lord Śiva and practising austerities. One day I saw a great light in the forest. With my insight I enquired into its nature. I saw that it was Lord Śiva himself.

I saluted the Lord and asked him: "Lord, what is the method of worshipping the Lord which destroys all sins and promotes all auspiciousness?"

THE LORD said:

Do you know who 'god' is? God is not Viṣṇu, or Śiva or Brahmā; not the wind, the sun or the moon; not the brāhmaṇa or the king; nor I nor you; not Lakṣmi nor the mind (intellect). **God is without form and undivided (not in the objects); that splendour (devanaṁ) which is not made and which has neither beginning nor end is known as god (deva) or Lord Śiva which is pure consciousness.** That alone is fit to be worshipped; and that alone is all.

If one is unable to worship this Śiva, then he is encouraged to worship the form. The latter yields finite results but the former bestows infinite bliss. He who ignores the infinite and is devoted to the finite abandons a pleasure-garden and seeks the thorny bush. However, sages sometimes worship a form playfully.

Now for the articles used in the worship: wisdom, self-control and the perception of the self in all beings are the foremost among those articles. The self alone is Lord Śiva who is fit to be worshipped at all times with the flowers of wisdom.

Indeed only the infinite consciousness (cid-ākāśa) which alone exists even after the cosmic dissolution, exists even now, utterly devoid of objectivity. All these mountains, the whole world, the firmament, the self, the jīva or the individuality and all the elements of which this world is constituted — all these are naught but pure consciousness. Before the so-called creation when only this pure consciousness existed, where were all these (heaven etc.)? Space (ākāśa), supreme or infinite space (paramākāśam), absolute space (brahmākāśam), creation, consciousness — are mere words and they indicate the same truth even as synonyms do. Even as the duality experienced in dream is illusory, the duality implied in the creation of the world is illusory. Even as the objects seem to exist and function in the inner world of consciousness in a dream, objects seem to exist and function in the outer world of consciousness during the wakeful state. Nothing really happens in both these states. Even as consciousness alone is the reality in the dream state, consciousness alone is the substance in the wakeful state too. That is the Lord, that is the supreme truth, that you are, that am I and that is all.

na sa dūre sthito brahman na duṣprāpaḥ sa kasyacit
saṁsthitaḥ sa sadā dehe sarvatraiva ca khe tathā (21)

The LORD continued:

The worship of that Lord is true worship and by that worship one attains everything. He is undivided and indivisible, non-dual and neither fashioned nor created by activity; he is not attained by external efforts. His adoration is the fountain-source of joy.

The external worship of a form is prescribed only for those whose intelligence has not been awakened, and who are immature like little boys. When one does not have self-control, etc. he uses flowers in worship; such worship is futile, even as adoring the self in an external form is futile. However, these immature devotees derive satisfaction by worshipping an object created by themselves; they may even earn worthless rewards from such worship.

I shall now describe to you the mode of worship appropriate to enlightened people like you. The Lord fit to be worshipped is indeed the one who upholds the entire creation, who is beyond thought and description, who is beyond the concepts of even the 'all' and the 'collective totality'. He alone is referred to as 'God' who is undivided and indivisible by space and time, whose light illumines all the objects, who is pure and absolute consciousness. He is that intelligence which is beyond all its parts, which is hidden in all that is, which is the being in all that is and which robs all that is of their being (i.e. which veils the truth). This Brahman is in the middle of being and non-being. It is God, and the truth that is indicated as 'OṀ'. It exists everywhere, like the essence in a plant. That pure consciousness which is in you, in me and in all the gods and goddesses, alone is God. Holy one, even the other gods endowed with form are indeed nothing but that pure consciousness. The entire universe is pure consciousness. That is God, that 'all' I am; everything is attained from and through him.

That God is not distant from anyone, O Holy One, nor is he difficult to attain: he is forever seated in the body and he is everywhere like space. He does everything, he eats, he holds everything together, he goes, he breathes, he knows every limb of the body. He is the light in which all these limbs function and in which all the diverse activities take place. He dwells in the cave of one's own heart. He transcends the mind and the five senses of cognition; therefore he cannot be comprehended or described by them — yet for the purpose of instruction he is indicated as 'consciousness'. Hence, though it appears as though he does everything, he does nothing. That consciousness is pure and seemingly engages itself in the activities of the world, to the same extent as the spring does in the flowering of trees.

śarīrapaṅkajabhrāntamanobhramarasaṁbhṛtāṁ
āsvādayati saṅkalpamadhusattāṁ cidīśvarī (34)

The LORD continued:

Somewhere this consciousness functions as space, somewhere as a jīva, somewhere as action, somewhere as substance and so forth, but without intending to do so. Even as all the 'different' oceans are but one indivisible mass of water, this consciousness, though described in different ways, is but one cosmic mass of consciousness. **In the body (which is like a lotus) it is the same consciousness that imbibes the experience — which is like honey gathered by the restless mind (which is like the bee).** In this universe all these various beings (the gods, the demons, mountains, oceans and so forth) flow within this infinite consciousness, even as eddies and whirlpools appear in the ocean. Even the wheel of ignorance, which causes the wheel of life and death to revolve, revolves within this cosmic consciousness whose energy is in constant motion.

It was consciousness, in the form of the four-armed Viṣṇu, that destroyed the demons, even as a thunderstorm equipped with the rainbow quenches the heat that rises from the earth. It is consciousness alone which takes the form of Śiva and Pārvati, of Brahmā the creator and the numerous other beings. This consciousness is like a mirror which holds a reflection within itself, as it were, without undergoing any modification thereby. Without undergoing any modification in itself, this consciousness appears as all these countless beings in this universe.

The infinite consciousness is like a creeper. It is sprinkled with the latent tendencies of countless jīvā. Desires are the buds. Past creations are the filaments. The sentient and the insentient beings are parts of the creeper. The one appears as many, but it has not become many.

It is by this infinite consciousness that all this is thought of, expressed and done. It is the infinite consciousness alone which shines as the sun. It is the infinite consciousness which appears as the bodies, which are in fact inert and which come into contact with one another and derive various experiences. This consciousness is like the typhoon which is unseen in itself but in which sand-particles and dust rise and dance as if by themselves. This consciousness casts a shadow in itself, as it were, and that is regarded as tamas or inertia.

In this body, thoughts and notions generate action in the light of this very consciousness. Surely, but for this consciousness even an object which is immediately in front of oneself cannot be experienced. The body cannot function or exist but for this consciousness. It grows, it falls, it eats. This consciousness creates and maintains all the movable and the immovable beings in the universe. The infinite consciousness alone exists, naught else exists. Consciousness alone has arisen in consciousness.

vāsanā vimalā yeṣāṁ hṛdayān nā 'pasarpati
sthiraikarūpajivās te jivanmukttāś cirāyuṣaḥ (32/35)

The LORD continued:

Even as there is no oil in a rock, the diversity of sight, seer and scene, or of doer, act and action, or of knower, knowledge and known, does not exist in pure consciousness. Similarly, the distinction between 'I' and 'you', between the one and the many, is verbal. On enquiry, all these disappear and only the unmodified pure consciousness remains. Consciousness does not undergo any modification nor does it become impure. This infinite consciousness, which is unmodified and non-dual, can be realised by one in the self-luminous inner light. It is pure and eternal, it is ever-present and devoid of mind.

Consciousness alone is the reality in all forms and all experiences. Action springs from thought, thought is the function of the mind, mind is conditioned consciousness, but consciousness is unconditioned! Jiva is the vehicle of consciousness, ego-sense is the vehicle of jīva, intelligence of ego-sense, mind of intelligence, prāṇa of the mind, the senses of prāṇa, the body of the senses, and motion is the vehicle of the body. Such motion is karma (action). Because prāṇa is the vehicle for the mind, when the prāṇa takes it the mind goes. But when the mind is merged in the spiritual heart, prāṇa does not move, and the mind attains a quiescent state.

The reflection of consciousness within itself is known as puryaṣṭaka. Mind alone is puryaṣṭaka, though others have described it more elaborately (as composed of the five elements, the inner instrument or antaḥkarana, the organs of action, the senses, ignorance, desire and karma). It is also known as the subtle body (liṅga śarīra). When the mind is divested of its support, it remains alone in the self. When the puryaṣṭaka is rid of all its supports, it attains a state of quiescence and falls motionless. When the lotus of the heart unfolds, the puryaṣṭaka functions; when that lotus folds, the puryaṣṭaka ceases to function. As long as the puryaṣṭaka functions the body lives; when it ceases to function, the body dies. This cessation can be caused by some form of inner conflict between the impurities and inner awakening. **If only pure vāsanā or tendencies fill one's heart, all conflicts cease and there are harmony, liberation and longevity.** Otherwise, when the body dies, the subtle body chooses another suited to fulfil the hidden vāsanā. Due to these vāsanā, the puryaṣṭaka forges new links with the new subtle body, forgetting its nature as pure consciousness.

Since the omnipresent infinite consciousness alone is present at all times, diversity is absurd and impossible. Belief in the existence of a goblin creates it. Belief in the diversity establishes it. When the non-dual being is known, the duality vanishes instantly. It is all, it is supreme blessedness and peace, it is beyond expression. It is purest OṀ. It is transcendent. It is supreme.

niyatir nityamudvegavarjitā 'parimārjitā
eṣā nṛtyati vai nṛtyaṁ jagajjālakanāṭakam (37/23)

The LORD continued:

In a manner of speaking, the supreme being (the infinite consciousness) is the father of Brahmā the creator, Viṣṇu the preserver, Śiva the redeemer and others. That infinite consciousness alone is fit to be adored and worshipped. However, there is no use inviting it for the worship; no mantrā are of any use in its worship for it is immediate (closest, one's own self) and hence does not need to be invited. It is the omnipresent self of all. The realisation of this infinite consciousness (which is totally effortless) is alone the best form of worship.

This infinite consciousness can be compared to the ultimate subatomic particle which yet hides within its heart the greatest of mountains. It encompasses the span of countless epochs, but does not let go of a moment of time. It is subtler than the tip of a single strand of hair, yet it pervades the entire universe. No one has seen its limits! It does nothing, yet it has fashioned the universe. Sustaining the entire universe, it does nothing at all. All substances are non-different from it, yet it is not a substance; though it is non-substantial it pervades all substances.

The supreme being is formless, and yet the following five are its aspects: will, space, time, order (or destiny) and the cosmic unmanifest nature. It has countless powers or energies or potencies. Chief among them are knowledge, dynamics, action and non-action.

All these are but pure consciousness; because they are called the potencies of consciousness, they are apparently regarded as distinct from consciousness, though in fact they are not.

This entire creation is like a stage on which all these potencies of consciousness dance to the tune of time. The foremost among these is known as 'order' (the natural order of things and sequences). It is also known as action, desire or will-to-do, time and so on. It is this potency that ordains that each thing should have a certain characteristic — from the blade of grass to the creator Brahmā. **This natural order is free from excitement but not purified of its limitation: that (natural order) is what dances a dance-drama known as the world-appearance.** It portrays various moods (compassion, anger and so on), it produces and removes various seasons and epochs, it is accompanied by the celestial music and the roaring of the oceans, its stage is illumined by the sun and the moon and the stars, its actors and actresses are the living beings in all the worlds — such is the dance of the natural order. The Lord who is the infinite consciousness is the silent but alert witness of this cosmic dance. He is non-different from the dancer (the cosmic natural order) and the dance (the happenings).

etadeva paraṁ dhyānaṁ pūjaiṣaiva parā smṛtā
yadanāratamantaḥstha śuddhacinmātravedanaṁ (25)

The LORD continued:

Such is the Lord who is fit to be worshipped constantly by holy ones. It is he indeed who is worshipped by wise men in various ways and in various forms such as Śiva, Viṣṇu, etc. Now listen to the ways in which he is to be worshipped.

First of all, one should abandon the body-idea (the notion that 'I am this body'). Meditation alone is true worship. Hence one should constantly worship the Lord of the three worlds by means of meditation. How should one contemplate him? He is pure intelligence, he is as radiant as a hundred thousand suns risen together, he is the light that illumines all lights, he is the inner light. The limitless space is his throat, the firmament is his feet, the directions are his arms, the worlds are the weapons he bears in his hands, the entire universe is hidden in his heart, the gods are hairs on his body, the cosmic potencies are the energies in his body, time is his gatekeeper, and he has thousands of heads, eyes, ears and arms. He touches all, he tastes all, he hears all, he thinks through all, though he is beyond thinking. He does everything at all times, he bestows whatever one thinks of or desires, he dwells in all, he is the all, he alone is to be sought by all. Thus should one contemplate him.

This Lord is to be worshipped by one's own consciousness, not by material substances — by waving of lamps, lighting incense, offering flowers or even food or sandalpaste. He is attained without the least effort; he is worshipped by self-realisation alone. **This is the supreme meditation, this is the supreme worship: the continuous and unbroken awareness of the indwelling presence, inner light or consciousness.** While doing whatever one is doing — seeing, hearing, touching, smelling, eating, moving, sleeping, breathing or talking — one should realise one's essential nature as pure consciousness. Thus does one attain liberation.

Meditation is the offering, meditation is the water offered to the deity to wash his hands and feet, self-knowledge gained through meditation is the flower — indeed all these are directed towards meditation. The self is not realised by any means other than meditation. If one is able to meditate even for thirteen seconds, even if one is ignorant one attains the merit of giving away a cow in charity. If one does so for one hundred and one seconds, the merit is that of performing a sacred rite. If the duration is twelve minutes, the merit is a thousandfold. If the duration is of a day, one dwells in the highest realm. This is the supreme yoga, this is the supreme kriyā (action or service). One who practises this mode of worship is worshipped by the gods and the demons and all other beings. However, this is external worship.

pāvanaṁ pāvanānāṁ yad yatsarvatamasāṁ kṣayaḥ
tad idānīṁ pravakṣye 'haṁ antaḥ pūjanam ātmanaḥ (1)

The LORD continued:

I shall now declare to you the internal worship of the self which is the greatest among all purifiers and which destroys all darkness completely. This is of the nature of perpetual meditation — whether one is walking or standing, whether one is awake or asleep, in and through all of one's actions one should contemplate this supreme Lord who is seated in the heart and who brings about, as it were, all the modifications within oneself. One should worship the 'bodha-liṅgaṁ' (the manifest consciousness or self-awareness) which sleeps and wakes up, goes about or stands, touches what is to be touched, abandons what should be abandoned, enjoys and abandons pleasures, engages in varied external activities, lends value to all actions and remains at peace in the vital organs in the body (deha-liṅgaṁ in the text may also refer to the three 'liṅgaṁ' associated with the psychic centres). This inner intelligence should be worshipped with whatever comes to one unsought. Remaining firmly seated in the stream of life and its experiences after having bathed in self-knowledge, one should worship this inner intelligence with the materials of self-realisation.

One should contemplate the Lord in the following manner: he is the light illumined by the solar force as well as the lunar force, his is the intelligence that eternally lies hidden in all material substances, he is the extrovert awareness that flows through the bodily avenues onto the external world, he is the prāṇa that moves in one's face (nose), he transforms contacts of the senses into meaningful experiences, he rides the chariot composed of prāṇa and apāna, he dwells in secret in the cave of one's heart. He is the knower of the knowable and the doer of all actions, the experiencer of all experiences, the thinker of all thoughts. It is he who knows all parts or limbs thoroughly, who is recognised by being and non-being and who illumines all experiences.

He is without parts but he is the all, he dwells in the body but he is omnipresent, he enjoys and does not enjoy, he is the intelligence in every limb. He is the thinking faculty in the mind. He rises in the middle of prāṇa and apāna. He dwells in the heart, in the throat, in the middle of the palate, the middle of the eyebrows and at the tip of the nose. He is the reality in all the thirty-six elements (or metaphysical categories), he transcends the internal states, he is the one who produces the internal sounds, and he brings into being the bird known as mind. He is the reality in what is described as imagination and non-imagination. He dwells in all beings as oil dwells in the seed. He dwells in the heart-lotus and again he dwells throughout the body. He shines as pure consciousness. He is immediately seen everywhere, for he is the pure experiencing in all experiences and apparently polarises himself when apprehending the objects of such experiences.

yathāprāptakramotthena sarvārthena samarcayet
manāgapi na kartavyo yatno 'trā 'pūrvavastuni (31)

The LORD continued:

One should contemplate that the Lord is the intelligence in the body. The various functions and faculties in the body serve that intelligence as consorts serve their lord. The mind is the messenger who brings and presents to the Lord the knowledge of the three worlds. The two fundamental energies, viz., the energy of wisdom (jñāna śakṭi) and the energy of action (kriyā śakṭi), are the consorts of the Lord. Diverse aspects of knowledge are his ornaments. The organs of action are the gates through which the Lord enters the outside world. 'I am that infinite self which is indivisible; I remain full and infinite' — thus the intelligence dwells in the body.

He who contemplates in this manner is equanimity itself, his behaviour is equanimous, guided by equal vision. He has reached the state of natural goodness and inner purity and he is beautiful in every aspect of his being. He worships the Lord who is the intelligence that pervades his entire body.

This worship is performed day and night perpetually, with the objects that are effortlessly obtained, and are offered to the Lord with a mind firmly established in equanimity and in the right spirit (for the Lord is consciousness and cares only for the right spirit). **The Lord should be worshipped with everything that is obtained without effort. One should never make the least effort to attain that which one does not possess.** The Lord should be worshipped by means of all the enjoyments that the body enjoys, through eating, drinking, being with one's consort and such other pleasures. The Lord should be worshipped with the illnesses one experiences and with every sort of unhappiness or suffering one experiences. The Lord should be worshipped with all of one's activities, including life and death and all of one's dreams. The Lord should be worshipped with one's poverty and prosperity. The Lord should be worshipped even with fights and quarrels as well as with sports and other pastimes, and even with the manifestations of the emotions of attraction and aversion. The Lord should be adored with the noble qualities of a pious heart: friendship, compassion, joy and indifference.

The Lord should be worshipped with all kinds of pleasures that are granted to one unsought, whether those pleasures are sanctioned by the scriptures, etc., or forbidden by them. The Lord should be worshipped with those that are regarded as desirable and others that are regarded as undesirable, with those that are considered appropriate and others that are considered inappropriate. For this worship one should abandon what is lost and one should accept and receive what has been obtained without effort.

samatākāśavadbhūtvā yattu syāllınamānasaṁ
avikāramanāyāsaṁ tadevā 'rcanamucyate (58)

The LORD continued:

One should engage oneself in this worship at all times, established in supreme equanimity in regard to all the percepts whether they be pleasant or unpleasant. One should regard everything as good and auspicious (or one should regard everything as a mixture of good and evil). Realising that everything is the one self, one should worship the self in this spirit. One should look with equal vision upon that which is pleasant and beautiful through and through and that which is unendurably unpleasant. Thus should one worship the self.

One should abandon the divisive notions of 'This I am' and 'This I am not' and realise that 'All this is indeed Brahman', the one indivisible and infinite consciousness. In that spirit one should worship the self. At all times, in all forms and their modifications, one should worship the self in and through all that one obtains. One should worship the self after having abandoned the distinction between the desirable and the undesirable, or even while relying on such a distinction (but using them as the materials for the worship).

Without craving and without rejecting, that which is effortlessly and naturally obtained may be enjoyed. One should not get excited or depressed when faced with insignificant and significant objects, just as neither sky nor space is affected by the diverse objects that exist and grow in it. One should worship the self, without psychological perversion, with every object that is obtained purely on account of the coincidence of the time, place and activity — whether they are popularly known as good or as not-good.

In this procedure for the worship of the self, whatever article has been mentioned as being necessary for the worship is of the same nature as all others, though the expressions used are different. Equanimity is sweetness itself and this sweetness is beyond the senses and the mind. Whatever is touched by that equanimity instantly becomes sweet, whatever its description or definition may be. **That alone is regarded as worship which is performed when one is in a state of equanimity like that of space, when the mind has become utterly quiescent without the least movement of thought, when there is effortless absence of perversity.** Established in this state of equanimity, the wise man should experience infinite expansion within himself while carrying out his natural actions externally without craving or rejection. Such is the nature of the worshipper of this intelligence. In his case delusion, ignorance and ego-sense do not arise, even in dream. Remain in this state, O sage, experiencing everything as a child does. Worship the Lord of this body (the intelligence that pervades it) with all that is brought to you by time, circumstance and environment, and rest in supreme peace, devoid of desire.

deśakālaparicchinno yeṣāṁ syāt parameśvaraḥ
asmākam upadeśyās te na vipaścid vipaścitāṁ (40/12)

The LORD continued:

Whatever you do and whenever you do it (or refrain from doing it) — all that is worship of the Lord who is pure consciousness. By regarding all that as the worship of the self who is the Lord; he is delighted.

Likes and dislikes, attraction and aversion are not found in the self independent of its essential nature; they are mere words. Even the concepts indicated by words like 'sovereignty', 'poverty', 'pleasure', 'pain', 'one's own' and 'others', are in fact worship of the self, for the conceiving intelligence is the self. Knowledge of the cosmic being alone is the proper worship of the cosmic being.

It is that self or cosmic consciousness alone which is indicated by expressions such as 'this world'. Oh, what a mysterious wonder it is that the self, which is pure consciousness or intelligence, somehow seems to forget its own nature and comes to regard itself as the jīva (the individual). In fact, in that cosmic being, which is the reality in everything, there is not even the division into worshipper, worship and the worshipped. It is impossible to describe that cosmic being which supports the entire universe without division; it is impossible to teach another concerning it. And, **we do not consider them worthy of being taught by us, who consider that god is limited by time and space.** Hence, abandoning all such limited concepts, abandoning even the division between the worshipper and the worshipped (Lord), worship the self by the self. Be at peace, pure, free from cravings. Consider that all your experiences and expressions are the worship of the self.

(In reply to Vasiṣṭha's request for a fuller explanation of Śiva, Brahmān, self, why they are so called and how such differences arose, the LORD continued:)

The reality is beginningless and endless and it is not even reflected in anything: that is the reality. However, since it is not possible to experience it through the mind and the senses, it is even regarded as if it were non-being.

(In reply to Vasiṣṭha's question: "If it is beyond the mind, how is it realised?" the LORD replied:)

In the case of the seeker who is eager to attain freedom from ignorance and who is therefore equipped with what is termed 'sātvika avidyā' (subtle ignorance), this sātvika avidyā, with the help of what are known as scriptures, removes the ignorance just as a washerman removes dirt with the help of another form of dirt (soap). By this catalytic action the ignorance is removed, the self realises the self and the self sees the self on account of its own self-luminous nature.

akāraṇānyapi prāptā bhṛśaṁ kāraṇatāṁ dvija
kramā gurūpadeśādyā ātmajñānasya siddhaye (13)

The LORD continued:

When a child is playing with charcoal, his hands become black. If he washes his hands but immediately plays again with charcoal, his hands become black again. However, if he does not handle charcoal again after washing, his hands can remain clean. Even so, if one enquires into the nature of the self and at the same time refrains from those actions which promote avidyā or ignorance, the darkness of ignorance vanishes. However, it is only the self that becomes aware of the self.

Do not look upon this diversity as the self. Do not entertain the feeling that self-knowledge is the result of the teaching of a preceptor. The guru or the preceptor is endowed with the mind and the senses; the self or Brahman is beyond the mind and the senses. That which is attained only after the other ceases, is not attained with its help while it still exists. However, **though the instructions of a preceptor and all the rest of it are not really the means for the attainment of self-knowledge, they have come to be regarded as the means for it.**

The self is not revealed either by the scriptures or by the instructions of a preceptor, and the self is not revealed without the instructions of a preceptor and without the help of the scripture. It is revealed only when all these come together. It is only when the scriptural knowledge, instructions of a preceptor and true discipleship come together that self-knowledge is attained.

That which IS after all the senses have ceased to function and all notions of pleasure and pain have vanished, is the self or Śiva, which is also indicated by expressions like 'that', 'truth' or 'reality'. However, that which IS when all these cease to be, exists even when all these are present, like the limitless space. Out of their compassion for the ignorant deluded ones, in an effort to awaken them spiritually and to awaken in them a thirst for liberation, the redeemers of the universe (known as Brahmā, Indra, Rudra and others) have composed scriptures like the veda and purāṇā (the legends). In these scriptures they have used words like 'consciousness', 'Brahman', 'Śiva', 'self', 'Lord', 'supreme self', etc. These words may imply a diversity, but in truth there is no such diversity.

The truth indicated by words like 'Brahman', etc., is indeed pure consciousness. In relation to it even the limitless space is as gross and substantial as a great mountain. That pure consciousness appears to be the knowable object and gives rise to the concept of intelligence or consciousness, though being the innermost self, it is not an object of knowledge. On account of a momentary conceptualisation, this pure consciousness gives rise to the ego-sense ('I know').

vāsanāvaśato duḥkhaṁ vidyamāne ca sā bhavet
avidyamānaṁ ca jagan mṛgatṛṣṇāmbubhaṅgavat (52)

The LORD continued:

This ego-sense then gives rise to the notions of time and space. Endowed with the energy of the vital air, it then becomes jiva or the individual. The individual thenceforward follows the dictates of the notions and slips into dense ignorance. Thus is the mind born in conjunction with the ego-sense and the different forms of psychological energy. All these together are known as the 'ātivāhika' body, the subtle body which moves from one plane to another.

After this, the substances (the objects of the world) corresponding to the subtle energies of the ātivāhika body were conceived of, and thus were the various senses (sight, touch, hearing, taste and smell), their corresponding objects and their connecting experiences brought into being. These together are known as the puryaṣṭaka and in their subtle state they are also known as the ātivāhika body.

Thus were all these substances created; but nothing was created in fact. All these are but apparent modifications in the one infinite consciousness. Even as dream-objects are within oneself, all these are non-different from the infinite consciousness. Even as when one dreams those objects they seem to become the objects of one's perception, all these, too, appear to be objective realities.

When the truth concerning them is realised, all these shine as the Lord. However, even that is untrue, for all these have never become material substances or objects. On account of one's own notions of their being substances which one experiences, they appear to have a substantiality. Thus conjuring up a substantiality, the consciousness sees the substantiality.

Conditioned by such notions it seems to suffer. **Conditioning is sorrow. But conditioning is based on thoughts and notions (or sensual and psychological experiences). However, the truth is beyond such experiences and the world is an appearance, like a mirage!** In that case, what is psychological conditioning, who conditions what and who is conditioned by such conditioning? Who drinks the water of the mirage? Thus, when all these are rejected the reality alone remains in which there is no conditioning, naught conditioned. It may be styled the being or the non-being, but it alone is. Mental conditioning is illusory non-being, like a ghost; when it is laid, the illusion of creation also vanishes. He who takes this ego-sense and this mirage known as creation to be real is unfit to be instructed. Preceptors instruct only a man endowed with wisdom, not foolish men. The latter pin their faith and hope on the world-appearance, like the ignorant man who bestows his daughter in marriage to the man seen only in his dream!

grāhyagrāhakasaṁbandhe sāmānye sarvadehināṁ
yoginaḥ sāvadhānatvaṁ yattadarcanam ātmanaḥ (43/8)

VASIṢṬHA continued:

The mountain seen in a dream only appears to exist in time and space. It does not occupy any space nor does it take time to appear and disappear. Even so is the case with the world. In whatever manner the omnipotent deity comes into being, in exactly the same manner a worm also comes into being within the twinkling of an eye. The jiva thinks of itself as Creator, Preserver and so on, but all this is nothing more than thought-form. However, this thought-form conceives and perceives other thought-forms and experiences them.

O Rāma, the unreal jiva perceives the unreal world on account of the unreal influence of the unreality. In all this what can be considered as real and what as unreal? An imaginary object is imaginatively described by someone; and one understands in one's own imagination and imagines that he understands it. Just as liquidity is in liquids, motion in wind, emptiness in space, even so is omnipresence in the self.

From the time the Lord instructed me, I have been performing the worship of the infinite self. By the grace of such worship though I am constantly engaged in the various activities I am free from sorrow. I perform the worship of the self, who is undivided though apparently divided, with the flowers of whatever comes to me naturally and whatever actions are natural to me.

To come into relationship (to possess and to be possessed) is common to all embodied beings; but the yogi is forever vigilant, and such vigilance is the worship of the self. Adopting this inner attitude and with a mind utterly devoid of any attachment, I roam in this dreadful forest of saṁsāra (world-appearance). If you do so, you will not suffer.

When great sorrow (like the loss of wealth and relatives) befalls you, enquire into the nature of truth, in the manner described. You will not be affected by joy or sorrow. You now know how all these things arise and how they cease, and you also know the fate of the man who is deluded by them, who does not enquire into their real nature. They do not belong to you, you do not belong to them. Such is the unreal nature of the world. Do not grieve.

Dear Rāma, you are pure consciousness which is not affected by the illusory perception of the diversity of creation. If you see this, how will notions of the desirable and the undesirable arise in you? Realising thus, O Rāma, remain established in the turiya (transcendental) state of consciousness.

RĀMA said:

By your grace, O Lord, I am free from the dirt of duality. I have realised that all this is indeed Brahman.

yadi tatpadamāpto 'si kadācit kālaparyayāt
tadahaṁbhāvanārūpe na maṅkttavyaṁ tvayā punaḥ (5)

VASIṢṬHA continued:

That is not considered action, O Rāma, which with an unattached mind you perform merely with the organs of action. The delight derived from sensual experience is fleeting. A repetition of that experience does not afford a repetition of the same delight. Who but a fool will entertain desire for such a momentary joy? Moreover, an object gives you pleasure only when it is desired. So the pleasure belongs to the desire — hence give up desire.

If in the course of time you attain the experience of that (the self), do not store it in your mind as a memory or ego-sense to be revived as desire once again. For when you rest on the pinnacle of self-knowledge it is unwise to fall into the pit of ego-sense again. Let hopes cease and let notions vanish, let the mind reach the state of no-mind, while you live unattached. You are bound only when you are ignorant. You will not be bound if you have self-knowledge. Hence, strive by every means to remain vigilant in self-knowledge.

When you do not engage yourself in sense-experiences and also when you experience whatever comes to you unsought, you are in a state of equanimity and purity, free from latent tendencies or memories. In such a state, like the sky, you will not be tainted even by a thousand distractions. When knower, known and knowledge merge in the one self, the pure experiencer does not once again generate a division within.

With the slightest movement in the mind (when the mind blinks) the saṁsāra (world-appearance) arises and ceases. Make the mind unwinking (free from movement of thought) by the restraint of the prāṇa and also the latent tendencies (vāsanā). By the movement (blinking) of prāṇa, the saṁsāra arises and ceases; by diligent practice make the prāṇa free from such movement. By the rise and cessation of foolishness (ignorance), self-binding action arises and ceases; restrain it by means of self-discipline and the instructions of the preceptor and the scriptures.

This world-illusion has arisen because of the movement of thought in the mind; when that ceases the illusion will cease, too, and the mind becomes no-mind. This can also be achieved by the restraint of prāṇa. That is the supreme state. The bliss that is experienced in a state of no-mind, that bliss which is uncaused, is not found even in the highest heaven. In fact, that bliss is inexpressible and indescribable and should not even be called happiness! The mind of the knower of truth is no-mind: it is pure satva. After living with such no-mind for some time, there arises the state known as turīya-atīta (the state beyond the transcendental, or the turīya state).

eṣaikikaiva vividheva vibhāvyamānā
naikātmikā na vividhā nanu saiva saiva
satyāsthitā sakalaśāntisamaikarūpā
sarvātmikā 'timahatī citirūpaśakttiḥ (36)

VASIṢṬHA continued:

In this connection, O Rāma, there is an instructive parable which I shall presently narrate to you.

There is a wood-apple fruit which is immeasurably large and which does not decay or perish, though it has existed for countless aeons. It is the source and support of the nectar of immortality and indestructibility. It is the abode of sweetness. Though it is most ancient, it is ever new, like the new moon. It is the very centre or heart of the universe, it is unmoving and it is not shaken even by the forces of cosmic dissolution. This wood-apple fruit, which is immeasurably large, is the original source of this creation.

Even when it is fully ripe it does not fall from its place. It is forever fully ripe, but it does not become overripe. Even the creator Brahmā, Viṣṇu, Rudra and the other gods do not know the origin of this wood-apple fruit. No one has seen the seed nor the tree on which this fruit grows. The only thing that can be said about it is that this fruit exists, without beginning, without middle and without end, without change and without modification. Even within this fruit there is no diversity; it is completely full, without emptiness. It is the fountain-source of all joys and delights, from the delight of an ordinary man to that of the highest of divinities. Thus, this fruit is none other than the manifestation of the energy of infinite consciousness.

This energy of the infinite consciousness, without even for a moment abandoning its true nature, has manifested this creation, as it were, by merely willing it in its own intelligence. In fact, even this (i.e. that it willed so) is not really true! The ego-sense that is implied in such willing is itself unreal; but out of this have proceeded all the elements and their corresponding subjective senses. In truth, that energy of the infinite consciousness itself is space, time, natural order, expansion of thought, attraction and repulsion, I-ness, you-ness and it-ness, above, below, the other directions, the mountains, the firmament and the stars, knowledge and ignorance — all, whatever is, was and ever will be. All that is nothing but the energy of the infinite consciousness.

Though it is one it is conceived of as diverse beings; it is neither one nor many. It is not even it! It is established in reality. It is of the nature of supreme, all inclusive peace. It is the one immeasurably great cosmic being or self. It is (cosmic) energy or the nature of (cosmic) consciousness.

bijaṁ puṣpaphalāntasthaṁ bījāntar nā 'nyadātmakaṁ
yādṛśī bījasattā sā bhavantī yātyathottaraṁ (30)

VASIṢṬHA continued:

There is yet another parable, O Rama, to illustrate this further. I shall now narrate that to you.

There is a great rock which is full of tenderness and affection, which is obvious and ever clearly perceived, which is soft, which is omnipresent and eternal. Within it countless lotuses blossom. Their petals sometimes touch one another, sometimes not; sometimes they are exposed and sometimes they are hidden from view. Some face downwards, some face upwards and some have their roots intertwined. Some have no roots at all. All things exist within it, though they do not.

O Rāma, this rock is indeed the cosmic consciousness; it is rock-like in its homogeneity. Yet within it all these diverse creatures of this universe appear to be. Just as one conceives or imagines different forms within the rock, this universe is also ignorantly imagined to exist in this consciousness. Even if a sculptor 'creates' different forms in the rock, it is still rock: even so in the case of this cosmic consciousness which is a homogeneous mass of consciousness. Even as the solid rock contains potentially diverse figures which can be carved out of it, the diverse names and forms of the creatures of this universe exist potentially in cosmic consciousness. Even as rock remains rock, carved or uncarved, consciousness remains consciousness whether the world appears or not. The world-appearance is but an empty expression; its substance is naught but consciousness.

In fact, even these manifestations and modifications are but Brahman, the cosmic consciousness — though not in the sense of manifestation or modification. Even this distinction — modification in the sense of modification, or any other sense — is meaningless in Brahman. When such expressions are used in relation to Brahman, the meaning is quite different, like water in the mirage. **Since the seed does not contain anything other than the seed, even the flowers and the fruits are of the same nature as the seed: the substance of the seed is the substance of subsequent effects, too.** Even so, the homogeneous mass of cosmic consciousness does not give rise to anything other than what it is in essence. When this truth is realised, duality ceases. Consciousness never becomes un-consciousness. If there is modification that too is consciousness. Hence, whatever there may be, wherever and in whatever form — all this is Brahman. All these exist forever in their potential state in the mass of homogeneous consciousness.

sa nānāto 'pyanānāto yathā 'ṇḍarasabarhiṇaḥ
advaitādvaitasattātmā tathā brahmajagadbhramaḥ (31)

VASIṢṬHA continued:

Time, space and other factors in this so-called creation (which is in truth another aspect of the same consciousness) are none other than consciousness. When it is realised that all these are but thoughts and notions, and that the self is one and indivisible, how then are these regarded as unreal? In the seed there is nothing but the seed — no diversity. At the same time there is the notion of potential diversity (of flowers, fruits) supposedly present in the seed. Even so, cosmic consciousness is one, devoid of diversity; yet the universe of diversity is said to exist only in notion.

The stone is single; the notion of numerous lotuses arises only in relation to that single stone. Even so the notion of diversity arises in consciousness without causing diversity. But just as water in mirage is and is not simultaneously, even so is diversity in relation to the infinite consciousness. All this is indeed Brahman, the infinite consciousness. Even as the notion of the existence of lotuses in the stone does not destroy the stone, Brahman is unaffected by world-appearance which exists as the very nature of Brahman in Brahman. There is no essential difference in truth between Brahman and the world: they are synonyms. When the reality is thus seen, Brahman alone is seen.

Even as all that is seen as water in the world is naught but hydrogen and oxygen gases, even so the world-appearance is but Brahman alone. The one consciousness appears as the mind, the mountains, etc., even as the multi-coloured feathers and the wings of the peacock are present in the egg of the peacock. This power or faculty is potentially present in the infinite consciousness. Whatever is now seen as the diverse objects of the universe, if it is seen with the eye of wisdom (the eye that is wisdom), then only Brahman or the infinite consciousness will be seen. **For that is non-dual though apparently diverse, just like the notion of diversity in the fluid in the peacock's egg. The notion of Brahman and the world is therefore both dual and non-dual.** That which is the substratum for all these notions of unity and diversity — that is the supreme state.

The infinite consciousness pervades the entire universe, and the universe exists in the infinite consciousness. The relationship is one of diversity and non-diversity — just as the numerous parts of the peacock are in the one egg-substance. Where is the diversity in all this?

**na dṛśyaṁ nopadeśārhaṁ nā 'tyāsannaṁ na dūragaṁ
kevalānubhavaprāpyaṁ cidrūpaṁ śuddhamātmanaḥ (10)**

VASIṢṬHA continued:

All these — the ego-sense and the space, etc. — have acquired the nature of real substances though they have not been created at all. Where nothing has arisen (been created) there everything is seen. Even so, the sages, gods and the perfected ones remain in their transcendental consciousness, tasting the bliss of their own nature. They have abandoned the illusion of duality of the observer and the object, and the consequent movement of thought. Their gaze is fixed and unwinking.

Though these sages are active here they do not entertain the least notion of illusory existence. They are firmly rooted in the abandonment of the relationship between the knower and the known (subject and object). Their life-force is not agitated. It is as if they were painted pictures; their mind does not move, even as the mind of painted figures does not move, for they have abandoned the conceptualising tendency of the consciousness.

They engage themselves in appropriate activity by a little movement of thought in consciousness (even as the Lord does). However, such movement of thought and the experiencing of the contact of the observer with the object also produce great joy in them. Their consciousness is absolutely pure, purified of all images (concepts and notions).

Such a state of purity of the self, the true nature of the infinite consciousness, is not a vision (an experience of the mind and the senses). It is incapable of being taught. It is not very easy nor is it far distant or impossible. It is attained by direct experience alone.

That alone exists, naught else: neither the body nor the senses and life-force, neither the mind nor the storehouse of memory or latent tendencies, neither the jiva nor even a movement in consciousness, neither consciousness nor the world. It is neither real nor unreal, nor something in between, neither void nor non-void, neither time nor space nor substantiality. Free from all these and free from a hundred veils in the heart, one should experience the self in all that is seen.

It is neither the beginning nor the end. Because it is ever present everywhere, it is taken for something else. Thousands are born and thousands die: but the self which is everywhere, inside and outside, is not affected. It remains in all these bodies, etc. as if it were just a little different from the infinite.

Though radiantly engaged in diverse activities, remain free from the sense of I-ness and mine-ness. For whatever is seen in this world is Brahman, free from characteristics and qualities; it is eternal, peaceful, pure and utterly quiescent.

samasyā ''dyantayor yeyaṁ dṛśyate vikṛtiḥ kṣaṇāt
saṁvidaḥ saṁbhramaṁ viddhi nā 'vikāre 'sti vikriyā (5)

RĀMA asked:

If Brahman does not undergo any modification at all, how does this world-appearance, which is and is not real, arise in it?

VASIṢṬHA replied:

True modification, O Rāma, is a transformation of a substance into another; like the curdling of milk, in which case the curd cannot once again return to its milk-state. Such is not the case with Brahman, which was unmodified before the world-appearance and which regains its unmodified state after the world-disappearance. **Both in the beginning and in the end it is unmodified homogeneous consciousness. The momentary and apparent modification in this is but a mild disturbance of consciousness, not a modification at all.** In that Brahman there is neither a subject nor an object of consciousness. Whatever a thing is in the beginning and in the end, that alone it is. If it appears to be something else in the middle, that appearance is regarded as unreal. Hence, the self is the self in the beginning and in the end and therefore in the middle, too! It never undergoes any transformation or modification.

RĀMA asked again: In that self, which is pure consciousness, how does this mild disturbance arise?

VASIṢṬHA replied:

I am convinced, O Rāma, that that infinite consciousness alone is real and that there is no disturbance at all in its nature. We use words like 'Brahman' just for the sake of communication or instruction, not to raise notions of one and two. You, I and all these things are pure Brahman: there is no ignorance at all.

RĀMA asked again: But at the end of the previous section, you exhorted me to enquire into the nature of this ignorance!

VASIṢṬHA replied:

Yes, at that time you were still not fully awakened. Such expressions as 'ignorance', 'jiva', etc., have been invented as aids to instructing the unawakened. One should use commonsense and suitable aids (yuktti also commonly means 'trick') to awaken the seeker before imparting the knowledge of the truth. If one declares, 'All this is Brahman' to an unawakened person, it is like a man petitioning a tree for relief from his suffering. It is by suitable aids that the unawakened is awakened. The awakened is enlightened by the truth. Thus, now that you are awakened, I declare the truth to you.

You are Brahman, I am Brahman, the whole universe is Brahman. Whatever you are doing, realise this truth at all times. This Brahman or the self alone is the reality in all beings, even as clay is the real substance in thousands of pots. Even as wind and its movement are non-different, consciousness and its internal movement (energy) which causes all these manifestations are non-different. It is the seed of notion falling on the soil of consciousness that gives rise to apparent diversity. If it does not so fall, mind does not sprout.

pūrṇāt pūrṇamidaṁ pūrṇaṁ pūrṇāt pūrṇaṁ prasūyate
purnena "pūritaṁ pūrṇaṁ sthitā pūrṇe ca pūrṇatā (2)

RĀMA said:

What is to be known is known, what is to be seen is seen. We are all filled with the supreme truth, thanks indeed to the nectarine wisdom of Brahman, imparted by you. **This fullness is filled with fullness. Fullness is born from fullness. Fullness fills fullness. In fullness, fullness is ever established.** However, for the further expansion of awareness, I ask again: pray bear with me. The sense-organs are obviously present in all: yet how is it that the dead person does not experience sensations, though while living he experienced their objects through those organs?

VASIṢṬHA continued:

Apart from the pure consciousness, there are neither the senses, the mind, nor even their objects. It is that consciousness alone which appears as the objects in nature and as the senses in the person. When that consciousness has apparently become the subtle body (puryaṣṭaka), it reflects the external objects.

The eternal and infinite consciousness is indeed free of all modifications; but when there arises the notion of 'I am' in it, that notion is known as the jīva. It is that jıva that lives and moves in this body. When the notion of 'I' arises (ahaṁbhāvanā), it is known as ego-sense (ahaṁkāra). When there are thoughts (mananā), it is known as mind (manas). When there is awareness (bodha), it is intelligence (buddhi). When seen (dṛś) by the individual soul (indra) it is known as the sense (indriya). When the notion of body prevails it appears to be body; when the notion of object prevails it appears to be the diverse objects. However, through the persistence of these notions, the subtle personality condenses into material substantiality. The same consciousness thereafter thinks 'I am the body', 'I am the tree', etc. Thus self-deluded it rises and falls until it attains a pure birth and is spiritually awakened. Then, by being devoted to the truth, it attains self-knowledge.

I shall now tell you how it perceives the objects. I said that on account of the notion of 'I am', consciousness abides as jıva in the body. When its senses descend upon similar bodies outside itself, there is contact between the two and there is desire to know (to become one with) them. When there is this contact the object is reflected within oneself and the jıva perceives this reflection, though it believes that the reflection is outside! The jiva knows only this reflection, which means it knows itself. This contact is the cause of the perception of external objects; hence it is possible only in the case of the ignorant one whose mind is deluded, and not in the case of the liberated sage. Of course, since the jıva (which is but a 'notion') and all the rest of it are inert and insentient, the reflection thus seen and experienced is in fact an optical illusion or intellectual perversion. The self is all-in-all all the time.

brahmapuryaṣṭakasyā ''davarthasaṁvidyathoditā
puryaṣṭakasya sarvasya tathaivodeti sarvadā (2)

VASIṢṬHA continued:

Just as the cosmic body (composed of the intelligence-energy and the cosmic elements) or the first puryaṣṭaka (cosmic subtle body) arose in the infinite consciousness as a notion, all the other bodies (puryaṣṭakā) also arise in the same manner. Whatever the jiva (which is the puryaṣṭaka or the subtle body) conceives of while still in the womb, that it sees as existent. Just as in the macrocosm the cosmic elements evolve, even so in the microcosm the senses corresponding to those elements evolve. Of course, they are not actually created. These expressions and descriptions are used merely for the sake of instruction. These ideas which are used in instruction are dispelled by the enquiry which they initially promote and prompt.

Even when you observe this ignorance very carefully and keenly you do not see it: it vanishes. The unreal is rooted in unreality. We only talk of water in the mirage. The water in the mirage, being unreal, has never been water at all. In the light of truth the reality of all things is revealed, and delusion or illusory perception vanishes.

The self is real. Jīva, puryaṣṭaka (the subtle body) and all the rest of it are unreal, and the enquiry into their nature is no doubt enquiry into their unreality! It is in order to instruct one in the real nature of the unreality that such expressions as 'jīva', etc., are used.

This infinite consciousness has, as it were, assumed the nature of the jiva, and oblivious of its true nature it experiences whatever it thinks of as being. Even as to the child the unreal ghost it visualises at night is truly real, the jīva conceives of the five elements which it sees as existing. These are nothing but notions of the jīva; however, the jīva sees them as if they are outside it. It thinks that some are within and others are outside of it. And so it experiences them.

Knowledge is inherent in consciousness, even as void is in space. However, consciousness now believes knowledge to be its own object. The diverse objects are limited by time and space, which are themselves but the notional division in consciousness brought about by this division (of consciousness and knowledge, as subject and object) within itself. Such division does not exist in the self, which transcends time and space.

However, the infinite consciousness with the knowledge inherent in it conceives of diverse creatures. Such is its power, which no-one can challenge. The inert space is unable to reflect itself within itself. But because its nature is infinite consciousness, Brahman reflects itself within itself and conceives of itself as a duality, though it is bodiless.

hematvakaṭakatve dve satyāsatyasvarūpiṇī
hemni bhāṇḍagate yadvaccittvācittve tathā ''tmani (36)

VASIṢṬHA continued:

Whatever this consciousness thinks of, that it sees as existing: its concepts and notions are never barren. **In a golden bracelet there are these two — gold and bracelet — one being the reality (gold) and the other being the appearance (of bracelet). Even so, in the self there are both consciousness and the notion of material (inert) substantiality.** Since consciousness is omnipresent, it is ever present in the mind in which the notion arises.

The dreamer dreams of a village which occupies his mind, and in which he lives for the time being; a little later he dreams of another situation and thinks he lives there. Even so, the jīva goes from one body to another; the body is but the reflection of the notion entertained by the jīva. The unreal (body) alone dies and it is the unreal that is born again, apparently in another body. Just as in the dream one experiences things seen and unseen, even so in the dream of the jiva it experiences the world and even sees what is to come in the future.

Even as an error yesterday can be rectified and turned into a good action by self-effort today, the habits of the past can be overcome by appropriate self-effort. However, the notion of jīva-hood and of the existence and functioning of the eyes, etc., cannot be abolished except by the attainment of liberation. Till then, they become alternately latent and patent.

A notion entertained by consciousness appears as the body. It has a corresponding subtle body (ātivāhika, which is also known as puryaṣṭaka) composed of mind, intellect, ego-sense and the five elements. The self is formless, but the puryaṣṭaka roams in this creation in sentient and insentient bodies until it purifies itself, lives as if in deep sleep and attains liberation. The subtle body exists all the time, during dreams and during sleep. It continues to exist in insentient 'bodies' (like inanimate objects) as if it were in deep sleep. All these are also experienced in this (human) body. Its deep sleep state is inert and insentient, its dream-state is the experience of this creation, its waking state is truly the transcendental (turīya) consciousness; and the realisation of the truth is liberation. The state of liberation-while-living is itself the turīya consciousness. Beyond that is Brahman which is turīya-atīta (beyond turīya). In every atom of existence there is naught else than the supreme being; wherever the world is seen, that is but an illusory world-appearance. This illusion, and therefore bondage, is sustained by psychological conditioning. Such conditioning is bondage and its abandonment is freedom. Dense and heavy conditioning is existence as inert objects, middling conditioning as animals and thin conditioning as humans. But enough of the perception of division: the whole universe is but the manifestation of the energy of infinite consciousness.

na puṁsa iva jīvasya svapnaḥ saṁbhavati kvacit
tenaite jāgrato bhāvā jāgratsvapnakṛto 'tra hi (2)

VASIṢṬHA continued:

What is known as this saṁsāra (world-appearance) is but the original dream of the jīva (the first person). **The dream of the jīva is not like the dream of a human being: the former's dream is experienced as the wakeful state. Hence it is that the wakeful state is considered a dream.** The jīva's long dream is instantly materialised, though it is unreal and unsubstantial. The jīva goes from one dream to another within that dream.

The entire universe appears in the one ocean of cosmic consciousness; in that universe dwell fourteen types of beings. This universe has already had Yama and others as its presiding deities. They have established the tenets of right conduct. However, when people become predominantly sinful, Yama the god of death sometimes engages himself in meditation for some years, during which the population increases and explodes.

The gods, frightened by this population explosion, resort to various devices to reduce it. All this has happened again and again countless times. The present ruler (Yama) is Vaivasvata. He, too, will have to perform meditation for some time. When, on account of that, the population of the earth will multiply very fast, all the gods will appeal to lord Viṣṇu to come to their aid. He will incarnate as lord Kṛṣṇa, along with his alter ego named Arjuna. His elder brother will be Yudhiṣṭhira or the son of Dharma, who will be the embodiment of righteousness. His cousin Duryodhana will fight a duel with Bhima, Arjuna's brother. In this battle between cousins eighteen divisions of armed forces will be killed; and thus will Viṣṇu dispose of the burden on the earth.

Kṛṣṇa and Arjuna will play the roles of simple human beings. When Arjuna sees that the armies on both sides are composed of his own kinsmen, he will become despondent and will refuse to fight. At that time, lord Kṛṣṇa will instruct him in the highest wisdom and bring about a spiritual awakening in him. He will tell Arjuna: "This (self) is neither born nor does it die, it is eternal and is not killed when this body is killed. He who thinks that it kills or that it is killed, he is ignorant. How, why and by whom is this infinite being, which is one without a second and which is subtler than space, destroyed? Arjuna, behold the self which is infinite, unmanifest, eternal and which is of the nature of pure consciousness and untainted. You are unborn and eternal!"

When the Lord will thus instruct Arjuna, the latter will say: "Lord, my delusion is gone. I have attained an awakening of intelligence through your grace." Arjuna will then engage himself in the conduct of the war, as if in a play.

Note: The very essence of the Bhagavad Gitā is found in these chapters — and many verses are quoted verbatim.

ciccamatkṛtireveyaṁ jagadityavabhāsate
nehā 'styaikyaṁ na ca dvitvaṁ mamādeśo 'pi tanmayaḥ (19)
vācyavācakaśiṣyehāguruvākyaiś camatkṛtaiḥ (20)

VASIṢṬHA continued:

Equip yourself with such an attitude, O Rāma, and remain unattached, endowed with the spirit of renunciation and with the realisation that whatever you do or you experience is an offering to the omnipresent being, Brahman. Then you will realise the truth, and that is the end of all doubts.

That is the supreme state, it is the guru of all gurū, it is the self, it is the light that illumines the world from within. It is the reality in all substances, that which endows the substances with their essential characteristic. The notion of 'world' arises only when the spirit of enquiry is absent. But, 'I' am before the world was. How then do the notions of world, etc., bind me? He who has thus realised the truth is free from all beginnings and all endings. He who is thus equipped with the spirit of non-duality (as if he is in deep sleep, though awake) is not disturbed though actively engaged in life. Such a person is liberated here and now.

What appears to be the world here is truly the magic (the work) of the infinite consciousness. There is no unity here, nor is there duality. My instructions, too, are of the same nature! The words, their meaning, the disciple, the wish (or the effort of the disciple) and the guru's ability in the use of the words — all these are also the play of the energy of the infinite consciousness! In the peace of one's own inner being, consciousness vibrates and the world-vision arises. If that consciousness does not vibrate, there will be no world-vision.

The mind is but the movement in consciousness. The non-realisation of this truth is world-vision! Non-realisation of this truth intensifies and aggravates the movement of thought in consciousness. Thus a cycle is formed. Ignorance and mental activity are perpetuated by each other.

When the inner intelligence is awakened the craving for pleasure ceases: this is the nature of the wise. In him this cessation of craving for pleasure is therefore natural and effortless. He knows that it is the energy of the self that experiences the experiences. He who, in order to please the public, refuses to experience what is to be experienced, he indeed beats the air with a stick! One attains self-knowledge by sometimes using appropriate means.

Desire for liberation interferes with the fullness of the self; absence of such desire promotes bondage! Hence, constant awareness is to be preferred. The sole cause for bondage and liberation is the movement in consciousness. Awareness of this ends this movement. The ego-sense ceases the very moment one observes it, for it has no support any longer. Then who is bound by whom, or who is liberated by whom?

tat sarvagatam ādyantarahitaṁ sthitamūrjitaṁ
sattāsāmānyamakhilaṁ vastutattvamihocyate (8)

VASIṢṬHA continued:

Such is the nature of the supreme being which is the infinite consciousness. They who are endowed with macrocosmic forms like Brahmā the creator, Viṣṇu and Śiva, are established in that supreme being; and they function here as the lords or kings of the world. Established in it, the perfected ones roam the heavens. Having attained it, one does not die nor does one grieve. The sage who dwells even for the twinkling of an eye in that pure being, which is of the nature of the illimitable and infinite consciousness and which is also known as the supreme self, is not again afflicted even though he continues to engage himself in the activities of this world.

RĀMA asked:

When the mind, the intellect and the ego-sense have all ceased to function, how does that pure being or infinite consciousness appear here?

VASIṢṬHA continued:

Brahman dwells in all bodies and experiences experiences — eats, drinks, speaks, gathers and destroys — but is free from the division of consciousness and its awareness. **That which is omnipresent and which is without beginning and end, and which is pure, unmodified, undifferentiated being — that is known as existence (vastu-tattvam) or reality.**

That exists as space in space, as sound in sound, as touch in touch, as skin in skin, in taste as taste, in form as form, in the eyes as sight, in smell as smell, in scent as scent, in the body as strength, in earth as the earth, in milk as milk, in wind as wind, in fire as fire, in intelligence as intelligence, in mind as mind, in the ego-sense as ego-sense. It rises as citta or mind in the mind. It is tree in tree. It is immobility in the immovable and mobility in the moving beings. It is insentience in the insentient and intelligence in the sentient. It is the divinity of gods and humanity in human beings. In animals it is bestial nature and in worms it is wormhood. It is the very essence of time and the seasons. It is dynamism in action and order in order. It is existence in the existent and death in the perishable. It is childhood, youth and age and also death.

It is undivided and indivisible, for it is the very essence of all things. Diversity is unreal, though it is real in the above sense (that the diversity is conceived of and pervaded by the infinite consciousness). Realise: 'All this is pervaded by me for I am omnipresent and devoid of body and such other limitation' and dwell in peace and supreme happiness.

VĀLMĪKI said:

As the sage Vasiṣṭha said this, the day came to an end and the assembly dispersed for their evening prayers.

tiryañco 'pi prapaśyanti svapne cittasvabhāvataḥ
dṛṣṭānāṁ ca śrutānāṁ ca cetaḥ smaraṇamakṣataṁ (62/18)

VASIṢṬHA continued:

In the self which is the infinite consciousness this creation appears but momentarily. During that moment itself the illusory notion that it is of a very long duration arises. The creation then appears to be solidly real. In this connection I shall narrate a legend to you, O Rāma. There once lived a mendicant who was devoted to meditation. His mind, having been purified by such meditation, came to possess the power to materialise its thoughts.

One day, being tired of continuous meditation, yet having his mind fully concentrated, he thought of doing something. He fancied birth as one who was illiterate and of a non-brāhmaṇa family. Instantly, he had become, as it were, a tribesman: there arose in him the feeling 'I am Jīvaṭa'. This dream-being roamed for sometime in the city also built of dream-objects. One day he got drunk and slept. He dreamt that he was a brāhmaṇa endowed with knowledge of the scriptures. While he was living a righteous life, one day this brāhmaṇa dreamt that he was a powerful king. He dreamt that he was a mighty emperor of unequalled glory. One day he indulged in royal pleasures and after that slept and dreamt of a celestial nymph.

Similarly, this nymph one day dreamt that she was a deer. And this deer dreamt that it was a creeper. Surely, **even animals behold dreams, for such is the nature of the mind which can recollect what has been seen and what has been heard.** The deer became a creeper. The inner intelligence in the creeper saw in its own heart a bee. It became a bee and the bee began to drink the nectar in the flowers on the creeper. It became attached to the nectar in one of those flowers, surely for its own destruction!

At night an elephant approached this creeper and plucked it, along with the bee, and crushed it in its mouth. However, the bee, having seen the elephant, contemplated the elephant and became an elephant. The elephant was captured by a king. One day it saw a hive of bees and on account of the memory of its own past birth it became a bee. It began to drink the nectar of the flowers in wild creepers. It became a creeper. The creeper was destroyed by an elephant, but because the creeper had seen swans in the nearby lake, it became a swan.

One day this swan was roaming in the company of many other swans. While the mendicant was meditating upon this swan, he was overcome by death. His consciousness therefore became embodied in the swan.

yadṛcchayā sthito jīvo bhūtatanmātrarañjitaḥ
kasminścidabhavat sarge bhikṣurakṣubhito 'bhitaḥ (9)

VASIṢṬHA continued:

That swan once beheld lord Rudra and in its heart there arose the conviction 'I am Rudra'. Instantly it abandoned its body as swan and became Rudra. And that Rudra dwelt in the abode of Rudra. However, since Rudra was endowed with true knowledge, he remembered all that had taken place!

RUDRA recollected thus:

Behold! How mysterious is this Māyā which deludes all the worlds: though it is unreal it appears to be real. First of all, in that infinite consciousness which was myself there arose the mind with objective consciousness, though yet cosmic and omniscient. **Then accidentally, I happened to be the jīva which felt attracted to and charmed by the finest part of the cosmic elements. Therefore during a certain creation-cycle I became the mendicant who remained totally unagitated.** He was able to overcome all distractions and remain immersed in the practice of contemplation.

However, every subsequent action is more powerful than a previous act. The mendicant considered himself Jīvaṭa and so did he become. After that he bethought he was a brāhmaṇa. Surely the more powerful thought-form overwhelms the weaker one. Then in course of time and on account of persistent contemplation, he became a king: surely, water imbibed by the plant becomes its fruit! Associated with royal pleasures are nymphs; contemplating them, the king became a nymph. Purely on account of infatuation, this nymph became a deer. The deer became a creeper which was obsessed with the idea that it would be pierced and a hole would be made. Contemplating the bee, it became a bee, which then pierced a hole in the creeper. The bee became an elephant.

I am Rudra who has been a Rudra during the past one hundred creation-cycles, and I roam this world-appearance which is nothing more than a psychological delusion. In one creation-cycle I was Jīvaṭa, in another I was the brāhmana, in another I was the king and in yet another I was the swan. Thus have I been revolving in this wheel known as the mind and the body.

It is aeons since I slipped from that supreme self or infinite consciousness. Soon after that fall I was that mendicant who was still endowed with knowledge of the truth. Then after passing through very many incarnations, through the grace of Rudra, whom I happened to behold, I have become Rudra. When the jīva by coincidence comes into contact with an enlightened person, then its impure vāsanā (tendencies) turn away. This happens to that person who constantly longs for such contact with an enlightened person. Such constant longing (or abhyāsa) itself materialises and becomes an accomplished fact.

yo yo 'bhitaḥ sa jīvasya saṁsāraḥ samudeti hi
tatrā 'prabuddhā jīva ghāḥ paśyanti na parasparaṁ (60)

RUDRA continued to recollect thus:

Surely it is because of one's inner conviction 'This body is my self' that this unreal perception expands. If one were to enquire into its true nature one would find that nothing remained! Enough of even such enquiry, which leads to nothing. This world is an optical illusion like the blueness of the sky. It is ignorance. Enough of even this effort to purify that ignorance! If this world-appearance which is unreal continues to appear, let it: it can do no harm. I shall retrace the chain of imaginary transformations and restore their underlying unity.

VASIṢṬHA continued:

Thus having resolved, Rudra went to where the body of the mendicant lay. He awakened it and inspired it to remember all that had taken place. The mendicant saw Rudra as his own self, and also recollected all that had happened.

Then both of them went to where Jīvaṭa lived in the same infinite consciousness. They revived his body. The three were indeed one. These three, who were wonder-struck at this mystery, then proceeded to the place of the brāhmaṇa who was asleep, embraced by his wife. They awakened his consciousness. Then they went to where the king was asleep in his royal bedchamber, surrounded by nymphs. They awakened his intelligence, too. He too was amazed at the realisation of the truth. Thus they went to where the swan lived — the swan that became Rudra.

They roamed the world of the one hundred Rudrā of the past. They realised that it was all one infinite consciousness in which all these diverse illusory events had apparently taken place. The one form had become many, as it were. These one hundred Rudrā pervaded the entire universe and were omnipresent.

On account of the fact that the jīva is surrounded on all sides by the world that arises from it, the unawakened jīvā do not see one another, do not understand one another. Just as all waves are of the same substance and are therefore one, the awakened jīvā realise their oneness and thus understand one another. Each jīva has its own illusory world-appearance. However, even as one finds empty space wherever one digs the ground, when this world-appearance of the jīva is enquired into, it invariably leads to the same infinite consciousness.

Differentiated consciousness is bondage; liberation is its absence. Whatever pleases you, affirm that and be firm in that. There is no difference between the two, for awareness is the same in both. Who will bemoan the loss of what exists only in ignorance? That which is gained by 'being still', exists already and has therefore already been 'gained'!

iha vidyādharo 'yaṁ syāmahaṁ syāmiha paṇḍitaḥ (23)
ityekadhyānasāphalyaṁ dṛṣṭānto 'syāṁ kriyāsthitau
ekatvaṁ ca bahutvaṁ ca maurkhyaṁ pāṇḍityameva vā (24)

VASIṢṬHA continued:

All of them attained awakening of their spiritual consciousness along with lord Rudra. Realising that they were part of Rudra, they were happy. Rudra saw the play of Māyā as it arose, and he inspired the others to play their roles in it once again, commanding them to return to him after such seemingly independent existence, and assuring them at the end of the world-cycle they would reach the supreme state. Rudra then vanished from sight, and Jīvaṭa and the others returned to their own respective abodes.

RĀMA asked:

Were Jīvaṭa and the others not mere dream-objects (imaginary entities) of the mendicant? How could they become real entities?

VASIṢṬHA replied:

Abandon the notion that imagination is something real! When thus the illusoriness of illusion is abandoned, what exists exists in the infinite consciousness. What is seen in dream and what is imagined to be real, appear as such at all times, even as to a traveller the temporal and spatial experiences are real, relative to the different places. In the heart of that infinite consciousness everything exists, and one experiences what one sees in it.

The dream-like nature of thought-form is realised only by the intense practice of yoga, not otherwise. It is by such practice that lord Śiva and others perceive everything everywhere. That which is in front of you and at the same time apprehended by your mind, is not realised if there is misapprehension in such perception or in such existence. Only when such misapprehension does not exist can that object be known and realised. Whatever one wishes is obtained only when one's inner being is wholly and solely devoted to it. He who is thus totally devoted to what is in front of him knows it perfectly; he who is totally devoted to an imaginary object knows it perfectly. If such one-pointed devotion is not there, then he destroys that object (is not aware of it). It was thus (by such one-pointed devotion) that the mendicant became Rudra and all the rest of it. Each one of them had his own world; hence, until the Rudra-consciousness was awakened in them they were unaware of one another. It was in fact by the will of Rudra that they were thus veiled, that they became of different forms and nature.

It is by one-pointed contemplation of 'May I become a celestial' or 'May I become a learned man' and as the fruit of such contemplation that one is enabled to become one or many or an ignoramus or a man of knowledge. It is possible by concentration and meditation to become a divinity or a human being and function accordingly.

sarvaśakttyaḥ svarūpatvājjīvasyā 'styekaśakttitā
anantaścā 'ntapṛkttaśca svabhāvo 'sya svabhāvataḥ (64/26)

VASIṢṬHA continued:

The infinite consciousness which is the true self of all is endowed with omnipotence, but the jīva (which is essentially non-different from the self) is endowed with one faculty (appropriate to its notion). Hence, depending upon the nature of the jīva, it enjoys endless powers or limited powers. The infinite consciousness is free from expansion and contraction: it is the jīva that gets what it seeks. The yogī who have acquired various faculties exist and manifest such faculties here and also elsewhere. However, since they are enjoyed here and there and in different places, such experiences appear to be many and varied — even as the famous Kārtavīrya generated fear in the hearts of many, though he remained at home! (A modern example is the radio: without leaving the studio, the speaker or singer enters countless drawing rooms. S.V.)

Similarly, lord Viṣṇu, without leaving his abode, incarnates as a human being on earth. Similarly, Indra (who presides over sacred rites), without leaving his heavenly abode, is present in a thousand places where such rites are performed. In response to the call of the devotees, lord Viṣṇu, who is one, becomes thousands and appears before the devotees. Even so, Jīvaṭa and the others, who were but the creatures of the mendicant's imagination or wish and who were animated by Rudra-consciousness, went to their various abodes and functioned as if independently. They played their different roles for sometime and then returned to the abode of Rudra.

All this was nothing but a momentary delusion which arose in the consciousness of the mendicant, though it was seen as if it were independent of the mendicant. Even so the birth and death of countless beings takes place in the one infinite consciousness, as it were. They imagine diversity in this world-appearance and then they seek unity in the self. At the time of their death they imagine within themselves another state of existence which appears to them as if outside! Until realisation of liberation the embodied being undergoes unfathomable sorrow. I told you the story to illustrate this truth. This is the fate not only of the mendicant, but of all beings. That being who forgets his inseparability from the supreme self imagines his own notions to be independent and utterly real and substantial. From one such dream he goes on to another dream, until he abandons the false notion 'I am the body'.

RĀMA asked:

O what a wonderful story! Lord, you said that all things that are conceived to be real are real and experienced as real. Pray, tell me, does this mendicant also exist somewhere?

VASIṢṬHA replied:

I shall contemplate this question and reply later. (At this stage the assembly rose for their noon prayers.)

pratyekamevamuditaḥ pratibhāsakhaṇḍaḥ
khaṇḍāntareṣvapi ca tasya vicitrakhaṇḍaḥ
sarve svayaṁ nanu ca te 'pi mitho na mithyā
sarvātmani sphurati kāraṇakāraṇe 'smin (28)

VASIṢṬHA continued:

O king, O Rāma! With the help of my eye of wisdom I searched for the mendicant. I entered into deep meditation, wishing to see that mendicant. I searched for him in this universe, but could not find him. How does one's imagination appear outside also as if real?

Then I proceeded north to the land of the Jinā. On top of an ant hill there exists a vihara (shrine? or Bihar) inhabited by people. There, in his own cottage, was a mendicant (bhikṣu) known as Dirghadṛśa whose head was yellow in colour. He was in deep meditation. Even his attendants did not enter his cottage, afraid to disturb his meditation. It was the twenty-first day of such meditation. It was destined to be his last day.

Though from one point of view he had been in meditation for only twenty-one days, from another point of view thousands of years had passed. For, such was the notion that arose in his mind. I knew that such a mendicant had lived in another epoch; and even in this epoch he is the second such mendicant. However, other than these two, I could not see a third mendicant. With all the wits at my disposal and all the faculties I could command, I entered into the very heart of this creation, looking for the third mendicant.

At last I found him, but he was not in this universe. He was in another universe which, however, was almost exactly like this universe, though created by another Brahmā. Even so have there been (and there will be in the future) countless beings. In this very assembly there are sages and holy brāhmaṇā who will thus entertain notions of other beings who will thereupon appear to be. Such is the nature of Māyā.

Some of these beings will be of natures similar to the one that imagines them. Others will be quite dissimilar. Yet others will partly resemble them. Thus is the great Māyā which baffles even great men. But it does not exist nor does it function here — for it is only delusion that causes all these to appear and disappear! Else, where is a short period of twenty-one days and where is a whole epoch? It is frightening even to think of the play of the mind.

All this is but appearance, which unfolds like the lotus in the morning and reveals diversity like a full-blown lotus. All this arises in the infinite consciousness which is pure; yet the appearance appears to be tainted by impurity. **Each thing appears as if fragmented and at the end of that fragmented existence it undergoes other strange fragmentation; all this is relatively real, not totally unreal. All of them manifest in the All — the cause is in the cause!**

eṣā guṇamayī māyā durbodhena duratyayā
nityaṁ satyāvabodhena sukhenaivā 'tivāhyate (7)

DAŚARATHA said:

O sage, tell me where that mendicant (bhikṣu) is meditating and I shall at once despatch my soldiers to wake him up from his meditation and bring him here.

VASIṢṬHA replied:

O king, that mendicant's body has already become lifeless and it cannot be revived. His jīva has attained enlightenment and liberation: it cannot be subjected to the experience of this world-appearance any more. His own attendants stand outside his cottage waiting to open the door at the end of one month, as instructed by him. They will find that by that time he has abandoned his body and will then install someone else in his place.

This Māyā (or world-appearance or delusion) is of the nature of limited and limiting qualities and attributes. It is said to be impossible to cross it by ignorance, but by the knowledge of truth it is easily crossed over.

It is wrong perception that sees a bracelet in gold. The mere appearance becomes the cause for such wrong perception. This Māyā (unreal appearance) is but a figure of speech, the appearance has the same relation to the supreme self that a wave has to the ocean. When one sees this truth the appearance ceases to be a delusion. It is on account of ignorance that this long-dream world-appearance appears to be real: thus does the jīva come into being. But when the truth is realised, it is seen that all this is the self.

Whatever be the notion that one entertains, it is the self alone that appears as that notion. This universe is the result of the notions thus entertained by countless such individuals. The original notion entertained by Brahmā has come to be experienced by the jīva as a solid reality. But when one attains the purity of consciousness similar to that of Brahmā, one sees all this as a long dream.

It is the notion of the object that becomes the mind and thus slips from infinite consciousness. It then undergoes varied experiences. But is this mind independent of the supreme self, is not the supreme self the mind, too? The jīva, the body and all the rest of it are but reflections or appearances of the supreme self! All these movements, etc., happen in the one infinite consciousness which is for ever infinite and consciousness, naught else: movement and so on are imaginary expressions. There is neither motion nor non-motion, neither one nor many — what is is as it is. Diversity arises in the unawakened state and it vanishes when one commences one's enquiry. The enquirer exists, but without any doubt — which indeed is the supreme state. Peace is known as the world, peace alone IS as this world-appearance. Ignorance is unreal: there is neither the seer, the seen nor the sight! The mind imagines a defect in the moon; it is not there as defect. The infinite consciousness has consciousness alone as its 'body' or manifestation or appearance.

ahamasmi jagatyasmin svasti śabdārthamātrakaṁ
sattāsāmānyameveti sauṣuptaṁ maunamucyate (26)

VASIṢṬHA continued:

O Rāma, remain forever firmly established in that state of utter freedom from movement of thought, resorting to the silence of deep sleep.

RĀMA said:

Sir, I have heard of silence of speech, silence of the eyes and other senses and I have also heard of the rigid silence of extreme asceticism. But what is this silence of deep sleep?

VASIṢṬHA replied:

Rāma, there are two types of muni (a sage who observes mouna or silence). One is the rigid ascetic and the other the liberated sage. The former forcibly restrains his senses and engages himself in dry (devoid of wisdom) kriyā (activities) with fanaticism. The liberated sage, on the other hand, knows what is what (the truth as truth and the unreal as unreal), he is endowed with self-knowledge and yet he behaves as any ordinary person here. What is regarded as silence or mouna is based on the nature and the behaviour of these muni.

Four types of silence have been described: (1) silence of speech, (2) silence of the senses (eyes, etc.), (3) violent restraint, as also (4) the silence of deep sleep. There is another known as silence of the mind. However, that is possible only in one who is dead or one who practises the rigid mouna (kāṣṭha mouna) or the silence of deep sleep (suṣupti mouna). Of these the first three involve elements of the rigid mouna. It is the fourth that is really conducive to liberation. Hence, even at the risk of incurring the displeasure of those who resort to the first three types of mouna, I say that there is nothing in those three which is desirable.

The silence of deep sleep is conducive to liberation. In it the prāṇa or life-force is neither restrained nor promoted, the senses are neither fed nor starved, the perception of diversity is neither expressed nor suppressed, the mind is neither mind nor non-mind. There is no division and hence no effort at abolishing it; it is called the silence of deep sleep, and one who is established in it may or may not meditate. There is knowledge of what IS as it is, and there is freedom from doubt. It is utter emptiness. It is supportless. It is of the nature of supreme peace, of which it can neither be said that it is real nor that it is unreal. That state in which one knows "There is no 'I', nor another, no mind nor anything derived from the mind", in which one knows "'I' is but an idea in this universe, and it is really pure existence" — that is known as the silence of deep sleep. In that pure existence which is infinite consciousness, where is 'I' or 'another'?

ajñastu ditacittatvāt kriyāniyamanaṁ vinā
gacchannyāyena mātsyena paraṁ duḥkhaṁ prayāti hi (9)

RĀMA asked:

How did the one hundred Rudrā come into being, O sage?

VASIṢṬHA replied:

The mendicant (bhikṣu) dreamt all the one hundred Rudrā. Whatever they whose minds are pure and unobscured by impurities, imagine or will-into-being, that alone they experience as being real. Whatever thoughtform thus arises in the one infinite consciousness appears to be so.

RĀMA asked again:

Why is it, O sage, that lord Śiva chose to appear as one unclad, inhabiting the cremation ground, garlanded with human skulls, smeared with ashes and as one who is easily overcome by lust?

VASIṢṬHA replied:

The conduct of the gods, the perfected beings and the liberated sages is not determined by rules and codes of conduct — these are invented by ignorant people. Yet, **since the mind of the ignorant is heavily conditioned, if they are not governed by such rules of conduct there will then arise disorder in which the big fish will eat the small fish.** The man of wisdom, on the other hand, does not drown himself in what is desirable and what is undesirable because he has his senses naturally in control and because he is awake and alert. He lives and works without intending to do so, without reacting to events on a causal basis, his actions being pure and spontaneous (as the cocoanut falling without any causal relation with the alighting of the crow on it); or he may not do anything at all!

Thus have even the members of the trinity (Brahmā, Viṣṇu and Śiva) engaged themselves in incarnation. In the case of the enlightened ones, their actions are beyond praise and reproach, beyond acceptance and rejection, for they have no notion of 'This is mine' and 'This is other'. Their actions are pure like the heat of fire.

I did not wish to elaborate on the other form of mouna, known as the silence of the disembodied, for you are still embodied. However, I shall briefly describe it now. They who are fully awakened, who are constantly engaged in samādhi and who are thoroughly enlightened, are known as sāmkhya-yogī. They who have reached the state of bodiless consciousness through prāṇāyāma, etc., are known as yoga-yogī. Indeed, the two are essentially the same. The cause of this world-appearance and bondage is indeed the mind. Both these paths lead to the cessation of the mind. Hence, by the devoted and dedicated practice of either the cessation of the movement of prāṇa or the cessation of thought, liberation is attained. This is the essence of all scriptures dealing with liberation.

ceto hi vāsanāmātraṁ tadabhāve paraṁ padaṁ
tattvaṁ saṁpadyate jñānaṁ jñānamāhur vicāraṇaṁ (38)

RĀMA asked:

O sage, if the cessation of the movement of prāṇa is liberation, then death is liberation! And all people attain liberation at death!

VASIṢTHA replied:

O Rāma, when prāṇa is about to leave the body it already makes contact with those elements with which the next one is to be fashioned. These elements are indeed the crystallisation of the vāsanā (psychological conditioning, memory-store, past impressions and predisposition) of the jīva, the reason why the jīva clings to those elements. When the prāṇa leaves the body it takes with it all the vāsanā of the jīva.

Not indeed until these vāsanā have been destroyed will the mind become no-mind. The mind does not abandon the life-force till self-knowledge arises. By self-knowledge the vāsanā are destroyed and thus the mind, too; it is then that the prāṇa does not move. That indeed is the supreme peace. It is by self-knowledge that the unreality of the concepts concerning worldly objects is realised. This puts an end to vāsanā and to the link between the mind and the life-force. Vāsanā constitute mind. **Mind is the aggregate of the vāsanā and naught else; if the latter cease, that itself is the supreme state. Knowledge is the knowledge of the reality. Vicāra or enquiry itself is knowledge.**

Total dedication to one thing, restraint of prāṇa and the cessation of the mind — if one of these three is perfected, one attains the supreme state. The life-force and the mind are closely related, like a flower and its fragrance or sesame seed and oil. Hence, if the movement of thought in the mind ceases, the movement of prāṇa ceases, too. If the total mind is one-pointedly devoted to a single truth, the movement of mind and therefore of life-force ceases. The best method is to enquire into the nature of the self which is infinite. Your mind will be completely absorbed — then both the mind and the enquiry will cease. Remain firmly established in what remains after that.

When the mind does not crave for pleasure it is absorbed into the self, along with the life-force. Ignorance is non-existence; self-knowledge is the supreme state! Mind alone is ignorance when it appears to be a reality; the realisation of its non-existence is the supreme state. If the mind remains absorbed even for a quarter of an hour it undergoes a complete change, for it tastes the supreme state of self-knowledge and will not abandon it. Nay, even if the mind has tasted it for a second, it does not return to this worldly state. The very seeds of saṁsāra (world-appearance or cycle of birth and death) are fried. With them, ignorance is dispelled and the vāsanā are utterly pacified; one who has reached this is rooted in satva (truth). He beholds the inner light and rests in supreme peace.

jīvo 'jīvo bhavatyāśu yati cittamacittatāṁ
vicārādityavidyānto mokṣa ityabhidhīyate (70/1)

VASIṢṬHA continued:

That is known as mokṣa or liberation when ignorance ceases through self-enquiry, when the jiva becomes no-jiva instantly and when the mind becomes no-mind. In this connection, O Rāma, listen to the following inspiring and enlightening questions asked by a vampire.

There lives a vampire in the Vindya forests. Once it entered a certain territory, desirous of appeasing its hunger. However, it would not kill anyone even when it was hungry, unless the victim deserved such treatment. Finding no such person in the forest, it entered a city and met the king.

The VAMPIRE said to the king: O king, I shall ask you a few questions. Give me the correct answers to them. What is that sun the particles of whose rays are these universes? In what mighty wind does this mighty space manifest? One goes from one dream to another dream ad infinitum, yet one does not abandon the self, though constantly abandoning the dream-reality. What is the self? The stem of a banana tree, when it is opened reveals layer after layer until you reach the pith. What is that subtle essence when this world-appearance is similarly enquired into? Of which atom are the universes themselves minuter atoms? In what formless 'rock' are the three worlds hidden (like an unsculpted figure in a rock)? Answer these questions. If you do not you certainly deserve to be eaten by me!

The KING answered: O vampire! This universe was once enveloped by a series of coverings, even as a fruit is enveloped by its skin. There was a branch on which there were thousands of such fruits. There was a tree with thousands of such branches, a forest with thousands of such trees, a hill with thousands of such forests, a country with thousands of such hills, a continent with thousands of such countries, a sphere with thousands of such continents, an ocean with thousands of such spheres, a being with thousands of such oceans within him and a supreme person who wears thousands of such beings as a garland. There is a sun in whose rays thousands of such supreme persons are found: that sun illumines all. That sun is the sun of consciousness, O vampire! In that light of that sun, these universes are but minutest atomic particles. It is because of the light of that sun that all these other things enumerated appear to be real.

In the supreme self shine as dust-particles substances (concepts or relative realities) known as time, space and motion which are conscious (movement in and of consciousness) and pure intelligence. This world-appearance is but the flesh in which the truth which is pure consciousness is clothed.

Having heard this answer from the lips of the king, the vampire became silent and deeply contemplative. O Rāma, like the king Bhagīratha you will achieve the impossible if you are able to remain firm in your knowledge of the truth and if you engage yourself in appropriate action in a life characterised by effortless experiencing of the natural course of events.

yena prāptena loke 'smin na prāpyam avaśiṣyate
tatkṛtaṁ sukṛtam manye śeṣam karma viṣūcikā (17)

At Rāma's request, VASIṢṬHA narrated the following story:

Once upon a time there was a king named Bhagīratha, who was devoted to dharma. He gave liberal gifts to the pious and holy ones and he was terror to the evil-doers. He worked tirelessly to eradicate the very causes of poverty. When he was in the company of the holy ones his heart melted in devotion.

Bhagīratha brought the holy river Gaṅgā from the heavens down to the earth. In this he had to encounter great difficulties and propitiate the gods Brahmā and Śiva and also the sage Jahnu. In all this he suffered frequent frustrations and disappointments.

He, too, was endowed with discrimination and dispassion even at an early age, O Rāma. One day while remaining alone he reflected thus: "This worldly life is really essenceless and stupid. Day and night chase each other. People repeat the same meaningless actions again and again. **I regard only that as proper action which leads to the attainment beyond which there is nothing to be gained; the rest is repeated foul excretion (as in cholera).**" He approached his guru Tritala and prayed, "Lord, how can one put an end to this sorrow and to old age, death and delusion which contribute to repeated birth here?"

TRITALA said:

Sorrow ceases, all the bondages are rent asunder and doubts are dispelled when one is fully established in the equanimity of the self for a long time, when the perception of division has ceased and when there is the experience of fullness through the knowledge of that which is to be known. What is to be known? It is the self which is pure and which is of the nature of pure consciousness which is omnipresent and eternal.

BHAGĪRATHA asked:

I know that the self alone is real and the body, etc. are not real. But how is it that it is not perfectly clear to me?

TRITALA said:

Such intellectual knowledge is not knowledge! Unattachment to wife, son and house, equanimity in pleasure and pain, love of solitude, being firmly established in self-knowledge — this is knowledge, all else is ignorance! Only when the ego-sense is thinned out does this self-knowledge arise.

BHAGĪRATHA asked:

Since this ego-sense is firmly established in this body, how can it be uprooted?

TRITALA replied:

By self-effort and by resolutely turning away from the pursuit of pleasure, and by the resolute breaking down of the prison-house of shame (false dignity), etc. If you abandon all this and remain firm, the ego-sense will vanish and you will realise that you are the supreme being!

samaḥ śāntamanā mauni vītarāgo vimatsaraḥ
prāptakāryaikakaraṇaḥ sa tirohitavismayaḥ (76/10)

VASIṢṬHA continued:

Having heard the precepts of the preceptor, Bhagīratha decided to perform a religious rite as a prelude to total renunciation of the world. In three days he had given away everything to the priests and to his relatives, whether they were endowed with good nature or not. His own kingdom he handed over to his enemies living across the borders. Clad in a small piece of loin-cloth he left the kingdom and roamed in countries and forests where he was totally unknown.

Very soon he had attained the state of supreme peace within himself. Accidentally and unknowingly he entered his own previous kingdom and solicited alms from the citizens there. They recognised him, worshipped him and prayed that he should be their king. But he accepted from them nothing but food. They bewailed, "This is king Bhagīratha. What a sad plight, what an unfortunate turn of events!" After a few days he left the kingdom again.

Bhagīratha once again met his preceptor and the two of them roamed the country, all the time engaged in spiritual dialogue: "Why do we still carry the burden of this physical body? On the other hand, why should it be discarded? Let it be as long as it will be!" They were devoid of sorrow and of rejoicing, nor could they be said to adhere to the middle path. Even if the gods and sages offered them wealth and psychic powers, they spurned them as blades of dry grass.

In a certain kingdom the king had died without an heir, and the ministers were in search of a suitable ruler. Bhagīratha, clad in a loin-cloth, happened to be in that kingdom. The ministers declared that he was the person fit to ascend the throne, and surrounded him. Bhagīratha mounted the royal elephant. Soon he was crowned king. While he was ruling that kingdom the people of his previous kingdom approached him once again and prayed that he should rule that kingdom also. Bhagīratha accepted. Thus he became the emperor of the whole world. **Remaining at peace within himself, with his mind silenced, free from desires and jealousy, he engaged himself in doing appropriate action in circumstances as they arose.**

Once he heard that the only way to propitiate the souls of his departed ancestors was to offer libation with the waters of the Gaṅgā. In order to bring the heavenly Gaṅgā down to earth he repaired to the forest to perform austerities, having entrusted the empire to his ministers. There he propitiated the gods and the sages and achieved the most difficult task of bringing the Gaṅgā down to earth so that all the people for all time to come might offer libations to their ancestors with the waters of the holy Gaṅgā. It is only from that time that this sacred Gaṅgā, which adorned the crown of lord Śiva's head, began to flow on the earth.

yadanyadbahuśo bhūtvā punarbhavati bhūriśaḥ
abhūtvaiva bhavatyanyaḥ punaśca na bhavatyalaṁ
anyatprāksaṁniveśāḍhyaṁ sādṛśyena vivalgati (7)

VASIṢṬHA continued:

Even so, Rāma, remain in a state of equanimity like king Bhagīratha. And, like Śikhidhvaja, having renounced everything, remain unmoved. I shall narrate to you the story of Śikhidhvaja. Pray, listen. Once there were two lovers who were reborn in a later age on account of their divine love for each other.

RĀMA asked:

O sage, how is it possible that the couple who lived together as husband and wife in one age is born again to be husband and wife in a later age?

VASIṢṬHA replied:

Such is the subtle nature of the world order, O Rāma. **Some things appear in abundance, and once again they manifest in abundance. Others are born now, having never been before; and having been now they are not born again. Others which have been before reappear in the same form now.** It is like the waves on the ocean: there are similar ones and there are dissimilar ones.

In the Mālva kingdom there was a king named Śikhidhvaja. He was endowed with every kind of royal excellence. He was righteous and noble, courageous and courteous. He lost his father very early in life. Though young, he was able to assert his sovereignty and he ruled the kingdom assisted by his able ministers.

The spring season set in. There was romance in the air. The young king began to dream of a partner. Day and night his heart longed for the beloved. The clever and wise ministers divined the state of their king's heart. They went to the Saurāstra kingdom and sought the hand of a princess for their king. Soon, the king Śikhidhvaja married Cūdālā.

Sikhidhvaja and Cūḍālā were so greatly devoted to each other that they were one jiva in two bodies. They shared many common interests and they played together in the pleasure-gardens. Even as the sun sends down his rays to make the lotus unfold, the king showered his beloved with his love and tried to please her in every way.

They shared their knowledge and their wisdom with each other so that both of them became highly learned in all branches of knowledge. Each dwelt in all radiance in the other's heart. In fact, it appeared as if the Lord Viṣṇu and his consort had come down on earth in order to accomplish a special mission!

asatyajaḍacetyāṁśacayanāc cidvapurjaḍaṁ
mahājalagato hyagniriva rūpaṁ svamujjati (26)

VASIṢṬHA continued:

Thus Śikhidhvaja and Cūḍālā enjoyed themselves for a number of years without a dull moment. No-one can arrest the passage of time. Life appears and disappears like a juggler's trick. Pleasure, when pursued, flies beyond reach even as an arrow which has left the bow. Sorrow preys upon the mind even as vultures prey upon a carcass. "What is there in this world, having attained which, the mind is never again subjected to sorrow?" Reflecting thus, the royal couple turned their attention to the study of spiritual texts.

They came to the conclusion that self-knowledge alone can enable one to overcome sorrow. They devoted themselves to self-knowledge with their heart and soul. They resorted to the company of sages of self-knowledge and adored them. They engaged themselves constantly in discussing self-knowledge and in promoting self-knowledge in each other.

Having thus constantly contemplated the means of self-knowledge, the QUEEN began to reflect thus:

Now I see myself and enquire "Who am I?" How could ignorance of self, and delusion arise? The physical body is surely inert and it is certainly not the self. It is experienced only on account of the movement of thought in the mind. The organs of action are but parts of the body and hence they too are inert, being parts of the body which is inert. The sense-organs are inert, too, for they depend upon the mind for their functioning. I consider even the mind to be inert. The mind thinks and entertains notions, but it is prompted to do so by the intellect, which is the determining agent. Even this intellect (buddhi) is surely inert, for it is directed by the ego-sense. Even this ego-sense is inert, for it is conjured up by the jīva, just as a ghost is conjured up by the ignorant child. The jīva is but pure consciousness clothed, as it were, by the life-force, and it dwells in the heart.

Lo and behold! I have realised that it is the self which is pure consciousness that dwells as the jīva because the consciousness becomes aware of itself as its own object. **This object is insentient and unreal; and because the self identifies itself with this object it apparently clothes itself with insentience, having apparently (but not in truth) abandoned its essential nature as consciousness.** For, such is the nature of consciousness: whatever it conceives itself to be, whether real or imaginary, that it becomes, apparently having abandoned its own nature. Thus, though the self is pure consciousness, it imagines itself to be insentient and unreal on account of its perception of objects.

Contemplating thus for a considerable time, Cūḍālā became enlightened.

na tasya janmamaraṇe na tasya sadasadgatī
na nāśaḥ sambhavatyasya cinmātranabhasaḥ kvacit (43)

VASIṢṬHA continued:

Delighted by this self-discovery, the queen exclaimed: "At last I have attained that which is to be attained (known). Now there is no loss. Even the mind and the senses are but the reflections of consciousness, though they are unreal independently of consciousness. This supreme consciousness alone exists. It is the supreme truth, untainted by any impurity, forever in a state of perfect equilibrium and devoid of ego-sense. Once this truth is realised, it shines constantly without setting.

"It is this consciousness that is known by various names — Brahman, supreme self, etc. In it there is no division into subject-object and their relationship (knowledge). Consciousness becomes conscious of its own consciousness; it cannot be realised otherwise (as an object of consciousness). It is this consciousness alone that is manifest as the mind, intellect and the senses. This world-appearance, too, is but consciousness, apart from which nothing is. Consciousness does not undergo any change; the only apparent change is the illusory appearance, which is illusory and therefore not real! In an imaginary ocean, imaginary waves arise. The mind-stuff itself is the ocean and the waves are of the mind-stuff, too. Even so the world-appearance arises in consciousness and is therefore non-different from it.

"I am pure consciousness, devoid of ego-sense and all-pervading. **There is neither birth nor death for this consciousness. It is not subject to destruction, for it is like space.** It cannot be cut or burnt. It is pure light of consciousness, without defect.

"I am free from all delusion. I am at peace. All these gods, demons and numerous beings are essentially unmade, for they are non-different from the consciousness. The appearance is illusory, even as soldiers made of clay are clay, not soldiers.

"The seer (subject) and the seen (object) are in reality the one pure consciousness. How has this delusion which gives rise to concepts like 'This is oneness' and 'There is duality' come into being? In whom does that delusion exist? Whose is it? I rest in nirvāṇa (liberation or enlightenment), without the least mental agitation, having realised that all that is (whether sentient or insentient) is pure consciousness. There is no 'this' or 'I' or 'the other'; there is no being or non-being. All this is peace."

Having thus realised, Cūḍālā rested in supreme peace.

idaṁ cā 'hamidaṁ nā 'haṁ satyā cā 'haṁ na cāpyahaṁ
sarvamasmi na kiñcicca tenā 'haṁ śrīmatī sthitā (28)

VASIṢṬHA continued:

Day by day the queen grew more and more introverted, rejoicing more and more in the bliss of the self. She was utterly free from craving and from attachment. Without abandoning anything and without seeking anything, she was natural in her behaviour and spontaneous in her actions. All her doubts were at rest. She had crossed the ocean of becoming. She rested in an incomparable state of peace.

Thus within a very short time she had reached the realisation that this world-appearance will also disappear in the same way in which it came into being! She shone radiant in the light of self-knowledge.

Seeing her thus radiant and peaceful, Śikhidhvaja asked her: "You appear to have regained your youthfulness and you shine with an extraordinary radiance, my beloved. You are not distracted by anything at all, and you have no craving. Yet, you are full of bliss. Tell me: is it that you have quaffed the nectar of the gods? Surely, you have attained something which is extremely difficult to attain."

CŪḌĀLĀ replied:

I have abandoned this emptiness which has assumed some sort of a form. I remain rooted in that which is truth, not in the appearance. Hence I am radiant. I have abandoned all these and I have resorted to something other than these, which is both real and unreal. Hence I am radiant. That is something and that is also not-something. I know that as it is. Hence I am radiant. I delight in the non-enjoyment of pleasures as if I have enjoyed them. I give way neither to joy nor to anger. Hence I am radiant. I experience the greatest joy in remaining established in the reality that shines in my heart. I am not distracted by the royal pleasures. Hence I am radiant. Even when I am in the pleasure-gardens, I remain firmly established in the self, neither in the enjoyment of pleasure nor in shyness, etc. Hence I am radiant.

I am the ruler of the universe. I am not the finite being. I delight in the self. Hence I am radiant. **This I am, I am not, in truth I am nor am I; I am the all, I am naught. Hence I am radiant.** I seek neither pleasure nor wealth nor poverty nor any other form of existence. I am happy with whatever is obtained without effort. Hence I am radiant. I sport with attenuated states of attraction and repulsion, with the insights gained through the scriptures. Hence I am radiant. Whatever I see with these eyes and experience with these senses, whatever I behold through my mind — I see nothing but the one truth which is seen clearly by me within myself.

jñasyopekṣātmakaṁ nāma mūḍhasyā "deyatāṁ gataṁ
heyaṁ sphāravirāgasya śṛṇu siddhikramaḥ kathaṁ (24)

Unable to understand the queen's words, ŚIKHIDHVAJA laughed at them and said:

You are childish and ignorant, my dear, and surely you are prattling! Having abandoned something for nothing, having abandoned real substances and attained the state of nothingness — how does one shine resplendent? Even as an angry man rejects a bed, if one abandons pleasures boasting, "I delight in unenjoyed pleasures", it is not conducive to delight! When one abandons everything (pleasures, etc.) and thinks he delights in emptiness, that does not make any sense. Nor does it make any sense if one thinks he is happy after having renounced clothes, food, bed, etc. 'I am not the body, nor am I anything else', 'Nothing is everything' — what else are these statements but sheer prattle? 'I do not see what I see' and 'I see something else' — these too are nothing but prattle.

Never mind; enjoy the pleasures that are afforded to you. I shall continue to sport with you; enjoy yourself.

VASIṢTHA continued:

Having said this, the king went away from the inner apartments. Cūḍālā thought, "It is a pity that the king is unable to understand" and she continued to go about her work. Thus they continued to live for a considerable time. Though Cūḍālā had no desires, a wish arose in her to move about in space. In order to acquire this power she sought solitude, and there exercised the vital air which has an upward tendency.

There are three types of attainable goals in this world, O Rāma: desirable, detestable and ignorable. What is desirable is sought with great effort; what is detestable is abandoned; between these two is that towards which one is indifferent. Normally, one regards that as desirable which promotes happiness, its opposite is considered undesirable and one is indifferent to those which bring neither happiness nor unhappiness. However, in the case of the enlightened ones these categories do not exist, for they look upon everything as a mere play and hence are utterly indifferent to everything seen or unseen.

I shall now describe to you the method of gaining what is attainable (siddhī or psychic powers), towards which the sage of self-knowledge is indifferent, which the deluded person considers desirable and which one who is intent on the cultivation of self-knowledge is keen to avoid.

sā coktā kuṇḍalīnāmnā kuṇḍalākāravāhinī
prāṇināṁ param śakttiḥ sarvaśakttijavapradā (42)

VASIṢṬHA continued:

All achievements are dependent upon four factors: time, place, action and means. Among these, action or effort holds the key because all endeavours towards the achievement are based on action or effort.

Some perverse practices also prevail, and they are said to make achievements possible. Especially in the hands of immature practitioners they are conducive to great harm. To this category belong the magic pill or unguent or wand, as also the use of gems, drugs, self-mortification and magic formulae. The belief that the mere dwelling in holy places like Śrīsaila or Meru enables one to attain spiritual perfection, is also defective.

Hence, in the context of the story of Śikhidhvaja I shall describe the technique of prāṇāyāma, or the exercise of the life force, and the achievements it brings about. Kindly listen.

In preparation, one should abandon all habits and tendencies that are unrelated to what one wishes to achieve. One should learn to close the apertures in the body and also learn the practice of the different postures. The diet should be pure. One should contemplate the meaning of holy scriptures. Right conduct and the company of holy ones are essential. Having renounced everything, one should sit comfortably. If one then practises prāṇāyāma for sometime without allowing anger, greed, etc., to rise within oneself, the life-force comes under one's perfect control.

Right from sovereignty over the earth to total liberation, everything is dependent upon the movement of the life-force. Hence all such achievements are possible through the practice of prāṇāyāma.

Deep within the body there is a nāḍī known as the āntraveṣṭikā. It rests in the vitals and it is the source of a hundred other nāḍī. It exists in all beings — gods, demons and humans, animals and birds, worms and fish. It is coiled at its source. It is in contact with all the avenues in the body, from the waist right up to the crown of the head.

Within this nāḍī dwells the supreme power. **It is known as kuṇḍalinī, because it is coiled in appearance. It is the supreme power in all beings and it is the prime mover of all power.** When the prāṇa or life-force which is in the heart reaches the abode of the kuṇḍalinī, there arises within oneself an awareness of the elements of nature. It is when the kuṇḍalinī unfolds and begins to move that there is awareness within oneself.

All the other nāḍī (radiating flow of energy) are tied to the kuṇḍalinī, as it were. Hence the kuṇḍalinī is the very seed of consciousness and understanding (or knowledge).

tatpañcadhā gataṁ dvitvaṁ lakṣase tvaṁ svasaṁvidaṁ
antarbhūtavikārādi dīpāddīpaśataṁ yathā (56)

RĀMA asked:

Is not the infinite consciousness forever indivisible? If so, how does this kuṇḍalinī arise and manifest itself, thus revealing this consciousness?

VASIṢTHA continued:

Indeed, there is the infinite consciousness alone everywhere at all times. However, it manifests as the elements here and there. The sun shines on everything, but it is reflected in a special way when its rays fall on a mirror. Similarly, the same infinite consciousness appears to be 'lost' in some, clearly manifest in some, at the height of its glory in yet others.

Even as space is (empty) space everywhere, consciousness is consciousness and naught else, whatever the appearance may be. It does not undergo any change. This consciousness itself is the five root-elements. **You behold with your consciousness the same consciousness which is the five root-elements, as if you were seeing another within yourself, even as with one lamp you see a hundred lamps.**

On account of a slight movement of thought, the same reality which is consciousness seems to become the fivefold elements, and thence the body. In the same way, the same consciousness becomes worms and other creatures, metals and minerals, earth and what is on it, water and other elements. Thus the whole world is nothing but the movement of energy in consciousness which appears as the fivefold elements. Somewhere this energy is sentient and elsewhere it appears as insentient, even as water when exposed to cold wind hardens and becomes solid. Thus is nature formed, and all things conform to nature.

However, all this is but the play of words, a figure of speech. What else is heat and cold, ice and fire? Again, these distinctions arise on account of conditioning and thought patterns. The wise man therefore enquires into the nature of such conditioning, whether it is latent or patent, good or evil. Such is fruitful quest; vain argumentation is like boxing with space.

Latent conditioning produces insentient beings; patent conditioning gives rise to gods, humans, etc. In some there is dense conditioning conducive to ignorance; in others there is attenuated conditioning conducive to liberation. Conditioning alone is responsible for the diversity in creatures.

For this cosmic tree known as creation, the first thought-form is the seed, with the various spheres for various parts of the tree and the past, present and future as the fruits. The fivefold elements of which the tree is formed arise of their own accord and cease of their own accord. Of their own accord they diversify and in due course they become unified and tranquil.

dehaduḥkhaṁ vidur vyādhimādhyākhyaṁ vāsanāmayaṁ
maurkhyamūle hi te vidyāttattvajñāne parikṣayaḥ (14)

VASIṢṬHA continued:

Kuṇḍalinī functions in the body composed of the five-fold elements, in the form of the life-force. It is this same kuṇḍalinī which is known variously as conditioning or limitation, as the mind, jīva, movement of thought, intellect (or the determining faculty) and ego-sense; for it is the supreme life-force in the body. As the apāna it constantly flows downward, as samāna it dwells in the solar plexus and as udāna the same life-force rises up. On account of these forces, there is balance in the system. If, however, the downward pull is excessive and the downward force is not arrested by appropriate effort, death ensues. Similarly, if the upward pull is excessive and it is not arrested by appropriate effort, death ensues. If the movement of the life-force is governed in such a way that it neither goes up nor down, there is an unceasing state of equilibrium and all diseases are overcome. Otherwise if there is malfunction of ordinary (secondary) nāḍī one is subject to minor ailments, and if the principal nāḍī are involved there is serious ailment.

RĀMA asked:

What are vyādhī (illnesses), what are ādhī (psychic disorders) and what are the degenerative conditions of the body? Pray, enlighten me on these.

VASIṢṬHA continued:

Ādhi and vyādhi are sources of sorrow. Their avoidance is happiness, their cessation is liberation. Sometimes they arise together, sometimes they cause each other and sometimes they follow each other. **Physical malady is known as vyādhi, and psychic disturbance caused by psychological conditioning (neuroses) is known as ādhi. Both these are rooted in ignorance and wickedness. They end when self-knowledge or knowledge of truth is attained.**

Ignorance gives rise to absence of self-control and one is constantly assailed by likes and dislikes and by thoughts like 'I have gained this, I have yet to gain that'. All this intensifies delusion; all these give rise to psychic disturbances.

Physical ailments are caused by ignorance and its concomitant total absence of mental restraint which leads to improper eating and living habits. Other causes are untimely and irregular activities, unhealthy habits, evil company, wicked thoughts. They are also caused by the weakening of the nāḍī or by their being cluttered or clogged up, thus preventing the free flow of the life-force. Lastly, they are caused by an unhealthy environment. All these are of course ultimately determined by the fruits of past actions performed either in the near or the distant past.

ātmajñānaṁ vinā sāro nā ''dhirnaśyati rāghava
bhūyo rajjvāvabodhena rajjusarpo hi naśyati (25)

VASIṢṬHA continued:

All these psychic disturbances and physical ailments arise from the fivefold elements. I shall now tell you how they cease. Physical ailments are twofold: ordinary and serious. The former arise from day-to-day causes and the latter are congenital. The former are corrected by day-to-day remedial measures and by adopting the proper mental attitude. **But the latter (serious) ailments, as also the psychic disturbances, do not cease until self-knowledge is attained: the snake seen in the rope dies only when the rope is again seen as rope.** Self-knowledge ends all physical and psychic disturbances. However, physical ailments that are not psychosomatic may be dealt with by medication, prayers and by right action, as also by baths. All these have been described in medical treatises.

RĀMA asked:

Pray, tell me: how does physical ailment arise from psychic disturbance and how can it be dealt with by means other than medical?

VASIṢṬHA continued:

When there is mental confusion one does not perceive one's path clearly. Unable to see the path in front of oneself, one takes a wrong path. The life-forces are agitated by this confusion and they flow haphazardly along the nāḍī. As a result, some nāḍī are depleted of energy and others are clogged.

Then there arise disturbances in the metabolism, indigestion, excessive appetite, as also improper functioning of the digestive system. Food eaten turns into poison. The natural movement of food in and through the body is arrested. This gives rise to various physical ailments.

Thus psychic disturbance leads to physical ailments. Just as myrobalan is capable of making the bowels move, even so certain mantrā like ya, ra, la, va, can also remedy these psychosomatic disorders. Other measures are pure and auspicious actions, service of holy men, etc. By these the mind becomes pure and there is great joy in the heart. The life-forces flow along the nāḍī as they should. Digestion becomes normal, diseases cease.

By the practice of pūraka or inhalation, if the kuṇḍalinī at the base of the spine is 'filled' and made to rest in a state of equilibrium, the body remains firm. When through the retention of the breath all the nāḍī are warmed up, the kuṇḍalinī rises up like a stick and its energies flood all the nāḍī of the body. On account of this the nāḍi are purified and made light. Then the yogi is able to travel in space. When the kuṇḍalinī arises through the brahmā-nāḍī and reaches the spot known as dvādaśānta (twelve finger-breadths from the crown of the head) during the recaka or exhalation, if the kuṇḍalinī can be held there for an hour, the yogi sees the gods and perfected beings who travel in space.

yadaccham śītalatvam ca tadasyā ''tmendurucyate
itīndorutthitaḥ so 'gniragniṣomau hi dehakaḥ (75)

RĀMA asked: How is it possible for these mortal eyes to behold the celestials?

VASIṢṬHA said:

Indeed, no mortal can behold the celestials with these mortal eyes. But through the eyes of pure intelligence the celestials are seen, as in a dream. The celestials are able to fulfil one's desires. Vision of celestials is non-different from dream, in fact, the only difference being that the effect of the vision is lasting. Again, if one is able to hold the life-force in the dvādaśānta (twelve finger-breadths from the body) for a considerable time after exhalation, the life-force is able to enter other bodies. This power is inherent in the life-force; though by nature unsteady, it can be steadied. Since the ignorance which envelops everything is insubstantial, such exceptions are often seen in the movement of energy in this world. Surely, all this is indeed Brahman, the diversity and diverse functions are mere figures of speech.

RĀMA asked:

In order to enter into minute spaces (nāḍī) and then in order to fill the inner space with the life-force, one's body has to be made both atomic and solid at the same time! How is it made?

VASIṢṬHA said:

When wood and the saw come together, wood is split. But when two pieces of wood come together, there is fire! All this is part of nature.

*In this physical body, two forces come together in the abdomen. Together they form a hollow stick. In it rests the kuṇḍalinī. This kuṇḍalinī stands midway between heaven and earth and is ever vibrant with life-force. Dwelling in the heart it experiences all. It keeps all the psychic centres in a state of constant vibration or motion. It digests or devours everything. It makes the psychic centres tremble by the movement of prāṇa. It sustains the fire in the body till all the essences have been exhausted.

By nature it is cool, but because of it the body becomes warm. It is spread throughout the body, though it dwells in the heart where it is contemplated by the yogī. It is of the nature of jñāna (knowledge) and in its light a distant object is seen as if near. **Whatever is cool is the moon, the self; from this moon arises fire. The body is made of this moon and this fire.** In fact, the entire world is made of these two, the cool moon and the warm fire. Or, you may consider that this world is the creation of knowledge and ignorance, the real and the unreal. In which case consciousness, light and knowledge are considered the sun or the fire, and inertness, darkness and ignorance are considered as the moon.

* The 'it' in this paragraph may refer to the gastric fire, life-force or even the kuṇḍalinī. Vasiṣṭha is surely not terribly keen on making and sustaining such distinctions!!

pıtvā mṛtopamaṁ śıtaṁ prāṇaḥ somamukhāgame
abhrāgamātpūrayati śarıraṁ pınatāṁ gataḥ (94)

VASIṢṬHA continued:

Fire and moon exist in a mutual causal relationship (in the body). In a way, theirs is the relationship of seed and tree, one giving birth to the other; in a way, it is like light and darkness in which one destroys the other. (One who questions all this, saying "Since there is no desire-motivation, such causality and such activity are illogical", should be quickly dismissed. For such activity is obvious and is the experience of all.)

The (fire) prāṇa drinks the nectarine coolness at the mouth of the cool moon, filling the entire space within the body. (It is the yogi's theory that nectar flows from the palate and is consumed by the gastric fire in the solar plexus — thus the cool moon is the cause of the burning fire — and he prescribes the viparītakaraṇī to prevent this loss of nectar. S.V.) Fire dies and becomes the moon, even as day ends and night arrives.

At the junction of the fire and the moon, of light and darkness, of night and day, there is the revelation of the truth which eludes the understanding of even wise men.

Even as a day consists of day and night, the jīva is characterised by consciousness and inertia. Fire and the sun symbolise consciousness and the moon symbolises darkness or inertia. Even as when the sun is seen in the sky darkness vanishes on earth, when the light of consciousness is seen, the darkness of ignorance and the cycle of becoming come to an end. And, if the moon (the darkness of ignorance or inertia) is seen for what it is, consciousness is realised as the only truth. It is the light of consciousness that reveals the inert body. Consciousness, being non-moving and non-dual, is not grasped. However it can be realised through its own reflection, the body.

Consciousness, when it becomes aware of itself, gains the world. When such objectification is abandoned there is liberation. Prāṇa is heat (fire), apāna is the cool moon, and the two exist like light and shade in the same body. The light of consciousness and the moon of description together bring about experience. The phenomena called the sun and the moon, which had existed from the beginning of world-creation, also exist in the body.

O Rāma, remain in that state where the sun has absorbed the moon into itself. Remain in that state in which the moon has merged with the sun in the heart. Remain in that state where there is the realisation that the moon is but the reflection of the sun. Know the junction of the sun and the moon within yourself. The external phenomena are utterly useless.

satyabhāvanadṛṣṭo 'yaṁ deho deho bhavatyalaṁ
dṛṣṭastvasatyabhāvena vyomatāṁ yāti dehakaḥ (27)

VASIṢṬHA continued:

Now I shall describe to you how the yogī make their bodies atomic, as also enormous.

There is a spark of fire that burns just above the heart-lotus. This fire is quickly augmented, but since it is of the nature of consciousness, it arises as the light of knowledge. When it thus grows in magnitude in a moment, it is able to dissolve the entire body; even the water-element in the body is evaporated by its heat. Then, having abandoned the two bodies (the physical and the subtle), it is able to go where it likes. The kuṇḍalinī-power rises up like smoke from fire and is merged in the space, as it were. Holding fast the mind, buddhi and the ego-sense, this kuṇḍalinī shines radiantly as a particle of dust. This spark or this particle is then able to enter into anything whatsoever. Then this kuṇḍalinī releases the water and the earth elements that had previously been absorbed into itself and the body resumes its original shape. Thus, the jīva is able to become as small as an atom and as big as a mountain.

I have thus described to you the yoga method, and shall now deal with the wisdom-approach.

There is but one consciousness which is pure, invisible, the subtlest of the subtle, tranquil, and which is neither the world nor its activities. It is aware of itself; hence this jīva-hood arises. This jīva perceives this unreal body as real, but when the jiva perceives it in the light of self-knowledge, this delusion vanishes and the body also becomes utterly tranquil. Then the jīva does not perceive the body. The confusion of the body with the self is the greatest delusion, which the light of the sun cannot dispel.

When the body is considered real, it becomes a real body. When it is perceived with the knowledge that it is unreal, it is merged in space. Whatever notion is firmly held concerning the body, that it becomes.

Another method is the practice of exhalation whereby the jīva is raised from the abode of the kuṇḍalinī and made to abandon this body, which then becomes inert like a log of wood. Then the jīva can enter into any other body, moving or non-moving and undergo the desired experience. After thus having acquired the experience it can re-enter the previous body or any other body at its will and pleasure. Or, it may remain as the all-pervading consciousness without entering into any particular body.

upadeśakramo rāma vyavasthāmātrapālanaṁ
jñaptestu kāraṇaṁ śuddha śiṣyaprajñaiva rāghava (13)

VASIṢṬHA continued:

Thus, the queen Cūḍālā came to be endowed with all the psychic powers (like the ability to make oneself atomic and enormous). She traversed the sky and entered into the deepest oceans and roamed the earth, without ever leaving the company of her husband. She entered into every type of substance — wood, rock, mountain, grass, sky and water, without any hindrance. She moved with the celestials and with the liberated sages and conversed with them.

Though she made every endeavour to enlighten her husband also, he was not only unresponsive but he laughed at her foolishness. He remained ignorant. She felt it unwise to exhibit her psychic powers before him.

RĀMA asked:

If even such a great siddha-yogini as Cūḍālā could not bring about the spiritual awakening and the enlightenment of king Śikhidhvaja, how does one attain enlightenment at all?

VASIṢṬHA said:

The instruction of a disciple by a preceptor is but a tradition; the cause of enlightenment is but the purity of the disciple's consciousness. Not by hearing nor by righteous acts is self-knowledge attained. Only the self knows the self, only the snake knows its feet! Yet, . . .

There was a wealthy villager in the Vindhya hills. Once when he was walking in the forest he lost a copper coin (one cent). He was a miser and so he began to search for it in the thick bush. All the time he was calculating. 'With that one cent I shall do some business, it will become four cents and then eight cents and so on'. For three days he searched, unmindful of the taunts of spectators. At the end of those three days he suddenly found a precious stone! (It was a philosopher's stone.) Taking it with him, he returned home and lived happily.

What was the cause of this miser finding the philosopher's stone? Surely, his miserliness and his searching the bush for the lost cent! Even so, in the case of the preceptor's instructions, the disciple looks for something but obtains something else! Brahman is beyond the mind and the senses; it cannot be known through someone else's instruction. Yet, without the instruction of the preceptor it is not known either! The miser would not have found the precious stone if he had not searched the bush for his one cent! Hence the instruction of the preceptor is considered the cause of self-knowledge — and yet he is not the cause! Look at this mystery of Māyā, O Rāma: one seeks something and obtains something else!

prāptakālaṁ kṛtaṁ kāryaṁ rājate nātha netarat
vasante rājate puṣpaṁ phalaṁ śaradi rājate (22)

VASIṢṬHA continued:

Devoid of self-knowledge, the king Śikhidhvaja became blinded by delusion. He was sunk in grief which nothing in the world could assuage. Soon he began to seek solitude, like you, O Rāma, doing just those royal duties which his ministers made him do. He gave plenty in charity. He performed various austerities. But there was no change in the delusion and in the sorrow. After considerable deliberation, one day

ŚIKHIDHVAJA said to the queen:

My dear, I have enjoyed sovereignty for a long time and I have enjoyed all the royal pleasures. Neither pleasure nor pain, neither prosperity nor adversity is able to disturb the mind of the ascetic. Hence I wish to go to the forest and become an ascetic. The beloved forest which resembles you in every respect (here he gives a romantic description of the forest, comparing it to the limbs of the queen) will delight my heart even as you do. So give me leave to go, for a good housewife does not obstruct her husband's wishes.

CŪḌĀLĀ replied:

Lord, that action alone shines as appropriate which is done at the appropriate time: flowers are appropriate to spring and fruits to the winter. Forest life is appropriate to old age, not for people of your age. At your age the household life is appropriate. When we grow old, both of us shall leave this household life and go to the forest! Moreover, your subjects will grieve over your untimely departure from the kingdom.

ŚIKHIDHVAJA said:

My dear, do not place obstacles on my path. Know that I have already left for the forest! You are but a child and it is not proper that you should go to the forest, too, and lead the hard ascetic life. Hence, remain here and rule the kingdom.

VASIṢṬHA continued:

That night, while the queen was still asleep, the king left the palace on the pretext of patrolling the city. He rode a whole day and reached a dense forest in the Mandara mountain. It was far, far from habitation and there were signs that the place had been inhabited previously by holy brāhmaṇā. There he built a cottage for himself and equipped it with whatever he considered necessary for the ascetic life — like a stick made of bamboo, eating utensil (plate), water vessel, a tray for flowers, a kamaṇḍalu, a rosary, a garment to protect him from the cold, a deer skin. There he commenced his ascetic life. The first part of the day he spent in meditation and japa (repetition of the holy mantra). The second part of the day he spent in gathering flowers, and this was followed by bath and worship of the deity. Thereafter he took a frugal meal consisting of fruits and roots. The rest of the time he spent in japa or the repetition of the mantra. Thus he spent a long time in that cottage without ever thinking of his kingdom, etc.

uvāca cā "tmanaivā 'ho yāvajjīvaṁ śarīriṇāṁ
na svabhāvaḥ śamaṁ yāti mamā 'pyutkaṇṭhitaṁ manaḥ (29)

VASIṢṬHA continued:

Cūḍālā awoke with a fright when she discovered that her husband had left the palace. She felt unhappy and decided that her place was by her husband's side. Quickly she also got out of the palace through a small window and flew in the sky, looking for her husband. Soon she found him wandering in the forest. But, before alighting near him, she considered future events through her psychic vision. She saw everything as it was destined to happen, to the smallest detail. Bowing to the inevitable, she returned to the palace by the same aerial route she had taken.

Cūḍālā announced that the king had left the palace on an important mission. From then on, she herself conducted the affairs of the state. For eighteen years she dwelt in the palace and he in the forest, without their seeing each other. He had begun to show signs of old age.

At that time, Cūḍālā 'saw' her husband's mind had ripened considerably and that it was time for her to help him attain enlightenment. Having thus determined, she left the palace at night and flew to where he was. She beheld the celestials and the perfected sages in the heavens. She flew through clouds, inhaling the heavenly perfume and looking forward with great eagerness to her reunion with her husband. She was excited and her mind was agitated. Becoming aware of this mental state, **she said to herself: "Ah, surely as long as there is life in the body, one's nature does not cease to be active. Even my mind is agitated so much!** Or perhaps, O mind, you are seeking your own consort. On the other hand my husband has surely forgotten all about his kingdom and me, after all these years of asceticism. In that case it is futile on your part, O mind, to get excited at the prospect of meeting him once again . . . I shall restore equilibrium to the heart of my husband in such a way that he will return to the kingdom, where we shall dwell together happily for a long time. That delight which is had in a state of utter equilibrium is superior to all other happiness."

Thinking thus, Cūḍālā reached the Mandara mountain. Still remaining in the sky she saw her husband as if he were another person, for the king who had always been clothed in royal robes, now appeared as an emaciated ascetic. Cūḍālā was depressed at this heart-breaking sight of her husband clad in coarse garment, with matted locks, quiet and lonely, with his colour darkened considerably as if he had had a bath in a river of ink. For a moment she thought: "Alas, the fruit of foolishness! For only the foolish reach such a condition as the king has reached. Surely it is on account of his own delusion that he has thus secluded himself in this hermitage. Here and now I shall enable him to attain enlightenment. I shall approach him in a disguise."

jīvitaṁ yāti sāphalyaṁ svamabhyāgatapūjayā
devādapyadhikaṁ pūjyaḥ satāmabhyāgato janaḥ (82)

VASIṢṬHA continued:

Afraid that Śikhidhvaja might once again spurn her teaching, considering that she was an ignorant girl, Cūḍālā transformed herself into a young brāhmaṇa ascetic and descended right in front of her husband. Śikhidhvaja saw the young ascetic and was delighted. The young ascetic was incomparably radiant, so that Śikhidhvaja took him to be a celestial. He worshipped the ascetic appropriately. Cūḍālā appreciatively accepted the worship and remarked: "I have travelled around the world but never have I been worshipped with such devotion! I admire your tranquillity and your austerity. You have chosen to tread the razor's edge, inasmuch as you have abandoned your kingdom and resorted to the forest life."

ŚIKHIDHVAJA replied:

Surely, you know everything, O son of the gods! By your very look you are showering nectar upon me. I have a lovely wife who is just now ruling my kingdom; you resemble her in some ways. And the flowers I have offered you in worship — may they be blessed. **One's life attains its fruition by the worship of the guest who arrives unsolicited; the worship of such a guest is superior even to the worship of the gods.** Pray, tell me who you are and to what I owe this blessing of your visit to me?"

THE BRĀHMAṆA (CŪḌĀLĀ) said:

There is a holy sage in this universe known as Nārada. Once he was engaged in meditation in a cave on the bank of the holy river Gaṅgā. At the end of his meditation, he heard the sound of bracelets apparently belonging to some people engaged in water sports. Out of curiosity he looked in that direction and saw a few of the foremost celestial nymphs sporting in water, naked. They were indescribably beautiful. His heart experienced pleasure and his mind momentarily lost its equilibrium, overcome by lust.

ŚIKHIDHVAJA asked:

Holy one, though he was a sage of great learning and a liberated one at that, though he was free from desire and from attachment and though his consciousness was as limitless as the sky, how was it that he was overcome by lust?

THE BRĀHMANA (CŪḌĀLĀ) said:

O royal sage, all beings in the three worlds, including the gods in heaven, have a body that is subject to the dual forces. Whether one is ignorant or one is wise, as long as one is embodied the body is subject to happiness and unhappiness, pleasure and pain. By enjoying satisfying objects, one experiences pleasure, and by deprivation (hunger etc.) one experiences pain. Such is nature.

svarūpe nirmale satye nimiṣamapi vismṛte
dṛśyamullāsamāpnoti prāvṛṣīva payodharaḥ (111)

THE BRĀHMAṆA (CŪḌĀLĀ) continued:

If the self which is the reality and which is pure is forgotten even for a moment, the object of experience attains expansion. If there is unbroken awareness, this does not happen. Even as darkness and light have come to be firmly associated with night and day, the experience of pleasure and pain has confirmed the existence of the body in the case of the ignorant. In the wise, however, even if such an experience is reflected in consciousness, it does not produce an impression. As in the case of a crystal, the wise man is influenced only by the object when it is actually and physically present nearby. But the ignorant person is so heavily influenced that he broods on the object even in its absence. Such are their characteristics, thinned out vulnerability is liberation, whereas dense colouring of the mind is bondage.

(In response to Śikhidhvaja's question: "How do pleasure and pain arise even in the absence of the concerned object?" the brāhmaṇa said:) The cause is the impression received by the heart through the body, the eyes, etc. Later this expands by itself. When the heart is agitated, the memory agitates the jīva in its kuṇḍalinī-abode. The nāḍī which branch out throughout the body are affected. Pleasure experiences and pain experiences affect the nāḍī differently. The nāḍī expand and blossom, as it were, in pleasure, not in pain.

When the jiva does not thus enter into the agitated nāḍī, it is liberated. Bondage is none other than subjection of the jīva to pleasure and pain: when such subjection does not exist there is liberation. The jīva gets agitated at the very 'sight' of pleasure and pain. However, if through self-knowledge it realises that pain and pleasure do not exist in truth, then it regains its equilibrium. Or, if it realises that these do not exist in itself nor does it (the jiva) exist in them, it realises total freedom. If it realises that all this is nothing but the one infinite consciousness, then again it attains equilibrium. Like a lamp without fuel, it does not get agitated again, for the jīva itself is then realised as a non-entity and it is reabsorbed in the consciousness of which it is but the first thought-emanation.

(Asked by Śikhidhvaja to elaborate on how the pleasure experience leads to the loss of energy, the brāhmaṇa said:) As I said, the jīva agitates the life-force. The movement of the life-force extracts the vital energy from the entire body. This energy then descends as the seminal energy which is discharged naturally.

(Asked "What is nature?" the brāhmaṇa said:) Originally, Brahman alone existed as Brahman. In it innumerable substances appeared like ripples on the surface of the ocean. This is known as nature. It is not causally related to Brahman, but it happened like a cocoanut accidentally falling when a crow happened to alight on it. In that nature are found diverse creatures endowed with diverse characteristics.

imāmakhaṇḍitāṁ samyak kriyāṁ sampādayannapi
duḥkhād gacchāmi duḥkhaughamamṛtaṁ me viṣaṁ sthitaṁ (87/14)

THE BRĀHMAṆA (CŪḌALĀ) continued:

It is by such nature of the self that this universe is born. It is sustained by self-limitation or conditioning on account of alternating order and disorder. When such self-limitation and such conflict between order and disorder cease, the beings will not be born again.

(Continuing the story of Nārada, the brāhmaṇa said:) Soon, Nārada regained his self-control. He gathered the seed which had been spilt, in a pot made of crystal. He then filled the pot with milk produced by his thought-force. In due course that pot gave birth to an infant which was perfect in every respect. Nārada named the baby and in course of time imparted the highest wisdom to it. The young boy was a peer to his father.

Later, Nārada took the boy to Brahmā the creator, the father of Nārada. Brahmā conferred upon the boy (whose name was Kuṁbha) the blessing of the highest wisdom. It is that boy, that Kuṁbha, that grandson of Brahmā, who is standing before you. I roam the world playfully, for I have nothing to gain from anyone. When I come into this world, my feet do not touch the earth.

(As Vasiṣṭha said this, the seventeenth day came to an end. The next day Vasiṣṭha continued.)

ŚIKHIDHVAJA said:

It is truly by the fruition of the good deeds done in many past incarnations that I have obtained your company today and am able to drink the nectar of your wisdom! Nothing in the world gives that peace which the company of the holy ones bestows on man.

THE BRĀHMAṆA (CŪḌALĀ) said:

I have told you my life story. Pray, now tell me who you are and what you are doing here. How long have you been here? Tell me everything truthfully, for recluses do not speak anything but the truth.

ŚIKHIDHVAJA replied:

O son of the gods, you know everything as it is. What else shall I tell you? I dwell in this forest on account of my fear of this saṁsāra (world-cycle or the cycle of birth and death). Though you know all this, I shall briefly relate my story to you. I am king Śikhidhvaja. I have abandoned my kingdom. I dread this saṁsāra in which one repeatedly and alternately experiences pleasure and pain, birth and death. However, though I have wandered everywhere and though I perform intense austerities, I have not found peace and tranquillity. My mind is not at rest. I do not indulge in activities nor do I seek to gain anything. I am alone here and unattached to anything; yet I am dry and devoid of fulfilment. **I have practised all the kriyā (yoga methods) uninterruptedly. But I only progress from sorrow to greater sorrow; and even nectar turns into poison for me.**

anupādeyavākyasya vaktuḥ pṛṣṭasya lilayā
vrajantyaphalatām vācastamasīvā 'kṣasaṁvidaḥ (42)

THE BRĀHMAṆA (CŪḌĀLĀ) SAID:

I once asked my grandfather, "Which is superior, kriya (action, the practice of a technique) or jñāna (self-knowledge)?" And he said to me:

"Indeed jñāna is supreme, for through jñāna one realises the one which alone is. On the other hand, kriyā has been described in colourful terms, as a pastime. If one does not have jñāna, then one clings to kriyā: if one does not have good clothes to wear, he clings to the sack.

"The ignorant are trapped by the fruits of their actions on account of their conditioning (vāsanā). When the latter is given up, action becomes no-action, whether it is conventionally regarded as good or evil. In the absence of self-limitation or volition, actions do not bear fruit. Actions by themselves do not generate reaction or 'fruit'; it is the vāsanā or the volition that makes action bear fruit. Just as the frightened boy thinks of a ghost and sees a ghost, the ignorant man entertains the notion of sorrow and suffers sorrow.

"Neither the vāsanā (self-limitation or conditioning) nor the ego-sense is a real entity! They arise because of foolishness. When this foolishness is abandoned, there is the realisation that all this is Brahman and there is no self-limitation. When there is vāsanā, there is mind; when the vāsanā ceases in the mind, there is self-knowledge. One who has attained self-knowledge is not born."

Thus, even the gods, Brahmā and others, have declared that self-knowledge alone is supreme. Why then do you remain ignorant? Why do you think, "This is the kamaṇḍalu" and "This is a stick" and remain immersed in ignorance? Why do you not enquire "Who am I?", "How has this world arisen?" and "How does all this cease?"? Why do you not reach the state of the enlightened by enquiring into the nature of bondage and liberation? Why are you wasting your life in these futile austerities and other kriyā? It is by resorting to the company of holy ones, by serving them and enquiring of them, that you will attain self-knowledge.

ŚIKHIDHVAJA said:

Aha, I have truly been awakened by you, O sage. I am freed of foolishness. You are my guru; I am your disciple. Pray instruct me in what you know, knowing which, one does not grieve.

THE BRĀHMAṆA (CŪḌĀLĀ) replied:

O royal sage, I shall instruct you if you are in a receptive mood and cherish my words. **If one playfully instructs another merely in answer to a query, when the latter does not intend to receive, cherish and assimilate the teaching, it becomes fruitless.** (After receiving such an assurance from Śikhidhvaja, Cūḍālā said:) Listen attentively: I shall narrate to you a story which resembles yours.

duḥkhāni maurkhyavibhavena bhavanti yāni
naivā 'pado na ca jarāmaraṇena tāni
sarvāpadāṁ śirasi tiṣṭhati maurkhyamekaṁ
kṛṣṇaṁ janasya vapuṣāmiva keśajālaṁ (27)

THE BRĀHMAṆA (CŪḌĀLĀ) said:

There was a man in whom there was the almost impossible combination of wealth and wisdom. He was endowed with all excellences, he was clever in his dealings, he achieved all his ambitions, but he was unaware of the self. He began to engage himself in austerities with the desire of acquiring the celestial jewel known as cintāmaṇi (the philosopher's stone which is supposed to be capable of fulfilling all the desires of its possessor). His effort was intense. So, within a very short period of time, this jewel appeared before him. Indeed, what is impossible for one who strives his utmost! One who applies himself to the task he has undertaken, unmindful of the effort and the difficulties, reaches the desired end even if he is poor.

This man saw the jewel in front of him, within his easy reach. But he was unable to reach any certainty concerning it. He began to muse with a mind confused by prolonged striving and suffering: "Is this the cintāmaṇi? Or is it not? Shall I touch it or not? Perhaps it will disappear if I touch it? Surely, it cannot be obtained within so short a period of time! The scriptures say that it can only be obtained after a whole lifetime of striving. Surely, because I am a poverty-stricken, greedy man, I am merely hallucinating the existence of this jewel before me. How could I be so lucky as to get it so soon? There may be some great ones who might obtain this jewel within a short time, but I am an ordinary person with just a little austerity to my credit. How is it possible for me to get this so soon?" Thus confused in his mind, he did not make any effort to take the jewel. He was not destined to get it. One gets only what he deserves, when he deserves it. Even if the celestial jewel stands in front of him, the fool ignores it! The jewel, thus ignored, disappeared. [Psychic attainments (siddhī) bestow everything on one whom they seek: after having destroyed his wisdom they go away.]

The man engaged himself further in austerities for the attainment of the cintāmaṇi. (The industrious do not abandon their undertaking.) After some time, he saw a glass-piece thrown playfully in front of him by the celestials. He thought it was the cintāmaṇi. Thus deluded he greedily picked it up. Confident that he could get whatever he sought with its help, he gave up all his wealth, family, etc. and went away to a forest. On account of his foolishness he suffered there. **Great calamities, old age and death are nothing in comparison to the suffering caused by foolishness. In fact, foolishness adorns the head of all sufferings and calamities!**

maurkhyaṁ hi bandhanamavehi paraṁ mahātman
baddho na baddha iti cetasi tadvimuktyai
ātmodayaṁ trijagadātmamayaṁ samastaṁ
maurkhye sthitasya sahasā nanu sarvabhūmiḥ (31)

THE BRĀHMAṆA (CŪḌĀLĀ) continued:

Listen, O king, to another story which also resembles yours. In the Vindhya forests there was an elephant which was extremely strong and equipped with strong and powerful tusks. The rider of this elephant had, however, imprisoned it in a cage. By this and the repeated use by the rider of weapons like the goad, the elephant was subject to great pain.

While the rider was away the elephant struggled to free itself from the cage. This effort went on for three whole days. Eventually it shattered the cage. Just at this time, the rider saw what the elephant had done. While the elephant was making good its escape, the rider climbed up a tree from which he planned to throw himself on its back and thus subdue it once again. However, he missed the elephant's head as he fell and landed right in front of it. The elephant saw its enemy (the rider) fallen in front of it: yet it was overcome by pity and therefore did not harm him. Such compassion is seen even in beasts. The elephant went away.

The rider got up, not seriously injured. (The evil-doer's body does not break down easily! Their evil deeds seem to strengthen their body.) The rider, however, was unhappy at the loss of the elephant. He continued to search the forest for the lost elephant. After a very long time he saw it standing in a thick forest. He gathered other elephant tamers and with their help dug a huge pit and covered it with foliage, eager to recapture that elephant.

Within the next few days that mighty elephant fell into the pit. Thus recaptured and bound by the wicked rider, the elephant still stands there!

The elephant had neglected to kill its enemy, though he had fallen right in front of it, and hence it had to undergo fresh suffering. One who does not, on account of his foolishness, act appropriately when the opportunity offers itself and thus remove all the obstacles, invites sorrow. By the false satisfaction 'I am free' the elephant fell into bondage: foolishness invites sorrow. **Foolishness is bondage, O holy one! One who is bound thinks he is free in his foolishness. Though all that exists in all the three worlds is but the self, to one who is firmly established in foolishness all that is but the expansion of foolishness.**

tyāgitā syāt kutastasya cintāmapyāvṛṇoti yaḥ
pavanaspandayukttasya niḥspandatvaṁ kutastaroḥ (14)

ŚIKHIDHVAJA said:

Holy one, explain the significance of these stories!

THE BRĀHMAṆA (CŪḌĀLĀ) said:

The wealthy learned man who went in search of the celestial jewel is you, O king! You have knowledge of the scriptures, yet you are not at rest within yourself as a stone rests in water. Cintāmaṇi is the total renunciation of everything, which puts an end to all sorrow. By pure total renunciation everything is gained. What is the celestial jewel in comparison? In as much as you were able to abandon the empire, etc. you have experienced such total renunciation.

After renouncing everything, you have come to this hermitage. However, one thing still remains to be renounced — your ego-sense. If the heart abandons the mind (the movement of thought) there is realisation of the absolute; but you are overcome by the thought of the renunciation which your renunciation has created in you. Hence, this is not the bliss that arises from total renunciation. **One who has abandoned everything is not agitated by worry: if wind can sway the branches of a tree, it cannot be called immovable.**

Such worries (or movements of thought) alone are known as mind. Thought (notion, concept) is another name for the same thing. If thoughts still operate, how can the mind be considered to have been renounced? When the mind is agitated by thoughts (worries, etc.) the three worlds appear to it instantly. As long as thoughts are still there, how can there be pure and total renunciation? Hence when such thoughts arise in your heart, your renunciation leaves your heart (like the cintāmaṇi leaving the man). Because you did not recognise the spirit of renunciation and cherish it, it left you — taking with it freedom from thoughts and worries.

When thus you were abandoned by the jewel (spirit of total renunciation), you picked up the glass-piece (austerities and all the rest of it). You began to cherish it, on account of your delusion. You have replaced the unconditioned and unattached infinite consciousness with the futile performance of austerities which alas, for your own sorrow, has a beginning and an end. One who abandons infinite joy which is easily attained, and engages himself in the acquisition of the impossible, is surely a pig-headed fool — and suicidal. You fell into the trap of this forest life and did not strive to sustain the spirit of total renunciation. You abandoned the bondage to kingdom and all the rest of it, but you have become bound again by what is known as the ascetic life. Now you are even more worried than before by cold, heat, wind, etc. and hence more firmly bound. Foolishly thinking, 'I have obtained the cintāmaṇi', you have really gained not even a piece of crystal!

This is the meaning of the first parable.

yadā vanaṁ prayātastvaṁ tadā 'jñānaṁ kṣataṁ tvayā
patitaṁ sanna nihataṁ manastyāgamahāsinā (14)

THE BRĀHMAṆA (CŪḌĀLĀ) continued:

Now listen to the significance of the second parable.

What was described as the elephant in the Vindhya hills, that you are on this earth. The two powerful tusks are viveka (discrimination, wisdom) and vairāgya (dispassion), which you possess. The rider who inflicted pain on the elephant is ignorance, which caused you sorrow. Though powerful, the elephant was overcome by the rider: though excellent in every way, you are overcome by this ignorance or foolishness.

The elephant's cage is the cage of desires in which you are imprisoned. The only difference is that the iron cage decays in course of time, but the cage of desire grows stronger with time. Even as the elephant broke out of its cage, you abandoned your kingdom and came here. However, psychological abandonment is not as easy as breaking out of a material cage.

Even as the rider was alerted by the escape, the ignorance and the foolishness in you tremble when the spirit of renunciation manifests in you. When the wise man abandons the pursuit of pleasure, ignorance flees from him. **When you went to the forest you had seriously wounded this ignorance, but you had failed to destroy it by the abandonment of the mind or movement of energy in consciousness,** even as the elephant failed to kill the rider. Therefore this ignorance has arisen once again and, remembering the way in which you overpowered the previous desires, it has trapped you in the pit known as asceticism.

If you had destroyed this ignorance once and for all when you renounced your kingdom, you would not have been trapped by this asceticism.

You are the king of the elephants, endowed with the powerful tusk of viveka or wisdom. However, alas, in this dense forest you have been trapped by the rider known as ignorance, and you lie imprisoned in the blind well known as asceticism.

O king, why did you not listen to the wise words of your wife, Cūḍālā, who is indeed a knower of the truth? She is the foremost among the knowers of the self and there is no contradiction between her words and her deeds. Whatever she says is true and is worth putting into practice. However, even if you did not in the past listen to her words and assimilate them, why did you not abandon everything in total renunciation?

dhanaṁ dārā gṛhaṁ rājyaṁ bhūmiśchatraṁ ca bāndhavāḥ
iti sarvaṁ na te rājan sarvatyāgo hi kastava (5)

ŚIKHIDHVAJA said:

I have renounced the kingdom, the palace, the country and my wife, too. How is it then that you think that I have not renounced everything?

THE BRĀHMAṆA (CŪḌĀLĀ) replied:

Wealth, wife, palace, kingdom, the earth and the royal umbrella and your relatives are not yours, O king: renouncing them does not constitute total renunciation! There is something else which seems to be yours and which you have not renounced, and that is the best part of renunciation. Renounce that totally and without any residue and attain freedom from sorrow.

ŚIKHIDHVAJA said:

If the kingdom and all that was in it are not mine, then I abandon this forest and all that is in it. (So saying, Śikhidhvaja mentally renounced the forest, etc.)

(On being told by the brāhmaṇa, "All these things are not yours, hence there is no meaning in renouncing them", Śikhidhvaja said:) Surely, this hermitage is everything for me. Right now, it is mine. I shall abandon that, too. (Thus resolved, Śikhidhvaja cleansed his heart of the very idea that the hermitage was his:) Surely, now I have completely renounced everything!

THE BRĀHMAṆA (CŪḌĀLĀ) repeated:

Surely, all these too are not yours. How then do you renounce them? There is something which you have not renounced and that is the best part of it. By renouncing that, attain freedom from sorrow.

ŚIKHIDHVAJA said:

If these, too, are not mine, then I shall abandon my staff, the deer skin, etc., and my cottage, too.

VASIṢṬHA said:

So saying, he sprang up from his seat. While the brāhmaṇa was passively looking on, Śikhidhvaja collected whatever there was in the cottage and made a bonfire of it. He threw away his rosary: "I am freed from the delusion that the repetition of a mantra is holy, and so I have no need for you". He reduced the deer skin to ashes. He gave away his water pot (kamaṇḍalu) to a brāhmaṇa (or threw it into the fire).

He said to himself, "Whatever is to be renounced must be renounced all at once and forever, otherwise it expands once again and is gathered once again. Hence, I shall once and for all burn everything up."

Thus having resolved, Śikhidhvaja, who had decided to give up all activities sacred and secular, collected all those articles that he had used till then and burnt them all up.

tavā 'styevā 'parityakttaḥ sarvasmād bhāga uttamaḥ
yaṁ parityajya niḥśeṣaṁ parāmāyāsyaśokatāṁ (13)

VASIṢṬHA continued:

Then, Śikhidhvaja set fire to the cottage which he had built unnecessarily, guided by his own previous (false) notions. After that, systematically he burnt whatever there was and whatever was left. He burnt or threw away everything, including his own clothes. Frightened by this bonfire even the animals ran away from that place.

ŚIKHIDHVAJA then said to the brāhamaṇa:

Awakened by you, O son of the gods, I have abandoned all the notions I had entertained for such a long time. I am now established in pure and blissful knowledge. From whatever proves to be the cause of bondage the mind turns away and rests in equilibrium. I have renounced everything. I am free from all bondage. I am at peace. I am blissful. I am victorious. The space is my dress; space is my abode and I am like space. Is there anything beyond this supreme renunciation, O son of the gods?

THE BRĀHMAṆA (CŪḌĀLĀ) replied:

You have not renounced everything, O king: hence, do not act as if you are enjoying the bliss of supreme renunciation! **You have something, as it were, which you have not renounced, that is the best part of renunciation. When that is also utterly abandoned without leaving a residue, then you will attain the supreme state, free from sorrow.**

After some thought, ŚIKHIDHVAJA said:

There is only one more thing left, O son of the gods: and that is this body which is the abode of the deadly snakes known as the senses, and which is composed of blood, flesh, etc. I shall now abandon that too and destroy it and thus achieve total renunciation.

As he was about to execute his resolve, THE BRĀHMAṆA said:

O king, why do you vainly endeavour to destroy this innocent body? Abandon this anger which is characteristic of the bull that sets out to destroy a calf! This ascetic body is inert and dumb. You have nothing to do with it. Therefore, do not attempt to destroy it. The body remains what it is, inert and dumb. It is motivated and made to function by some other power or energy. The body is not responsible for the experience of pleasure and pain. Further, destroying the body does not mean total renunciation. On the other hand, you are throwing away something which is an aid to such renunciation! If you are able to renounce that which functions through this body and which agitates the body, then you have truly abandoned all sin and evil and then you will have become a supreme renouncer. If that is renounced, everything (including this body) is renounced. Otherwise, the sin and evil, even if they remain submerged temporarily, will arise again.

sthitaṁ sarvaṁ parityajya yaḥ śete 'snehadīpavat
sa rājate prakāśātmā samaḥ sasnehadīpavat (52)

THE BRĀHMAṆA (CŪḌĀLĀ) said:

That alone is total renunciation which is the renunciation of that which is all, which is the sole cause of all these and in which all these abide.

ŚIKHIDHVAJA prayed:

Holy sir, please tell me what that is which should be renounced.

THE BRĀHMAṆA (CŪḌĀLĀ) said:

O noble one! It is the mind (which also goes by the names 'jīva', 'prāṇa', etc.) or the citta, which is neither inert nor non-inert and is in a state of confusion which is the 'all'. It is this citta (mind) which is confusion, it is the human being, it is the world, it is all. It is the seed for the kingdom, for the body, wife and all the rest of it. When this seed is abandoned there is total renunciation of all that is in the present and even in the future!

All these — good and evil, kingdom and forest — cause distress in the heart of one who is endowed with the citta, and great joy in one who is mindless. Just as the tree is agitated by the wind, this body is agitated by the mind. The diverse experiences of beings (old age, death, birth and so on) and also the firmness of the holy sages are verily the modifications of the mind. It is the mind alone which is referred to variously as buddhi, the cosmos, ego-sense, prāṇa, etc. Hence its abandonment alone is total renunciation. Once it is abandoned, the truth is experienced at once. All notions of unity and diversity come to an end. There is peace.

On the other hand, by renouncing what you consider not-yours, you are creating a division within yourself. If one renounces everything, then everything exists within the void of the one infinite consciousness. **When one rests in that state of total renunciation like the lamp without fuel, he shines with supreme brilliance like a lamp with fuel.** Even after renouncing the kingdom etc., you exist. Similarly, even after the mind has been renounced, that infinite consciousness will exist. Even when all these have been burnt, you have not undergone any change; even when you have totally abandoned the mind, there will be no change. One who has totally renounced everything is not afflicted by fear of old age, death and such other events in life. That alone is supreme bliss. All else is terrible sorrow. OṀ! Thus assimilate this truth and do what you wish to do. In that total renunciation does the highest wisdom or self-knowledge exist: the utter emptiness of a pot is where precious jewels are stored. It is by such total renunciation that the Śākya Muni (Buddha) reached that state beyond doubt in which he was firmly established. Hence, O king, having abandoned everything, remain in that form and in that state in which you find yourself. Abandon even the notion 'I have renounced all' and remain in a state of supreme peace.

tyāgastasyā 'tisukaraḥ susādhyaḥ spandanādapi
rājyādapyadhikānandaḥ kusumādapi sundaraḥ (6)

ŚIKHIDHVAJA said:

Pray, tell me the exact nature of this citta (mind) and also how to abandon it so that it does not arise again and again.

KUṀBHA (THE BRĀHMAṆA — CŪḌĀLĀ) replied:

Vāsanā (memory, subtle impressions of the past, conditioning) is the nature of this citta (mind). In fact they are synonymous. **Its abandonment or renunciation is easily accomplished, more delightful than even the sovereignty over a kingdom and more beautiful than a flower.** It is certainly very difficult for a foolish person to renounce the mind, even as it is difficult for a simpleton to rule the kingdom.

The utter destruction or extinction of the mind is the extinction of saṁsāra (the creation-cycle). It is also known as the abandonment of the mind. Therefore uproot the tree whose seed is the 'I'-idea with all its branches, fruits and leaves, and rest in the space in the heart.

What is known as 'I' arises in the absence of the knowledge of the mind (self-knowledge); this 'I' is the seed of the tree known as mind. It grows in the field of the supreme self which is also pervaded by the illusory power known as Māyā. Thus a division is created in that field and experience arises. With this, the determining faculty known as the buddhi arises. Of course it has no distinct form, as it is but the expanded form of the seed. Its nature is conceptualisation or notional; and it is also known as the mind, jiva and void.

The trunk of this tree is the body. The movement of energy within it that results in its growth, is the effect of psychological conditioning. Its branches are long and they reach out to great distances; they are the finite sense-experiences which are characterised by being and non-being. Its fruits are good and evil (pleasure and pain, happiness and unhappiness).

This is a vicious tree. Endeavour every moment to cut down its branches and to uproot it. Its branches, too, are of the nature of conditioning, of concepts and of percepts. They (the branches) are endowed with the fruits of all these. If you remain unattached to them, unconcerned about them and without identifying yourself with them, through the strength of your intelligence (consciousness) these vāsanā are greatly weakened. You will then be able to uproot the tree altogether. The destruction of the branches is secondary; the primary thing is to uproot it.

How is the tree to be uprooted? By engaging oneself in the enquiry into the nature of the self — 'Who am I?' This enquiry is the fire in which the very seed and roots of the tree known as citta (mind) are burnt completely.

kāraṇaṁ yasya kāryasya bhūmipāla na vidyate
vidyate neha tatkāryaṁ tatsaṁvittistu vibhramaḥ (54)

ŚIKHIDHVAJA said: I know that I am pure consciousness. How this impurity (ignorance) arose in it, I do not know. I am distressed because I am unable to get rid of this impurity which is not-self and unreal.

KUṀBHA asked: Tell me if that impurity (ignorance), on account of which you are an ignorant man bound to this saṁsāra, is real or unreal?

ŚIKHIDHVAJA replied: That impurity is also the ego-sense and the seed for this big tree known as citta (mind). I do not know how to get rid of it. It returns to me even when it is renounced by me!

KUṀBHA said: The effect arising from a real cause is self-evident at all times everywhere. Where the cause is not real, the effect is surely as unreal as the second moon seen in diplopia. The sprout of saṁsāra has arisen from the seed of ego-sense. Enquire into its cause and tell me now.

ŚIKHIDHVAJA replied: O Sage, I see that experience is the cause of ego-sense. But, tell me how to get rid of it.

KUṀBHA asked again: Ah, you are able to find the causes of effects! Tell me then the cause of such experience. I shall then tell you how to get rid of the cause. When consciousness is both the experiencing and the experience, and when there was no cause for the experience-as-the-object to arise, how did the effect (experience) arise?

ŚIKHIDHVAJA replied: Surely on account of the objective reality, such as the body? I am unable to see how such objective reality is seen as false.

KUṀBHA said: If experience rests on the reality of objects like the body, then if the body etc. are proved to be unreal, on what will experience rest? **When the cause is absent or unreal, the effect is non-existent and the experience of such an effect is delusion.** What then is the cause of objects like the body?

ŚIKHIDHVAJA asked: The second moon is surely not unreal because it has a cause which is eye-disease. The barren woman's son is never seen — and that is unreal. Why, is not the father the cause for the existence of the body?

KUṀBHA replied: But then that father is unreal: that which is born of unreality is unreal, too. If one says that the first Creator is the original cause of all subsequent bodies, in fact even that is not true! The Creator himself is non-different from the reality; hence his appearance as other than the reality (this creation, etc.) is delusion. The realisation of this truth enables one to get rid of the ignorance and ego-sense.

evaṁ jagadbhramasyā 'sya bhāvanaṁ tāvadātataṁ
śilībhūtasya śītena salilasyeva rūkṣatā (2)

ŚIKHIDHVAJA asked:

If all this: from the Creator to the pillar, is unreal; how has this real sorrow come into being?

KUṀBHA replied:

This delusion of the world-existence attains expansion by its repeated affirmation: when water is frozen into a block it serves as a seat! Only when ignorance is dispelled does one realise the truth; only then does the original state manifest itself. When the perception of diversity is attenuated, the saṁsāra ceases to be experienced and you shine in your own original glory.

Thus, you are the supreme primordial being. This body, this form, etc., have come into being on account of ignorance and misunderstanding. All these notions of a creator and of a creation of diverse beings have not been proved to be real. When the cause is unproven how can one take the effect to be real? All these diverse creatures are but appearance, like water in the mirage. Such a deceptive appearance ceases on being enquired into.

ŚIKHIDHVAJA asked:

Why can it not be said that the supreme self or the infinite consciousness (Brahman) is the cause whose effect is the Creator?

KUṀBHA replied:

Brahman or the supreme self is one without a second, without a cause and without an effect, for it has no reason (motivation or need) to do anything, to create anything. It is therefore not the doer, neither is there any action, instrument nor seed for such activity. Hence it is not the cause for this creation or the Creator. Hence, there is no such thing as creation. You are therefore neither the doer of actions nor the enjoyer of experiences. You are the all, ever at peace, unborn and perfect. Since there is no cause (reason for creation), there is no effect known as the world; the world-appearance is but delusion.

When thus the objectivity of the world is seen to be unreal, what is experience and of what? When there is no experience, there is no experiencer (the ego-sense). Thus, you are pure and liberated. Bondage and liberation are mere words.

ŚIKHIDHVAJA said:

Lord, by the wise and well-reasoned words which you have uttered I have been fully awakened. I realise that since there is no cause, Brahman is neither the doer of anything nor the creator of anything. Hence, there is neither mind nor an ego-sense. Such being the case, I am pure, I am awakened. I salute my self. There is naught which is the object of my consciousness.

tatsāramekameveha vidyate bhūpate tataṁ
ekamekāntacitkāntaṁ naikamapyadvitāvaśāt (24)

VASIṢṬHA continued:

Thus awakened, spiritually, Śikhidhvaja entered into deep meditation from which he was playfully awakened by Kuṁbha, who said: "O king, you have been duly awakened and enlightened. What has to be done now has to be done, regardless of whether this world-vision ceases or does not cease. Once the light of the self has been seen, you are instantly freed from the undesirable and from mental modifications, and you remain as one liberated while still living."

Śikhidhvaja, who was now radiant with self-knowledge, asked the brāhmaṇa Kuṁbha 'for further understanding': "When the reality is one indivisible, infinite consciousness, how could this apparent division of the seer, the seen and sight arise in it?"

KUṀBHA replied:

Well asked, O king. This is all that remains for you to know. Whatever there is in this universe will cease to be at the end of this world-cycle, leaving only the essence, which is neither light nor darkness. That is pure consciousness which is supreme peace and infinite. It is beyond logic and intellectual comprehension. It is known as Brahman or nirvāṇa. It is smaller than the smallest, larger than the biggest and the best among the excellent. In relation to it, what now appears to be is but an atomic particle!

That which shines as the I-consciousness and which is the universal self, is what exists as this universe. There is indeed no real distinction between that universal self and the universe, as there is no distinction between air and its movement. One may say that between the waves and the ocean there is a causal relationship in terms of time and space: but in the universal self or infinite consciousness there is no such relationship, and hence the universe is without a cause. In that infinite consciousness this universe floats as a particle of dust. In it the word 'world' comes to be endowed with substantiality or reality.

That (infinite consciousness) alone is the essence here. It pervades all. It is one. It is consciousness. It holds everything together. Yet, one cannot say it is one because of the total absence of divisibility or duality. Hence, it is sufficient to know that the self alone is the truth, and not let the notion of duality arise. That alone is everywhere at all times in all the diverse forms. It is not seen (not experienced through the senses and the mind) nor is it an object to be attained. Hence, it is neither the cause nor the effect. It is extremely subtle. It is pure experiencing (neither the experiencer nor the experience). Though it is thus described, it is beyond description. Hence one cannot say that it is nor that it is not. How then can it be the cause of this creation?

kevalaṁ paramevetthaṁ paramaṁ bhāsate śivaṁ
ato jagadahantādi praśna evātra nocitaḥ (41)

KUṀBHA said:

That which has no seed (cause) and which is indescribable is therefore not the cause of another — naught is born of that. Hence, the self is neither the doer, nor the action nor the instrument. It is the truth. It is the eternal absolute consciousness. It is self-knowledge. There is no creation in the supreme Brahman. One may theoretically establish the arising and the existence of a wave in the ocean on the basis of time (of its arising) and space (in which it seems to exist as a wave). But, who has tried to establish even such a relationship between Brahman and the creation? For, in Brahman time and space do not exist. Thus, the world has no basis at all.

ŚIKHIDHVAJA said:

Surely, one can rationalise the existence of waves in the ocean. But I do not understand how it is that the world and the ego-sense are uncaused.

KUṀBHA said:

Now you have correctly understood the truth, O king! That is because there is in fact no reality which corresponds to the words 'world' and 'ego-sense'. Just as emptiness (or the notion of distance) exists, non-different from space, even so this world-appearance exists in the supreme being or infinite consciousness — whether in the same form or with another form.

When thus the reality of this world is well understood, then it is realised as the supreme self (Śiva). When rightly understood, even poison turns into nectar. When it is not thus rightly understood, it becomes evil (aŚivam), the world of sorrow. For whatever this consciousness realises itself to be, that it becomes. It is because of a confusion in the self that this consciousness sees itself as embodied and as the world.

It is that supreme self alone that shines here as the supreme being (Śivam). Hence, the very questions concerning the world and the ego-sense are inappropriate. Surely, questions are appropriate only concerning those substances that are real, not with regard to those whose existence is unproved. The world and the ego-sense have no existence independent of the supreme self. Since there is no reason for their existence, the truth is that it is the supreme self alone that exists. It is the energy of Brahman (Māyā) that has created this illusion by the combination of the five elements. But consciousness remains consciousness and is realised by consciousness; diversity is perceived by the notion of diversity. The infinite raises infinity within itself, the infinite creates infinity; infinite is born of infinity and infinity remains infinite. Consciousness shines as consciousness.

upalambhastu yaścā 'yameṣā cittacamatkṛtiḥ
cittatvamātrasattā 'sti dvitvamaikyaṁ ca nāstyalaṁ (15)

KUṀBHA said:

In the case of gold it may be said that at a certain time and at a certain place it gave rise to an ornament. But from the self (which is absolute peace) nothing is created and nothing ever returns to it. Brahman rests in itself. Hence it is neither the seed nor the cause for the creation of the world, which is a matter of mere experience. Apart from this experience, nothing exists which could be referred to as the world or the ego-sense. Therefore the infinite consciousness alone exists.

ŚIKHIDHVAJA said:

I realise, O sage, that in the Lord there is neither world nor the ego-sense. But how do the world and the ego-sense shine as if they exist?

KUṀBHA replied:

Indeed, it is the infinite which, beginningless and endless, exists as pure experiencing consciousness. That alone is this expanded universe — which is its body, as it were. There is no other substance known as the intellect, nor is there an outside nor void. The essence of existence is pure experiencing which is therefore the essence of consciousness. Just as liquidity exists inseparable from water, consciousness and unconsciousness exist together. There is no rationale for such existence, for what is, is as it is. Since there is neither a contradiction nor a division in consciousness it is self-evident.

If the infinite consciousness is the cause of something else, then how can it be regarded as indescribable and incomparable? Hence, Brahman is neither a cause nor a seed. What then shall we regard as the effect? It is therefore inappropriate to associate the creation with Brahman and to associate the inert with the infinite consciousness. If there appears to be a world or ego-sense, these are but empty words meant to entertain.

Consciousness is not destroyed. However, if such destruction can be comprehended, the consciousness that comprehends it is free from destruction and creation. **If such destruction can be comprehended, it is surely the trick of consciousness. Hence consciousness alone exists, neither one nor many! Enough of this discussion.**

When thus there is no material existence, thinking does not exist either. There is neither a world nor the ego-sense. Remain well established in peace and tranquillity, free from mental conditioning, whether you are embodied or disembodied. When the reality of Brahman is realised, there is no room for worry and anxiety.

yatkiñcitparamākāśa iṣatkacakacāyate
cidādarśena jātatvānna cittam no jagatkriyā (15)

ŚIKHIDHVAJA said:

Holy one, pray instruct me in such a way that it will be perfectly clear to me that the mind is non-existent.

KUMBHA said:

O king, indeed there is not and there never has been an entity known as the mind. That which shines here and is known as the mind is indeed the infinite Brahman (consciousness). It is ignorance of its true nature that gives rise to the notion of a mind and the world and all the rest of it. When even these are insubstantial notions, how can 'I', 'you', etc. be considered real? Thus, there is no such thing as the 'world', and whatever appears to be is uncreated. All this is indeed Brahman. How can that be known and by whom?

Even in the beginning of the present world-cycle this world was not created. It was described as creation by me only for your comprehension. In the total absence of any causative factors, all these could not have been created at all. Therefore, whatever there is is Brahman and naught else. It is not even logical to say that the Lord who is nameless and formless created this world! It is not true. When thus the creation of this world is seen to be false, then surely the mind that entertains the notion of such a creation is false, too.

Mind is but a bundle of such notions which limit the truth. But then, division implies divisibility. When the infinite consciousness is incapable of division, there is no divisibility and hence there is no division. How can mind, the divider, be real? Whatever appears to be here is perceived in Brahman, by Brahman, and such perception is, by courtesy, known as the mind! It is the infinite consciousness alone that is spread out as the universe. Why then call it the universe? **In this plane or dimension of infinite consciousness whatever slight appearance there seems to be is but the reflection of consciousness in itself: hence there is neither a mind nor the world.** Only in ignorance is all this seen as 'the world'. Hence the mind is unreal.

Only creation is negated by this, not what IS. The reality that is seen as this world is beginningless and uncreated. Hence, the scriptural declarations and one's own experiences concerning the appearance and the disappearance of substances here cannot be considered invalid, except by an ignoramus. One who denies the validity of such declarations and experiences is fit to be shunned. The transcendental reality is eternal; the world is not unreal (only the limiting adjunct, the mind, is false). Therefore, all this is the indivisible, illimitable, nameless and formless infinite consciousness. It is the self-reflection of Brahman, which is of infinite forms, that appears to be the universe with its creation-dissolution cycle. It is this Brahman itself which knows itself for a moment as this universe and appears to be such. There is no mind.

ahamityeva saṅkalpo bandhāyā 'tivināśine
nā 'hamityeva saṅkalpo mokṣāya vimalātmane (11)

ŚIKHIDHVAJA said:

My delusion is gone. Wisdom has been gained by your grace. I remain free from all doubts. I know what there is to be known. The ocean of illusion has been crossed. I am at peace, without the notion of 'I', but as pure knowledge.

KUṀBHA said:

When the world does not exist as such, where is 'I' or 'you'? Hence, remaining at peace within yourself, engage yourself in non-volitional actions as are appropriate from moment to moment. All this is but Brahman which is peace; 'I' and 'the world' are words without substance. When the insubstantiality of such expressions is realised, then what was seen as the world is realised as Brahman.

The creator Brahmā is but an idea or notion. Even so is 'self' or 'I'. In their right or wrong comprehension lies liberation or bondage! **The notion 'I am' gives rise to bondage and self-destruction. The realisation 'I am (is) not' leads to freedom and purity.** Bondage and liberation are but notions. That which is aware of these notions is the infinite consciousness which alone is. The notion 'I am' is the source of all distress. The absence of such a feeling is perfection. Realise 'I am not that ego-sense' and rest in pure awareness.

When such pure awareness arises, all notions subside. There is perfection. In the pure awareness, perfection or the Lord, there is neither causality nor the resultant creation or objects. In the absence of objects, there is no experience or its concomitant ego-sense. When the ego-sense is non-existent, where is saṁsāra (the cycle of birth and death)? When thus saṁsāra does not exist, the supreme being alone remains. In it the universe exists as carvings in uncarved stone. He who thus sees the universe, without the intervention of the mind and therefore without the notion of a universe, he alone sees the truth. Such a vision is known as nirvāṇa.

Even as the ocean alone exists when the word 'wave' is deprived of its meaning, Brahman alone exists when the word 'creation' is seen as meaningless. This creation is Brahman; Brahman alone is aware of this creation. When the word-meaning of 'creation' is dropped, the true meaning of 'creation' is seen as the eternal Brahman. When one enquires into the word 'Brahman', the All is comprehended. When one similarly enquires into the word 'creation', Brahman is comprehended. However, that consciousness which is the basis and the substratum for all such notions and their awareness is known by the word 'Brahman'. When this truth is clearly realised and when the duality of knowledge and known is discarded, what remains is supreme peace, which is indescribable and inexpressible.

cittaṁ nāśasvabhāvaṁ tadviddhi nāśātmakaṁ nṛpa
kṣaṇanāśo yataḥ kalpacittaśabdena kathyate (11)

ŚIKHIDHVAJA said:

If the supreme being is real and the world is real, then I assume that the supreme being is the cause and the world the effect!

KUṀBHA replied:

Only if there is causality can the effect be assumed. But, where there is no causality, how can the effect arise from it? There is no causal relationship between Brahman and the universe: whatever there is here is Brahman. When there is no seed even, then how is something born? When Brahman is nameless and formless, there is surely no causality (seed) in it. Hence, Brahman is non-doer, in whom causality does not exist. Therefore, there is no effect which can be called the world.

Brahman alone thou art and Brahman alone exists. When that Brahman is comprehended by unwisdom, it is experienced as this universe. This universe is, as it were, the body of Brahman. When that infinite consciousness considers itself as other than it really is, that is said to be self-destruction or self-experience. **That self-destruction is the mind. Its very nature is the destruction (veiling) of self-knowledge. Even if such self-destruction is momentary, it is known as the mind that lasts for a world-cycle.**

Such a notional existence ceases only by the dawn of right knowledge and the cessation of all notions. Since the notional existence is unreal it ceases naturally when the truth is realised. When the world exists only as a word but not as a real independent substance, how then can it be accepted as a real existence? Its independent existence is like water in the mirage. How can that be real? The confused state in which this unreality appears to be real is known as the mind. Non-comprehension of the truth is ignorance or the mind; right comprehension is self-knowledge or self-realisation. Even as the realisation 'This is not water' brings about the realisation of the mirage as mirage, the realisation that 'This is not pure consciousness but kinetic consciousness which is known as the mind' brings about its destruction.

When thus the non-existence of the mind is realised, it is seen that the ego-sense, etc. do not exist. One alone exists — the infinite consciousness. All notions cease. The falsity which arose as the mind ceases when notions cease. I am not, nor is there another, nor do you nor do these exist; there is neither mind nor senses. One alone is — the pure consciousness. Nothing in the three worlds is ever born or dies. The infinite consciousness alone exists. There is neither unity nor diversity, neither confusion nor delusion. Nothing perishes and nothing flourishes. Everything (even the energy that manifests as desire and desirelessness) is your own self.

vāsanātmasu yāteṣu maleṣu vimalaṁ sakhe
yadvaktti gururantastadviśatīṣur yathā bise (14)

KUṀBHA said:

I hope that you have been inwardly awakened spiritually, and that you know what there is to be known and see what there is to be seen.

ŚIKHIDHVAJA replied:

Indeed Lord, by your grace I have seen the supreme state. How was it that it eluded my understanding so far?

KUṀBHA said:

Only when the mind is utterly quiet, when one has completely abandoned all desire for pleasure and when the senses have also been rid of their colouring or covering, are the words of the preceptor rightly comprehended. (The previous efforts were not wasted, for) the various efforts made so far have attained fruition today and the impurities in the bodies have dropped away. **When thus one is freed from psychological conditioning and the impurities have been removed or purified, the words of the guru enter directly into the innermost core of one's being just as an arrow enters the stalk of the lotus.** You have attained that state of purity and therefore you have been enlightened by my discourse and your ignorance has been dispelled.

By our satsaṅga (holy company) your karmā (actions and their residual impressions) have been destroyed. Till this very forenoon you were filled with the false notions of 'I' and 'mine' on account of ignorance. Now that on account of the light of my words the mind has been abandoned from your heart, you have been awakened fully, for ignorance lasts only so long as the mind functions in your heart. Now you are enlightened, liberated. Remain established in the infinite consciousness, freed from sorrow, from striving and from all attachment.

ŚIKHIDHVAJA said:

Lord, is there a mind even for the liberated person? How does he live and function here without a mind?

KUṀBHA replied:

Truly, there is no mind in the liberated ones. What is mind? The psychological conditioning or limitation which is dense and which leads to rebirth is known as mind: this is absent in the liberated sages. The liberated sages live with the help of the mind which is free from conditioning and which does not cause rebirth. It is not mind at all but pure light (satva). The liberated ones live and function here established in this satva, not in the mind. The ignorant and inert mind is mind; the enlightened mind is known as satva. The ignorant live in their mind, the enlightened ones live in satva.

brahmacinmātramamalaṁ sattvamityādi nāmakaṁ
yadgītaṁ tadidaṁ mūḍhāḥ paśyantyaṅga jagattayā (101/55)

KUṀBHA continued:

You have attained to the state of satva (the unconditioned mind) on account of your supreme renunciation. The conditioned mind has been totally renounced, of this I am convinced. Your mind has become like pure infinite space. You have reached the state of complete equilibrium which is the state of perfection. This is the total renunciation in which everything is abandoned without residue.

What sort of happiness (destruction of sorrow) does one gain through austerities? Supreme and unending happiness is attained only through utter equanimity. What sort of happiness is that which is gained in heaven? He who has not attained self-knowledge tries to snatch a little pleasure through the performance of some rituals. One who does not have gold clings to copper!

O royal sage, you could easily have become wise with the help of Cūḍālā. Why did you have to indulge in this useless and meaningless austerity? It has a beginning and an end, and in the middle there is an appearance of happiness. However, your austerity has in a way led to this spiritual awakening. Now remain rooted in wisdom.

It is in the infinite consciousness that all these realities and even the unreal notions arise and into it they dissolve. Even ideas like 'This is to be done' and 'This is not to be done' are 'droplets of this infinite consciousness'. Abandon even these and rest in the unconditioned. All these (austerity, etc.) are indirect methods. Why should one not adopt the direct method of self-knowledge.

That which has been described as satva should be renounced by the satva itself — that is, by total freedom from it or by non-attachment to it. Whatever sorrow arises in the three worlds, O king, arises only from mental craving. If you are established in that state of equanimity which treats of both movement and non-movement of thought as non-different, you will rest in the eternal.

There is only one infinite consciousness. **That Brahman which is pure consciousness is itself known as satva. The ignorant see it as the world.** Movement (agitation) as also non-movement in that infinite consciousness are only notions in the mind of the spectator: the totality of the infinite consciousness is all these but devoid of such notions. Its reality is beyond words!

VASISTHA continued:

Having said this, Kumbha vanished from sight even while the king was about to offer flowers in adoration. Reflecting over the words of Kumbha, Śikhidhvaja entered into deep meditation, completely free from all desires and cravings and firmly established in the unconditioned state.

prabodhakāraṇaṁ yasya durlakṣyāṇuvapurhṛdi
vidyate sattvaśeṣontarbije puṣpaphalaṁ yathā (24)

VASIṢṬHA continued:

While Śikhidhvaja was thus engaged in deep meditation utterly free from the least mental modification or movement in consciousness, Cūḍālā abandoned her disguise and returned to the palace, and in her own female form conducted the affairs of the state. She returned to where Śikhidhvaja was after three days and was delighted to see that he was still absorbed in meditation. She thought, "I should make him return to world-consciousness; why should he abandon the body now? Let him rule the kingdom for sometime and then both of us can simultaneously abandon the body. Surely the instructions I have given him will not be lost. I shall keep him alert and awake through the practice of yoga".

She roared like a lion again and again. Still he did not open his eyes. She pushed the body down. Yet he remained immersed in the self. She thought, "Alas, he is completely absorbed in the self. How shall I bring him back to body consciousness? On the other hand, why should I do so? Let him reach the disembodied state and I shall also abandon this body now!"

While she was getting ready to abandon her body, she again thought, "Before I abandon my body, let me see if there is the seed of mind (vāsanā) somewhere in his body. If there is, he can be awakened and then both of us can live as liberated beings. If there is not and if he has attained final liberation, I shall also abandon this body." She examined his body and found that the seed of individuality was still present in him.

RĀMA asked:

Lord, when the body of the sage lies like a log of wood, how can one know that there is still a trace of satva (purified mind) in him?

VASIṢṬHA said:

In his heart, unseen and subtle, there is the trace of satva which is the cause for the revival of body-consciousness. It is like the flower and the fruit which are potentially present in the seed. In the case of the sage whose mind is totally free from the movement of thought, who is devoid of the least notion of duality or unity, whose consciousness is utterly firm and steady like a mountain — his body is in a state of perfect equilibrium and does not show signs of pain or pleasure; it does not rise or fall (live or die) but remains in perfect harmony with nature. It is only as long as there are notions of duality or unity that the body undergoes changes as the mind does. It is the movement of thought that appears as this world. Because of that the mind experiences pleasure, anger and delusion, which thus remain irrepressible. But when the mind is firmly established in equanimity, such disturbances do not arise in one. He is like pure space.

dehe yasminstu no cittaṁ nā 'pi sattvaṁ ca vidyate
sá tāpe himavadrāma pañcatvena vilīyate (33)

VASIṢṬHA continued:

When the satva is in a state of total equilibrium, then no physical or psychological defects are experienced. It is not possible to abandon satva, it reaches its end in course of time. **When there is neither the mind nor even the satva in the body, then, like snow melting in the heat, the body dissolves in the elements.** Śikhidhvaja's body was free from the mind (movement of thought) but was endowed with a trace of satva. Therefore it did not thus dissolve into the elements. Noticing this, Cūḍālā decided, "I shall enter into the pure intelligence which is omnipresent, and endeavour to awaken body consciousness in him. If I do not do so, he will surely awaken after sometime. But, why should I remain alone till then?"

Cūḍālā thereupon left her body and entered into the pure mind (satva) of Śikhidhvaja. She agitated that pure mind and quickly re-entered her own body, which she instantly transformed into that of the young ascetic Kuṁbha. Kuṁbha began to sing the Sāma Veda hymns gently. Listening to this, the king returned to body consciousness. He saw Kuṁbha once again in front of him. He was happy. He said to Kuṁbha: "Luckily, we have once again arisen in your consciousness, O Lord! And you have come here again merely to shower your blessings on me!"

KUṀBHA said:

Since the time I left you and went away, my mind (heart) has been here with you. There is no desire to go to heaven but only to be near you. I do not have a relative, friend, trustworthy person or disciple like you in this world.

ŚIKHIDHVAJA replied:

I consider myself supremely blessed that, though you are perfectly enlightened and unattached, you wish to be with me. Pray, do stay with me here in this forest!

KUṀBHA asked:

Tell me: did you rest in the supreme state for a while? Have you abandoned notions like 'This is different', 'This is unhappiness' etc? Has your craving for pleasure ceased?

ŚIKHIDHVAJA replied:

By your grace, I have reached the other shore of this saṁsāra (world-appearance). I have gained what there is to be gained. There is naught but the self — neither the known nor what is yet to be known (unknown), neither attainment nor what is renounced and what should be renounced, neither an entity nor the other, nor even satva (a pure mind). Like the limitless space, I remain in the unconditioned state.

yāvattilaṁ yathā tailaṁ yāvaddehaṁ tathā daśā
yo na dehadaśāmeti sacchinattyasinā 'mbaraṁ (42)

VASIṢṬHA continued:

After spending an hour at that place, the king and Kuṁbha went into the forest where they roamed freely for eight days. Kuṁbha suggested that they should go to another forest and the king consented. They observed the normal rules of life and performed appropriate religious rites to propitiate ancestors and the gods. False notions like 'This is our home' and 'This is not' did not arise in their hearts. Sometimes they were clad in gorgeous robes, at others in rags. Sometimes they were anointed with sandal-paste, at others with ashes. After a few days the king also shone with the same radiance as Kuṁbha.

Seeing the radiance of the king, Kuṁbha (Cūḍālā) began to think: "Here is my husband who is noble and strong. The forest is delightful. We are in a state in which fatigue is unknown. How then does desire for pleasure not arise in the heart? The liberated sage welcomes and experiences whatever comes to him unsought; if he is caught up in conformity (rigidity) it gives rise to foolishness (ignorance). She whose passions are not aroused in the proximity of her noble and strong husband when they dwell surrounded by a garden of flowers, is as good as dead! What does the knower of the truth or the sage of self-knowledge gain by abandoning what is obtained without effort? I should make it possible for my husband to enjoy conjugal pleasures with me." Having thus decided, Kuṁbha said to Śikhidhvaja: "Today is an auspicious day when I should be in heaven to see my father. Give me leave to go and I shall return this evening."

The two friends exchanged flowers. Kuṁbha left. Soon Cūḍālā abandoned the disguise, went to the palace and discharged the royal duties. She returned to where Śikhidhvaja was, again in the disguise of Kuṁbha. Noticing a change in Kuṁbha's facial expression, the king asked: "O son of the gods, why do you look so unhappy? Holy ones do not allow any external influence to disturb their equilibrium."

KUṀBHA said:

They who, though remaining established in equilibrium, do not let their organs function naturally as long as the body is alive, are obstinate and stubborn people. **As long as there is sesame there is oil; as long as there is the body there are the different moods also. He who rebels against the states that the body is naturally subject to, cuts space to pieces with a sword.** The equilibrium of yoga is for the mind, not for the organs of action and their states. As long as the body lasts, one should let the organs of action perform their proper function, though the intellect and the senses remain in a state of equanimity. Such is the law of nature to which even the gods are subject.

suhṛdyāveditaṁ duḥkhaṁ paramāyāti tānavaṁ
ghanaṁ jaḍaṁ kṛṣṇamapi mukttavṛṣṭirivā 'mbudaḥ (3)

KUṀBHA continued:

Now, O king, please listen to what misfortune has befallen me. For, **if one confides his unhappiness to a friend, it is greatly ameliorated, even as the heavy and dark cloud becomes light by shedding rain.** The mind also becomes clear and peaceful when a friend listens to one's fate, even as water becomes clear when a piece of alum is dropped into it.

After I left you I went to heaven and performed my duties there. As evening approached, I left heaven to return to you. In space en route I saw the sage Durvāsa flying in haste to be in time for his evening prayers. He was clad, as it were, in the dark clouds and adorned with lightning. This made him look like a woman rushing to meet her lover. I saluted him and said so, in fun. Enraged by my impudence, he cursed me: "For this insolence, you will become a woman every night." I am grieved at the very thought that every night I shall become a woman. It is indeed a tragedy that the sons of god who are easily overcome by lust, thus suffer the consequences of insulting holy sages. However, why should I grieve, for this does not affect my self.

ŚIKHIDHVAJA said:

What is the use of grief, O son of the gods? Let come what may, for the self is not affected by the fate of the body. Whatever be the joy or sorrow that is allotted to one, it affects the body, not the indweller. If even you yield to grief, what about the ignorant people! Or, perhaps, while narrating an unfortunate incident you are merely using appropriate words and expressions!

VASIṢṬHA continued:

Thus they consoled each other, for they were inseparable friends now. The sun had set and the darkness of the night was creeping on the earth. They performed their evening prayers. Soon, Kuṁbha's body began to show a creeping change. Fighting back his tears and in a choked voice, he said to Śikhidhvaja: "Alas, see, I feel as if my body is melting away and that it is pouring down on earth. My chest is sprouting breasts. My skeletal structure undergoes changes appropriate to a woman. Look, dress and ornaments appropriate to a woman spring from the body itself. O what shall I do, how shall I hide my shame, for I have truly become a woman!"

Śikhidhvaja replied: "Holy one, you know what there is to be known. Do not grieve over the inevitable. One's fate affects only the body, not the embodied one." Kuṁbha also agreed: "You are right. I do not now feel any sorrow. Who can defy the world order or nature?"

Thus conversing, they went to bed (slept in the same bed). Thus Cūḍālā lived with her husband as a young male ascetic during the day and as a woman at night.

**kṛtenā 'nena kāryeṇa na śubhaṁ nā 'śubhaṁ sakhe
paśyāmi tanmahābuddhe yathecchasi tathā kuru (8)**

VASIṢṬHA continued:

After a few days of such companionship, Kuṁbha (Cūḍālā in disguise) said to Śikhidhvaja: "O king, listen to my submission. For sometime now I have been a woman by night. I wish to fulfil the role of a woman at night. I feel that I should live as the wife of a worthy husband. In the three worlds there is none who is as dear to me as you are. Hence, I wish to marry you and enjoy conjugal pleasure with you. This is natural, pleasant and possible. What fault is there in it? We have given up both desire and rejection and we have total equal vision. Hence, let us do what is natural, without desire and aversion."

Śikhidhvaja replied: "**O friend, I do not see either good or evil in doing this. Therefore, O wise one, do what you wish to do.** Because the mind rests in perfect equilibrium, I see only the self everywhere. Hence do what you wish to do."

Kuṁbha replied: "If that is how you feel, O king, then today itself is the most auspicious day. The celestial bodies shall witness our wedding."

Both of them then gathered all the articles necessary for the wedding rite. They bathed each other with holy water in preparation for the sacred rite. They offered worship to the ancestors and gods.

By this time, the night-time had arrived. Kuṁbha became transformed into a lovely woman. 'He' said to the king: "O dear friend, now I am a woman. My name is Madanikā. I salute you. I am your wife." Śikhidhvaja then adorned Madanikā with garlands, flowers and jewels. Admiring her beauty, the king said: "O Madanikā, you are radiant like goddess Lakṣmī. May we be blessed to live together like the sun and the shadow, Lakṣmi and Nārāyaṇa, Śiva and Pārvatī. May we be blessed with all auspiciousness."

The couple themselves tended the sacred fire and performed the nuptial rite, in strict accord with the injunctions of the scriptures. The altar had been decorated with flowery creepers and with precious and semi-precious stones. Its four corners were decorated with cocoanuts and there were also pots full of holy water of the Gaṅgā. In the centre was the sacred fire. They went round this fire and offered the prescribed oblations into it with the appropriate sacred hymns. Even while so doing the king frequently held Madanikā's hand, thus revealing his fondness for her and his joy on that occasion. They then circumambulated the sacred fire thrice, performing what is known as the Laja Homa. Then they retired to the nuptial chamber (a cave specially prepared for the occasion). The moon was showering cool rays. The nuptial bed was made of fragrant flowers. They ascended this bed and consummated their wedding.

niyataṁ kiñcidekatra sthitaṁ svargakamidṛśaṁ
śakra gantuṁ na jānāmi tvadājñāṁ na karomyahaṁ (28)

VASIṢṬHA continued:

As the sun rose, Madanikā became Kuṁbha. Thus, this pair lived as friends during the day and as husband and wife during the night. While Śikhidhvaja was asleep one night, Kuṁbha (Cūḍālā in disguise) slipped away to the palace and discharged the royal duties there and quickly returned to the king's bedside.

For a month they lived in the caves of the Mahendra mountain. They then roamed in different forests and migrated from one mountainside to another. For sometime they lived in the garden of the gods known as the Pārijāta forest on the southern slopes of the Maināka mountain. They also roamed the Kuru territory and the Kosala territory.

After they had enjoyed themselves in this manner for a number of months, Cūḍālā (disguised as Kuṁbha) thought: "I shall test the maturity of the king by placing before him the pleasures and delights of heaven. If he is unaffected by them, surely he will never again seek pleasure."

Having thus decided, Cūḍālā created by her magic powers the illusion in which Śikhidhvaja saw the chief of the gods (Indra) accompanied by the celestials standing right in front of him. Unruffled by their sudden appearance, the king offered them due worship. Then he asked Indra: "Pray, tell me: what have I done to deserve this, that you have taken all this trouble to come here today?"

Indra replied: "Holy one, we have all come here drawn irresistibly to your presence. We have heard your glories sung in heaven. Come, come to heaven: having heard of your greatness the celestials long to see you. Pray accept these celestial insignia which will enable you to traverse the space even as the perfected sages do. Surely, O sage, liberated beings like you do not spurn happiness that seeks them unsought. May your visit purify the heaven." Śikhidhvaja said: "I know the conditions that prevail in heaven, O Indra! But to me heaven is everywhere and also nowhere. I am happy wherever I am because I desire nothing. However, **I am unable to go to the kind of heaven which you describe and which is limited to one place! Hence I am unable to fulfil your command**". "But," said Indra, "I think it is proper that liberated sages should suffer to experience the pleasures allotted to them." Śikhidhvaja remained silent. Indra was getting ready to leave. Śikhidhvaja said, "I shall not come now for now is not the time."

Having blessed the king and Kuṁbha, Indra and all his retinue disappeared.

ahametena cā 'rthena nodvegaṁ yāmi mānini
yadyadiṣṭatamaṁ loke tattadevaṁ vijānatā (22)

VASIṢṬHA continued:

After withdrawing that magical display, Cūḍālā said to herself: "Luckily, the king is not attracted by temptations of pleasure. Even when Indra visited him and invited him to heaven, the king remain unaffected and pure like space. I shall now subject him to another test to see if he is swayed by the twin forces of attraction and repulsion."

That very night, Cūḍālā created by her magic powers a delightful pleasure garden and an extraordinarily beautiful bed in it. She created a young man, physically more attractive than even Śikhidhvaja. There on that bed she appeared to be seated with her lover in close embrace.

Śikhidhvaja had concluded his evening prayers and he looked for his wife Madanikā. After some search, he discovered the secret hiding place of this couple. He saw them completely immersed in their love play. Her hair encircled him. With her hands she held his face. Their mouths were joined to each other in a fervent kiss. They were obviously very excited with passionate love for each other. With every movement of their limbs they expressed their extreme love for each other. On their faces danced the delight of their hearts. The chest of one was beating against the chest of the other. They were utterly oblivious of their surroundings.

Śikhidhvaja saw all this but was unmoved. He did not wish to disturb them and so turned to go. But his presence had been noticed by the couple. He said to them, "Pray, let me not disturb your happiness."

After a time, Madanikā came out of the garden and met Śikhidhvaja, feeling ashamed of her own conduct. But the king said: "My dear, why did you come away so soon? Surely all beings live in order to enjoy happiness. And it is difficult to find in this world a couple who are in such harmony. **I am not agitated on this account for I know very well what people like very much in this world.** Kuṁbha and I are great friends, Madanikā is but the fruit of Durvāsa's curse!"

Madanikā pleaded: "Such is the nature of women, O lord! They are wavering in their loyalty. They are eight times as passionate as men. They are weak and so cannot resist lust in the presence of a desirable person. Hence, please forgive me and do not be angry." Śikhidhvaja replied: "I am not at all angry with you, my dear. But it is appropriate that I should henceforth treat you as a good friend and not as my wife." Cūḍālā was delighted with the king's attitude which conclusively proved that he had gone beyond lust and anger. She instantly shed her previous form as Madanikā and resumed her original form as Cūḍālā.

sakhā bhrātā suhṛdbhṛtyo gurur mitraṁ dhanaṁ sukhaṁ
śāstramāyatanaṁ dāsaḥ sarvaṁ bhartuḥ kulāṅganāḥ (27)

ŚIKHIDHVAJA said:

Who are you, O lovely lady, and how did you come here? How long have you been here? You look very much like my wife!

CŪḌĀLĀ replied:

Indeed, I am Cūḍālā. I myself assumed the form of Kuṁbha and the others in order to awaken your spirit. I myself also assumed the form of this small illusory world with all this garden, etc. which you saw just now. From the very day you unwisely abandoned your kingdom and came here to perform austerities, I have been endeavouring to bring about your spiritual awakening. It is I, assuming the form of Kuṁbha, who instructed you. The forms you perceived, of Kuṁbha and others, were not real. And now you have been fully awakened and you know all that there is to know.

VASIṢṬHA continued:

Śikhidhvaja entered into deep meditation and inwardly saw all that had happened from the time he left the palace. He was delighted and his affection for his wife increased greatly. Coming back to body-consciousness he embraced Cūḍālā with such fervour that is impossible to describe. Their hearts overflowing with love for each other, they remained for sometime as if in a superconscious state.

ŚIKHIDHVAJA then said to Cūḍālā:

O how sweet is the affection of a dear wife which is sweeter than nectar! To what discomfort and pain you have subjected yourself for my sake! The way in which you have redeemed me from this dreadful ocean of ignorance has no comparison whatsoever. Tradition has given us several great women who have been exemplary wives, but they are nothing compared to you. You excel them all in all the virtues and noble qualities. You have struggled hard and brought about my enlightenment. How shall I recompense you for this? Indeed, loving wives thus strive to liberate their husbands from this ocean of saṁsāra. In this they achieve what even the scriptures, guru and mantra are unable to achieve, on account of their love for their husbands. **The wife is everything to her husband — friend, brother, well-wisher, servant, guru, companion, wealth, happiness, scripture, abode (vessel), slave.** Hence, such a wife should at all times and in all ways be adored and worshipped.

My dear Cūḍālā, you are indeed the supreme among women in this world. Come, embrace me again.

VASIṢṬHA said:

Having said so, Śikhidhvaja again fondly and fervently embraced Cūḍālā.

na rājan mama bhogeṣu vāñchā nā 'pi vibhūtiṣu
svabhāvasya vaśādeva yathāprāptena me sthitiḥ (68)

CŪḌĀLĀ said:

Lord, when I saw that you were performing meaningless austerities, my heart was greatly pained. I relieved myself of that pain by coming here and striving to awaken you. It was indeed for my own joy and delight. I do not deserve any praise for that!

ŚIKHIDHVAJA replied:

From now on may all the wives fulfil their own selfish ends by awakening their husbands' spirit, as you have done!

CŪḌĀLĀ said:

I do not see in you now the petty cravings, thoughts and feelings that tormented you years ago. Pray, tell me, what are you now, in what are you established and what do you see?

ŚIKHIDHVAJA replied:

My dear, I rest in that which you, within me, bring about. I have no attachment. I am like the infinite, indivisible space. I am peace. I have attained that state which is difficult even for the gods like Viṣṇu and Śiva to reach. I am free from confusion and delusion. I experience no sorrow nor joy. I cannot say, 'This is' nor 'The other is'. I am freed of all coverings and I enjoy a state of inner well-being. What I am that I am — it is difficult to put into words! You are my guru, my dear: I salute you. By your grace, my beloved, I have crossed this ocean of saṁsāra; I shall not once again fall into error.

CŪḌĀLĀ asked:

In that case, what do you wish to do now?

ŚIKHIDHVAJA answered:

I know no prohibitions nor injunctions. Whatever you do, that I shall know as appropriate. Do what you think appropriate and I shall follow you.

CŪḌĀLĀ said:

Lord, we are now established in the state of liberated ones. To us, both desire and its opposite are the same. Of what use is the discipline of prāṇa or the practice of infinite consciousness? Hence, we should be what we are in the beginning, in the middle and in the end and abandon the one thing that remains after this. We are the king and the queen in the beginning, in the middle and in the end. The one thing to be abandoned is delusion! Hence, let us return to the kingdom and provide it with a wise ruler.

ŚIKHIDHVAJA asked:

Then, why should we not accept Indra's invitation to heaven?

CŪḌĀLĀ replied:

O king, I do not desire pleasure nor the glamour of a kingdom. I remain in whatever condition I am placed by my very nature. When the thought 'This is pleasure' is confronted by the thought 'This is not', they both perish. I remain in that peace that survives this.

The two liberated ones then spent the night in conjugal delight.

bhuktvā bhogānanekān bhuvi sakalamahīpālacūḍāmaṇitve
sthitvā vai dīrghakālaṁ paramamṛtapadaṁ prāptavān satvaśeṣaḥ
evaṁ rāmā "gataṁ tvaṁ prakṛtamanusaran kāryajātaṁ viśokas
tiṣṭhottiṣṭha svayaṁ vā prasabhamanubhavan bhogamokṣādilakṣmīḥ (110/30)

VASIṢṬHA continued:

At daybreak the couple arose and performed their morning duties. Cūḍālā materialised by her thought-power a golden vessel containing the sacred waters of the seven oceans. With these waters she bathed the king and crowned him emperor. She said: "May you be endowed with the lustre of the eight divine protectors of the universe."

In his turn, the king re-established Cūḍālā as his queen. He suggested to her that she could create an army by her thought-power. She did so.

Headed by the royal couple mounted on the most stately elephant, the entire army marched towards their kingdom. On the way, Śikhidhvaja pointed out to Cūḍālā the various places associated with his ascetic life. They soon reached the outskirts of their city where they were given a rousing welcome by the citizens.

Assisted by Cūḍālā, Śikhidhvaja ruled the kingdom for a period of ten thousand years, after which he attained nirvāṇa (liberation, like a lamp without oil) from which there is no rebirth. **After enjoying the pleasures of the world because he was the foremost among kings, and after having lived for a very long time he attained the supreme state, because in him there was but a little residue of satva. Even so, O Rāma, engage yourself in spontaneous and natural activity, without grief. Arise. Enjoy the pleasures of the world and also final liberation.**

Thus have I told you, O Rāma, the story of Śikhidhvaja. Pursuing this path, you will never grieve. Rule as Śikhidhvaja ruled. You will enjoy the pleasures of this world and attain final liberation, too. Even so did Kaca who was the son of Bṛhaspati, the preceptor of the gods.

RĀMA asked:

Lord, please tell me how Kaca, the son of Bṛhaspati, attained enlightenment.

VASIṢṬHA said:

While Kaca was still young, he was eager to attain liberation from saṁsāra. One day he went to his father Bṛhaspati, and asked: "Lord, you know everything. Please tell me how one can free oneself from this cage known as saṁsāra."

cittaṁ nijamahaṅkāraṁ viduścittavido janāḥ
antaryo 'yamahaṁbhāvo jantostaccittamucyate (28)

BṚHASPATI said:

Liberation from this prison-house known as saṁsāra is possible only by total renunciation, my son!

VASIṢṬHA continued:

Hearing this, Kaca went away to the forest, having renounced everything. Bṛhaspati was unaffected by this turn of events. Wise ones remain unaffected by union and separation. After eight years of seclusion and austerity, Kaca happened to meet his father once again and asked him: "Father, I have performed austerities for eight years after renouncing everything; how is it I have not attained the state of supreme peace?"

Bṛhaspati merely repeated his previous commandment, "Renounce everything", and went away. Taking it as a hint, Kaca discarded even the bark with which he covered his body. Thus he continued his austerities for three years. Again he sought the presence of his father and after worshipping him, asked: "Father, I have renounced even the stick and clothes, etc. I have still not gained self-knowledge!"

Bṛhaspati thereupon said: "By 'total' is meant only the mind, for mind is the all. Renunciation of the mind is total renunciation." Having said so, Bṛhaspati vanished from sight. Kaca looked within in an effort to find the mind in order that it might be renounced. However much he searched, he could not find what could be called the mind! Unable to find the mind, he began to think: "The physical substances like the body cannot be regarded as mind. Why, then, do I vainly punish the innocent body? I shall go back to my father and enquire into the whereabouts of the terrible enemy known as the mind. Knowing it, I shall renounce it."

Having thus resolved, Kaca sought his father's presence and asked, "Please tell me what the mind is so that I may renounce it." Bṛhaspati replied: "**They who know the mind say that the mind is the 'I'. The ego-sense that arises within you is the mind.**" "But, that is difficult, if not impossible," said Kaca. Bṛhaspati responded: "On the other hand, it is easier than crushing a flower which is in your hand, easier than closing your eyes! For that which appears to be because of ignorance, perishes at the dawn of knowledge. In truth there is no ego-sense. It seems to exist on account of ignorance and delusion. Where is this ego-sense, how did it arise, what is it? In all things at all times there is but the one pure consciousness! Hence this ego-sense is but a word. Give it up, my son, and give up self-limitation or psychological conditioning. You are the unconditioned, never conditioned by time, space, etc."

ahaṅkāramasadviddhi mainamāśraya mā tyaja
asataḥ śaśaśṛṅgasya kila tyāgagrahau kutaḥ (112/3)

VASIṢṬHA continued:

Thus instructed in the highest wisdom, Kaca became enlightened. He remained free from ego-sense and possessiveness. Live like him, O Rāma. **The ego-sense is unreal. Do not trust it and do not abandon it. How can the unreal be grasped or renounced?** When the ego-sense is itself unreal, what are birth and death? You are that subtle and pure consciousness which is indivisible and free from ideation, but which encompasses all beings. It is only in the state of ignorance that the world is seen as an illusory appearance; in the vision of the enlightened, all this is seen as Brahman. Abandon the concepts of unity and diversity and remain blissful. Do not behave like the deluded man, and suffer!

RĀMA said:

I derive supreme bliss from your nectarine words. I am now established in the transcendental state. Yet, there is no satiety. Though I am satisfied, again I ask you, for no one will be satiated with nectar. Who is the deluded man you referred to?

VASIṢṬHA said:

Listen to this humorous story of the deluded man, O Rāma. There is a man who was fashioned by the machinery of delusion. He was born in a desert and grew up in the desert. There arose a deluded notion in him: "I am born of space, I am space, the space is mine. I should therefore protect that space." Having thus decided, he built a house to protect space. Seeing the space safely enclosed in the house he was happy. But in course of time, the house crumbled. He wept aloud, "O my space! Where have you gone? Alas it is lost."

Then he dug a well and felt that the space in it was protected. It, too, was lost in time. One after the other, he built a pot, a pit and also a small grove with four sal trees. Each of them perished after a short time, leaving the deluded man unhappy.

Listen to the meaning of this story, O Rāma. The man fashioned by delusion is the ego-sense. It arises as motion arises in wind. Its reality is Brahman. Not knowing this, the ego-sense looks upon space around it as itself and its possession. Thus it identifies itself with the body, etc. which it desires to protect. The body, etc. exist and perish after some time. On account of this delusion the ego-sense grieves repeatedly, thinking that the self is dead and lost. When the pot, etc. are lost, the space remains unaffected. Even so, when the bodies are lost the self remains unaffected. The self is pure consciousness, subtler than even space, O Rāma. It is never destroyed. It is unborn. It does not perish. And it is the infinite Brahman alone that shines as this world-appearance. Knowing this, be happy forever.

ekadeśagatā viṣvagvyāpya karmāṇi kurvate
yoginastriṣu kāleṣu sarvāṇyanubhavantyapi (124/8)

VASIṢṬHA continued:

The whole universe is pure consciousness, but as an object it is inert appearance. Everything, including you and I, though alive is dead. Abandon the world-idea in the world and the I-you idea in ourselves, and engage yourself in appropriate action.

Once upon a time there was a king known as Vipaścit. His four ministers guarded the four borders of his kingdom. One day a wise man visited him and announced: "The minister guarding the eastern border is dead. The one guarding the south attempted to cover the eastern side, too; and he was also killed. When the minister guarding the west rushed to the south, he was killed." At that moment the minister from the north entered, saluted the king and said: "The city is surrounded by the enemy. Only you have the power to destroy the enemy."

The king worshipped the sacred fire before he joined his forces on the battlefield. He prayed: "Lord, today I offer my own head as a sacrifice. May four powerful beings emerge to ensure victory over the enemy." The king beheaded himself, and instantly four radiant beings emerged from the sacred fire. It was obvious that they could not be overcome by any warlike device that the enemy might adopt, whether it be missiles or mantrā, drugs etc. They prayed to the god of fire that they should see everything in the universe that they could see.

The king in his four forms proceeded to the battlefield. The enemy fell. The survivors fled. The fourfold Vipaścit pursued them, proceeding in four directions. Each one of them reached an ocean. They had all reached the boundaries of earth.

Though consciousness is one, non-dual and omnipresent, it seems to become diverse like the mind of the dreamer. Thus the diverse appears to be one, but it is both diverse and non-diverse. Therefore whatever appeared before each of the four Vipaścit reflected in his consciousness and was experienced by him. **Yogī can perform actions everywhere and experience all things in all the three periods of time, though apparently remaining in one place.**

The Vipaścit who went east slept for seven years on the slopes of the sunrise mountain on the continent known as Śāka; having drunk of the water that was in the rock, he had become like stone. The Vipaścit who went west to the sunset mountain fell a victim to the charms of a nymph. The Vipaścit who went east remained incognito in a forest for some time. On account of the charm of a celestial he lived as a lion for ten days; overpowered by a goblin, he lived as a frog for ten years. The Vipaścit who went north dwelt for a hundred years in a blind well. The one who went west learnt the method of becoming a celestial and lived as such for fourteen years.

They were eventually rescued by one another by appropriate means.

prabodhamanugacchantyā aprāptāyāḥ paraṁ padaṁ
ekasyā apyanekasyāḥ sarvaṁ sarvatra yujyate (125/18)

VASIṢṬHA continued:

The four Vipaścit were neither enlightened nor were they ignorant: in such people the signs of enlightenment are seen, as also the signs of ignorance and bondage. In a state in which there is both awakening and non-awakening, all these things are possible. It is when there is such partial awakening that one enjoys psychic powers. Thus, the four Vipaścit experienced the states that the others had. Yogī who practice contemplation and who attain various psychic powers through grace or boons, are subject to ignorance. Even in the case of those liberated sages who are still alive, there is comprehension of materiality while they are engaged in day-to-day activity. Mokṣa or liberation is also a state of the mind. The natural function of the body adheres to it and does not cease. However, whether his body is cut into a thousand pieces or he is crowned an emperor, the liberated one is liberated even if he apparently weeps and laughs. Within himself he is neither elated nor depressed.

Later the four Vipaścit were killed, one after the other in different situations. Remaining in their subtle bodies, they saw their own previous history. On account of past mental impressions they thought they were once again clothed in physical bodies in order to witness the magnitude of the world, in accordance with a boon they had obtained from the god of fire. They kept roaming.

The western Vipaścit had the good fortune to meet Lord Viṣṇu. He attained nirvāṇa. The eastern Vipaścit attained the realm of the moon. The southern Vipaścit destroyed his enemies and even now rules the country, because he clung to his memory. The northern Vipaścit was eaten by a crocodile. When it died, he became one. Later he died in the realm of the gods and became a god. He reached the boundaries of the earth-plane, which he remembered from his past experiences. When he died he had no desire to take another body, but he had not been enlightened. He wished to engage himself in pure mental activity, for the sake of which he assumed a subtle body. Though he began to investigate the nature of the subtle body, he did not investigate the illusory nature of ignorance; hence he rests in it. Another of the Vipaścit also fell into a similar predicament. Yet another Vipaścit became a deer after abandoning his body, and lives on a mountain.

Though they had the same vāsanā (impulse) to start with, they were drawn in different directions. The vāsanā of beings becomes either dense or light by repeated exercise and repetition of its effects. It is also subject to the influence of time, place and activity. The Vipaścit who roamed from one country to another saw an illusory creation. That Vipaścit realised the truth; his ignorance (and his body) ceased to be. Ignorance, too, is infinite even as Brahman is infinite. It is the infinite consciousness alone that sees countless universes here and there. When this truth is not realised, it is known as ignorance; when it is realised the very same consciousness is known as Brahman. There is no division between the two.

yenaivā 'bhyuditā yasya tasya tena vinā gatiḥ
na śobhate na sukhadā na hitāya na satphalā (130/2)

VASIṢṬHA continued:

Even as one who is endowed with limbs knows them, I know everything which exists in Brahman, as Brahman is my own self. The two Vipaścit who wander in distant universes are not seen in our consciousness. But the one who became a deer is within the field of our understanding. It is the deer that was presented to you as a gift by the king of Trigartha.

(Amazed, Rāma had the deer brought to the court.)

King Vipaścit had adored the sacred fire. That was the original cause for the coming into being of this deer. By entering into fire this deer will regain its former state. **Redemption is the reversal of the original cause which gave rise to the fall. No other path is fruitful or adequate or laudable.** (The sage Vasiṣṭha raised the sacred fire and prayed that the deer might be restored to its former state. The deer jumped into the fire and a shining being — Bhāsa — arose from it. He narrated his story.)

BHĀSA (VIPAŚCIT) said:

I saw many things and I wandered a lot without experiencing fatigue. I experienced many things in many different ways. All this I remember. I experienced many pleasures and much sorrow in many bodies over a long period of time and in distant places in this limitless space. I was determined to see and experience everything. This was the original boon which I obtained from the fire-god.

For a thousand years I lived as a tree. My mind was totally centred within myself, and without mental activity I produced flowers and fruits. For a hundred years I was a deer. For fifty years I was a śarabha (an eight-footed animal more powerful than the lion). After that I became a celestial, then a swan, a jackal, a nymph in another world and then an ascetic and so on. I saw a world made entirely of water. Elsewhere I saw a woman in whose body the three worlds were reflected as in a mirror. She said: "I am pure consciousness and all the worlds are my limbs. Till you see everything with the same bewilderment with which you see me, you cannot know their real nature."

I saw worlds and universes of diverse nature. There is no world I have not seen, nothing I have not experienced. Once I was asleep with a nymph in a garden. Suddenly I woke up to find myself floating downstream. She explained: "There is a moonstone mountain nearby which melts when the moon rises and causes such a flood." We flew away from there and lived elsewhere. Even after all this I had not seen the end of the manifestation of ignorance known as 'the objective universe', for it was an illusion which had somehow got itself firmly rooted in my heart, just as the fear of a ghost gets hold of the heart of a child. However well I realise 'This is not real' after intense enquiry, the feeling 'This is' does not cease. From moment to moment new experiences of pleasure and pain arise and cease, like the flowing stream of a river.

brahmādīnāṁ tṛṇāntānāṁ dvidhā bhavati saṁbhavaḥ
eko brahmamayo 'nyastu bhrāntijastāviman śṛṇu (136/22)

BHĀSA continued:

While I was roaming a shining world in space, one day a gigantic shadow enveloped that earth. Soon I saw an enormous thing falling upon it. I was afraid and so entered into the fire and sought the protection of the fire-god. With his help we bored a small hole in that huge body and emerged in outer space. From there we saw the colossal form. It agitated and shattered all the celestial bodies including this earth while it fell. The siddhā, sages and celestials prayed to Kālarātri who appeared in front of them, accompanied by goblins. She was dry and bloodless. The siddhā said to her: "O divine mother, this is our offering to you. Pray consume it quickly." She began to eat that body up. Her own lean body grew in size. She began to dance.

When Kālarātri had eaten that body, the earth became visible again. Its very bones became the mountains on earth. Because the earth was made of the flesh of that being it is called 'medinī'. The FIRE-GOD narrated the following story concerning that huge being:

In a certain universe there lived a gigantic person named Asura. Once he destroyed the hermitage of a sage who cursed him: "You are proud of your gigantic body. Become a mosquito!" The Asura (demon) was burnt by the curse. There arose in him self-awareness, just as a seed sprouts in favourable conditions. In that self-awareness lay the sage's curse and the notion of a mosquito. Therefore he became a mosquito. (VASIṢṬHA explained: **From Brahmā down to the blade of grass all beings are subject to two forms of birth: the first is Brahmā's creation and the other is illusory creation.**) The mosquito dwelt on a blade of grass which was eaten by a deer. Because he died looking at the deer, he became a deer. The deer was killed by a hunter; hence he was born as a hunter. While roaming the forest he met a sage who awakened him with the question: "Why do you engage yourself in this cruel life of a hunter? Abandon this and seek to attain nirvāṇa."

In a matter of days the hunter entered into the wisdom of the scriptures, just as a flower enters a man's body as its fragrance. One day he asked the sage, "How is it that dream which takes place within, appears to be outside?"

THE SAGE replied:

To find the answer to this question, I once practised contemplation. I exhaled the mind, with the prāṇa, outside the body. The prāṇa entered the body of another being which appeared in front of me. I followed it into that being. I saw all the organs. I entered the heart of that being. I attained the principle of light in which the three worlds are reflected. Remaining there I saw the entire universe as if I were seeing it from my own vitality.

yadā svakarmaṇi spande vyagraḥ prāṇo bhṛśaṁ bhavet
tadā tadihitavyagraḥ prāṇo nā ''tmodyamī bhavet (139/12)

THE SAGE continued:

In that dream-world, too, there were the sun, the mountains and oceans, as also gods, demons and human beings. I realised: "This surely is the divine form of the truth concerning consciousness. Whatever that consciousness manifests in itself is known as the world." I have now realised that this world, which is said to be the dream-object, is the perception of this infinite consciousness. The expression of this perception is the waking state. Dream is dream only in relation to the waking state, but a dream is waking state in itself. They are two aspects of the waking state. Then, what is sleep? 'Let me rest in peace' — when this one notion prevails in the mind, there is sleep; this can arise even in the waking state. The fourth (turīya) state is perfect illumination when the world-appearance ceases.

I left that being's vitality and entered into its consciousness. Initially there was dual awareness; since, however, the two perceiving intelligences were similar, the two mixed well, like water and milk. I then absorbed into myself the consciousness of the other being; I began to experience the world as he did. After some time he retired to sleep. He collected the rays of his mind. Even as a tortoise draws its limbs into itself, his senses were drawn into his heart along with their functions. His sense organs became as if they were dead. I was within him and I followed the course of his mind and entered into his heart. All the channels within him were dense and congested on account of fatigue; and on account of food, drink, etc., the life-breath flowed slowly through the nostrils. The self is its own object now and there is no other externalising activity. Hence it shines in itself as itself.

Mind is the creator of the world. Prāṇa was brought into being by the mind which thinks "Prāṇa is my movement and I shall not be without prāṇa." **When the prāṇa is busily engaged in its own movement, it is unable to exert in self-knowledge.**

The relationship between the mind and prāṇa is that of a rider and the vehicle. When the mind and the prāṇa function in harmony, the person engages himself in various activities. When there is disturbance there is disharmony. When both are at rest there is sleep. When the nāḍī are clogged by food or when there is weakness or fatigue, there is sleep, because the prāṇa is unable to move properly.

When darkness fell, the being into whose heart I had entered fell asleep. I slept too. When the food he had eaten had been digested and when the nāḍī were clear, the life-force began to move and sleep weakened. Then I saw the world with its sun and so on, as if it arose in the heart. I saw all this where I was. This world was overwhelmed by a flood. I, too, was swept away in a flood. Luckily, I obtained a foothold on a rock. But a huge wave knocked me into the waters again.

sargādāvatha dehānte bhātaṁ yadvedanaṁ yathā
tattathā "mokṣamevā "ste tadidaṁ sarga ucyate (143/17)

THE SAGE continued:

What I have described so far was but a dream — what is impossible in or irreconcilable with a dream? After the previous events, I said to myself: "I am sixteen years of age and I am living in a hermitage in a village." All this became real to me. The memory of the previous experience began to fade. I considered the body to be my only hope. Wisdom was far from me. Vāsanā or mental conditioning was the very essence of my being and I was devoted to wealth. I observed all my social and religious duties. I knew what to do and what not to do.

One day a sage came to me as my guest. I served him. He described the universe in great detail, and concluded that all that was the one infinite consciousness. I was spiritually awakened. At once I recollected that I had entered into another body. I became one with the other person's prāṇa and with it I came out. I realised that I was seated in samādhi. My disciples revealed that only one hour had passed since I entered into samādhi. The person into whose heart I had entered was another traveller. Out of curiosity, I re-entered the other person's heart while he was still asleep. In it the cosmic dissolution had just concluded.

But, where is body, where is the heart, what is dream, where are water, flood and so on, where is awakening or the cessation of such awakening, where is birth and where is death? There is only pure consciousness. In the presence of this consciousness even the smallest and the subtlest of space appears macrocosmic. The persons seen in a dream have no past karma. Even so, the jīvā that arose in the beginning of 'creation' have no karma because they are pure consciousness. It is only when one becomes firmly rooted in the notion of this world-appearance as the reality, that the notion of karma arises. Then the jīvā roam here, bound by their karma. If it is realised that this creation itself is no-creation and that Brahman alone exists, then where is karma, who is karma and who belongs to that karma?

That awareness or experience which arises in the beginning of creation (sargādi) and at the end of the life-span of the body (dehānta), continues to exist till it ceases to be (or till liberation is attained), and that is known as creation. This creation is in the heart of the infinite consciousness, even as the dream is in your heart, both as the cause and the effect.

Dharma (virtue), adharma (sin), vāsanā (latent tendency), the active self and jīva— all these are synonyms which are notions with no corresponding reality. The one pure consciousness appears as the diverse dream-objects in a dream. All these millions of objects which appear in the dream become one again in deep sleep. Similarly, when this dream-world appears in the infinite consciousness that itself is called creation; when this itself enters into the equivalent of the deep sleep state, it is known as cosmic dissolution.

svapne tu jāgratsaṁskāro yastajjāgratkṛtaṁ navaṁ
ajāgrajjāgradā "bhāsaṁ kṛtamityeva tadvidaḥ (19)

THE SAGE continued:

All that exists and all that does not exist are like dream-experiences. Such being the truth, what is bondage and who is liberated? The cloud-formations in the sky throw up ever-changing forms and patterns — even so is the world-appearance ever changing. It seems to be stable and unchanging on account of ignorance. In this infinite space there are countless worlds even as we have our own world: one man's world is not experienced by another person. The measure and experience of frogs living in a well, lake and ocean are different from one another. They do not share one another's knowledge. People sleeping in one house have different dreams in which they experience life in different worlds, as it were: even so, some people have different worlds in the same space, while others may not have. All this is but the mysterious and efficient work of the infinite consciousness.

Consciousness has the faculty of holding on to something; a notion so held is known as saṁskāra. But when it is realised that the notion is only reflected in consciousness, it is seen that there is no saṁskāra independent of consciousness. In dream there is no previous memory but only the experience of the objects that are experienced for the time being. One may even experience in a dream one's own death, as also objects that appear to be like those seen before.

This creation was but a mirror-reflection in the indivisible consciousness in the beginning, and hence it was non-different from that consciousness. Brahman (the infinite consciousness) alone shines as this world, which is not something new. The cause alone is the effect. The cause was there before the effect and will remain even after the effect ceases to be. Because the cause 'acts efficiently' (saṁyak karoti) in bringing about the effect, it itself is known as saṁskāra.

That which existed before the arising of the dream but which shines as that which was seen before, is known as saṁskāra. There is no other external factor known as saṁskāra (popularly translated into 'latent impressions of past experiences and actions'). Things seen and unseen exist in the consciousness which shines in its own light and experiences all those things as if already seen. **In dream the saṁskārā created in the waking state arise; but in the waking state itself they are created anew. But they who know the truth declare that they were in fact created in a state that appeared to be the waking state but which in fact is not.** Just as movement arises in air spontaneously, even so notions arise in consciousness: where is the need for saṁskāra to create them? When the experience of a thousand things arises in consciousness, it is known as creation; and when the experience of the thousand things ceases in consciousness, that is known as the cosmic dissolution. Thus the pure consciousness (cid ākāśa) brings into being this diversity with all its names and forms without ever abandoning its indivisibility, just as you create a world in your dream.

**bhātyakāraṇakaṁ brahma sargātmā 'pyabudhaṁ prati
taṁ pratyeva ca bhātyeṣa kāryakāraṇadṛgbhramaḥ (49)**

THE SAGE continued:

The perception or the experience of 'the world' exists within the atomic particle of infinite consciousness. Just as the reflection in a mirror is only mirror, however, it is non-different from the infinite consciousness. This infinite consciousness is beginningless and endless; that itself is called creation. Wherever this consciousness shines there this creation exists, non-different from it, even as a body is non-different from its limbs. You and I are consciousness, the entire world is consciousness: by this realisation the creation is seen as an integral part of consciousness, and therefore uncreated. Hence, I am that atomic particle of consciousness and as such I am infinite and omnipresent. Therefore, wherever I am I see everything from there itself. I am a particle of consciousness but I am one with the infinite consciousness on account of the realisation of this truth, even as water is the same as water.

Therefore, by entering into the 'ojas' I experienced the three worlds. All this happened within it, and within it I saw the three worlds — not outside. Whether it is called dream or waking, inside or outside, all this is within the infinite consciousness.

THE HUNTER asked:

If this creation is causeless, how does it come into being? If it has a cause, what is the cause of the dream-creation?

THE SAGE replied:

In the beginning, creation had no cause whatsoever. Since the objects of this creation had no cause whatsoever, conflicting diversity of objects opposed to one another does not arise. The one absolute Brahman alone shines as all this and is denoted by words like 'creation', etc. Thus, this causeless creation is Brahman but it appears to be part of that which has no parts, to be diverse in the indivisible, to have a form in the formless. Because it is pure consciousness it appears to assume various forms like the mobile and immobile objects. And as the gods and the sages it creates and sustains a world order with all the injunctions and prohibitions. Existence, non-existence, the gross and the subtle, etc. do not in any way affect the omnipresent consciousness.

However, from there on effects do not arise without a cause. The world order and its lord (Brahman) act on one another just as one arm restrains the other, though both belong to the same person.

Thus, this creation arises without desire and without psychological causation. The world order (niyati) exists within Brahman; Brahman does not exist without niyati. Thus, this creation has a cause, but only in relation to the one whose creation it is, and as long as that creation lasts in relation to him. **The ignorant think that Brahman shines or appears as this creation without a cause; and it is again the ignorant that are caught up in this cause-and-effect tangle or deluded notion that causality is inviolably real.** The creation takes place as a coincidence — the ripe cocoanut falls accidentally just when a crow alights on it. Then niyati determines 'This is this' and 'That is that'.

yadendriyāṇi tiṣṭhanti bāhyataśca samākulaṁ
tadā mlānānubhavanaḥ saṁkalpārtho 'nubhūyate (2)

THE SAGE continued:

The jīva knows and experiences the external world with the externalised senses and the inner dream world with the inner senses. **When the senses are engaged in the experience of the external world, then the field of internal notions is vague and unclear.** But when the senses are turned within then the jīva experiences the world within himself with the greatest clarity. There is no contradiction in this world-appearance whatsoever at any time; it is as one sees it is. Therefore, when the eyes are extroverted the jīva experiences the world as if it were outside in the infinite consciousness. The aggregate of the senses of hearing, touch (skin), sight (eyes), smell (nose), taste (tongue) and desire is known as the jīva, which is of the nature of pure consciousness endowed with life-force. This jīva exists, therefore, in everything everywhere as everything, and hence he experiences everything everywhere.

When the jīva (the 'ojas' or the vital essence) is filled with 'phlegm' (śleṣma or kapha, one of the three humours that constitute the vital essence of the body), he sees its effects there and then. He 'sees' himself rising from the ocean of milk; he sees the moon floating in the sky; he sees lakes and lotuses, gardens and flowers, rejoicing and festivals in which women sing and dance, feasts with a lot of food and drink, rivers flowing into the ocean, huge palaces painted white, fields covered with fresh snow, parks with deer resting in them, and mountain ranges.

When the jīva is filled with 'bile' (pitta, which is another humour) he experiences its effects there and then. He 'sees' flames which are beautiful, which produce sweating of the nerves and which throw up black smoke that darkens the sky, suns which are dazzling in their brilliance and scorching in their heat, oceans and mist rising from them, impassable forests, mirages with swans swimming in them; he sees himself running along the road in fear and covered with hot dust, he sees the earth scorched dry and hot. Wherever the eyes see, they see everything on fire, even the clouds rain fire, and because of this pervasive fire everything looks brilliant.

When the jīva is filled with 'wind' (vāta, which is another humour) he experiences the following effects. He sees the world as if it is new, he sees himself and even rocks and mountains flying; everything revolving and rotating, flying angels and celestials, and the earth and all that is in it quakes. He sees himself as having fallen into a blind well or a dreadful calamity, or as standing perilously on top of a tree of great height or a mountain peak.

kṣubdhairantarbahiścaiva svalpaiḥ svalpaṁ prapaśyati
samaiḥ samamidaṁ dṛśyaṁ vātapittakaphādinā (59)

THE SAGE continued:

When the jīva is filled with vāta, pitta and śleṣma (wind, bile and phlegm), he comes under the influence of the wind, and experiences distress. He sees a shower of mountains and of rocks, he hears dreadful sounds with which trees revolve in the bowels of the earth. Whole forests whirl around with all the animals in the forests. All the trees are on fire and there is the sound of burning issuing from all the caves. He sees the collision of mountains. He sees the oceans rising to fill the entire sky and carrying away whole forests and even clouds, lifting them up to the region of Brahmā the creator. The whole sky seems to be clear and clean because of all this friction and rubbing within it. The three worlds appear to be filled with the battle cries of soldiers and warriors.

When thus the jīva is agitated and distressed by all this dreadful vision, he becomes unconscious. Like a worm which lies buried in the earth, like a frog hidden in a rock, like a foetus in the womb, like the seed within the fruit, like the unborn sprout in a seed, like an atom in a molecule, like an uncut figure in a rock, he rests within himself. He is undisturbed by the movement of prāṇa because in his resting place there are no 'holes' or outlets. He enters into deep sleep, which is like resting inside a rock or inside a blind well.

When mental effort makes a hole in that resting place, then he knows the world of dreams, having been made aware of it by the movement of the life-force or prāṇa. When this life-force falls from one nāḍī (nerve-channel) on to another, there is a vision of a shower of mountains. If there is too much of such movement caused by vāta, pitta and ślesma, there is a lot of such experience; if it is less, the experience is less.

Whatever the jīva experiences within (in dream, etc.) on account of the vāta, pitta and śleṣma, that he experiences outside, too, and in that field his own organs of action function appropriately. **When agitated or disturbed inside and outside, he (the jīva) experiences a little disturbance if the disturbance of the vāta, pitta and kapha (ślesma) is slight, and he experiences equanimity if they are in a state of balance or equilibrium.** The jīva experiences all these outside when the three humours are agitated or disturbed: burning, drowning, moving in air, resting on rocks and mountains, hell, rising and falling from the sky, hallucinations like drowning in a playground, sunshine at midnight, perversion of intelligence in which one's own appear to be strangers and enemies appear like friends. With closed eyes these are all seen within oneself and with open eyes these are seen outside: but all these delusions are brought about by the disturbed equilibrium of the three humours. When they are in a state of equilibrium, the jīva residing within them sees the whole world as it is, as it really IS, non-different from Brahman.

tadevaṁ svapna evā 'yaṁ jāgradbhāvamupāgataḥ
sarve vayamiha svapnapuruṣāstava suvrata (151/9)

THE SAGE continued:

When I saw, while still in the heart of the other person, my own relations and so on, I momentarily forgot that they were the product of my own notions, and I lived with them for a period of sixteen years, until I met the ascetic who awakened my intelligence. He revealed to me: "All of us are in the heart of a macrocosmic being who is regarded as such by all of us. Even so, there will be other macrocosmic beings for others. This macrocosmic being is the cause for the experiences of pleasure and pain and for the diverse types of actions.

When the 'ojas' of this macrocosmic being is disturbed, it is agitated, and that effect is experienced by all of us who are in his heart. We are affected by natural calamities which cease when his heart regains equanimity. Therefore, this macrocosmic being is the reality of this particular creation. By coincidence, when some people engage themselves in evil actions, the resultant unhappiness befalls all.

Consciousness bestows reward on one when the actions arise from one's own personal notion 'I do this'; when the consciousness is freed from such a notion, such action is not followed by its fruits. As in a dream, the effect of an action is not governed by a definite cause. At times the dream-experience has a cause; and at other times it has no cause. It is simply accidental coincidence."

Thus instructed by the ascetic I was instantly enlightened. I could not leave him. At my request he lived with me. (That very ascetic is sitting right next to you.) I wanted to see my own body as well as the body which I had begun to investigate. However much I tried, I could not get out of the heart of the person where I was. I was puzzled. But the ascetic explained the mystery: "Surely you will know everything if you see it with your inner vision. You are not this little personality; you are the macrocosmic person himself. Once you desired to enter into the heart of a being in order to experience a dream. That into which you entered is this creation. While you were in that body, a great fire arose and it destroyed your body as well as the body of the other person. You continued to vibrate as just consciousness. You could not find an exit. Not finding the two bodies, you exist in this 'world'. **Thus, your dream has materialised into the waking state reality. All of us here are your own dream-objects.** Similarly, you are our dream-objects. That in which all this happens is the pure consciousness which exists everywhere at all times."

The ascetic had referred to me as 'the teacher of the hunter'. When questioned by me, he revealed the future: "After some years a great famine will arise here. All your relatives will perish. However, you and I shall know no sorrow, since we are knowers of the truth. In course of time a nice forest will grow here. One day a hunter will come to that place in pursuit of game. You will enlighten him with your talks and stories. Thus you will become the teacher of the hunter."

avaśyaṁ bhavitavyo 'rtho na kadacana kenacit
vidhātumanyathā śakyastanna kṣarati yatnataḥ (155/53)

THE HUNTER asked:

How shall I ever rest in the self?

THE SAGE replied:

You have no doubt set out to attain self-knowledge, but you have not found your foothold on sound wisdom. You wish to get out of this world-appearance, and with this end in view you wish to know its extent. In order to ascertain this, you are engaged in penance. You will continue to perform such penance for several world-cycles. Then the Lord will appear before you. He will grant you the boon of a long life in good health, and the ability to travel at will in space in order to explore the extent of creation. You will see countless universes and then realise that just as all this is unreal and diverse in the eyes of the ignorant, they are real and indivisible to the enlightened. You will then abandon your body. **That which is inevitable cannot be averted by anyone at any time. It is not altered by any amount of effort.** Your body will fall crushing the earth by its sheer size and weight. The goddess known as 'Dryness' (Kālarātri) will consume that body and thus purify the earth.

Your jīva will behold the entire world as you see the world in your dream. It will then regard itself as king Sindhu, whose kingdom is invaded by king Vidūratha. On account of this thought there will be a fierce battle between you two. You will kill Vidūratha and become the king of the whole world. Your minister will reveal to you that Vidūratha did not win the battle because he had prayed for liberation, and that you did not pray for liberation because your impure heart had craved for victory over enemies and so on. The minister will exhort you: "Yesterday's evil action is transformed into good action by today's noble deeds. Therefore, strive to be good and do good now." When you hear this you will renounce the world, and through the association of holy ones you will attain the highest wisdom and liberation.

BHĀSA continued:

The fire-god disappeared after narrating the story of that being whose corpse fell down. However, I was still caught in the deer-body. I met Indra the king of heaven who revealed to me my true identity. Once a hunter pursued me, overpowered me and brought me to you to serve as your pet, O Rāma! Limitless is this ignorance with countless branches in all directions: it cannot come to an end by any means other than self-knowledge.

Strange and wonderful is this Māyā which is perplexing and which gives rise to delusion in the mind, and in which thesis and antithesis exist together without conflict or contradiction. Every inch of space is filled with the creations of 'dead' jīvā. Such worlds are countless. They are unseen. They exist all together, without any contradiction or conflict. This universe appears in Brahman and ceases to be the next moment, for Brahman alone is real.

jantoryathā manorājyaṁ vividhārambhabhāsuraṁ
brāhmaṁ tathedaṁ vitataṁ manorājyaṁ virājate (21)

VASIṢṬHA continued:

From the supreme Brahman, the mind first arose with its faculty of thinking and imagination. And this mind remains as such in that Brahman, even as fragrance in a flower, as waves in the ocean and as rays of light in the sun. Brahman, which is extremely subtle and invisible, was forgotten, as it were, and thus arose the wrong notion of the real existence of the world-appearance.

If one thinks that the light rays are different and distinct from the sun, to him the light rays have a distinct reality. If one thinks that a bracelet made of gold is a bracelet, to him it is indeed a bracelet and not gold.

But if one realises that the light rays are non-different from the sun, his understanding is said to be unmodified (nirvikalpa). If one realises that the waves are non-different from the ocean, his understanding is said to be unmodified (nirvikalpa). If one realises that the bracelet is non-different from gold, his understanding is said to be unmodified (nirvikalpa).

He who sees the display of sparks does not realise that it is but fire. His mind experiences joy and sorrow as these sparks fly up and scatter on the ground. If he sees that the sparks are but fire and non-different from it, he sees only fire and his understanding is said to be unmodified (nirvikalpa).

He who is thus established in the nirvikalpa is indeed a great one. His understanding does not diminish. He has attained whatever is worth attaining. His heart does not get enmeshed in the objects. Hence, O Rāma, abandon this perception of diversity or objectification and remain established in consciousness.

Whatever the self contemplates is materialised on account of the inherent power in the consciousness. That materialised thought then shines as if independent! Thus, whatever the mind (which is endowed with the faculty of thought) contemplates, materialises instantly. This is the origin of diversity. Hence, this world-appearance is neither real nor unreal. **Even as sentient beings create and experience diverse objects in their own day-dreams, this world-appearance is the day-dream of Brahman.** When it is realised as Brahman, then the world-appearance is dissolved; for from the absolute point of view this world is non-existent. Brahman remains as Brahman and it does not create something which was not already in existence!

O Rāma, whatever you do, know that it is nothing but pure consciousness. Brahman alone is manifest here as all this, for naught else exists. There is no scope for 'this' and the 'other'. Therefore, abandon even the concepts of liberation and bondage. Remain in the pure, egoless state, engaging yourself in natural activity.

teṣāmantarjanāḥ santi janaṁ prati punarmanaḥ
punarmanaḥ prati jagajjagatprati punarjanaḥ (63/33)

VASIṢTHA continued:

Once upon a time I desired to renounce all the activities of the world and to meditate in total seclusion. Where could I find a suitable place? Having abandoned the forests, cities, oceans and caves which are full of distractions, I went into outer space, but found that it was also subject to distractions by celestials. I went further to a lonely spot in which I imagined a hermitage. A hundred years passed in a twinkling of an eye, for when one is deeply absorbed in contemplation the passage of time is not noticed.

As I returned to body-consciousness I heard a sigh. In order to discover its nature, I entered into samādhi again. In the infinite consciousness I saw reflected the image of countless universes, which were diverse in composition and time-space structure. In one of them I saw a woman, the source of the sound, who saluted me; I ignored her and continued to investigate the diversity of the universes. I saw that space and consciousness alone existed, in which you look at something and say "This is such and such" and experience it as such! On account of this there is infinite diversity. In some universes moonlight is hot, sunlight cool; there is sight in darkness and blindness in daylight; good is destructive and evil constructive; poison promotes health and nectar kills, in accordance with the notions that arise in consciousness. In some there are no women; in some the beings do not possess one or more of the senses and there are only one or two elements.

It cannot be said that I remained at one spot or that I roamed about; for I had attained infinite consciousness. I witnessed all this within the self which had assumed the form I witnessed, just as you 'see' different parts of your body at night with eyes closed. The lady and I had bodies made of pure imaginary space. This is true of all bodies! Yet we experience them as if they are real and solid, even as we experience substantiality of dream-objects. It is because of the very nature of the infinite consciousness that these space-bodies seem to exist; their reality is of course the sole reality, Brahman. Everything exists everywhere at all times as the pure indivisible consciousness. In the infinite play of the infinite there are infinite minds with infinite worlds in them. In every one of them there are continents and mountains, villages and cities inhabited by people who have their own time-space scale and life-span. When these jīvā reach the end of their life-span, if they are not enlightened they continue to exist in infinite space, creating their own dream-worlds. **Within them are other people within whom are minds; within those minds are worlds in which there are more beings, ad infinitum.**

This illusory appearance has no beginning and no end; it is Brahman and Brahman alone. O Rāma, in all these diverse objects there is nothing but pure consciousness.

iṣṭavastvarthinām tajjñasūpadiṣṭena karmaṇā
paunaḥpuṇyena karaṇānnetaraccharaṇam mune (67/23)

VASIṢṬHA continued:

In response to my question concerning her identity, the woman celestial said: "In a corner of this universe you live. Beyond that are universes of diverse phenomena, very different from this. On the slopes of a far-distant mountain range there is a solid rock within which I dwell. The world within this rock is just like yours: it has its own inhabitants, angels and demons, heavens and hells, the sun and the moon and all the rest of it. I have been in it for countless aeons, along with my husband. Since we are intensely attracted to each other, we have not attained liberation. However, my husband is a brāhmaṇa and celibate from birth, educated but lazy. He wished to have a wife who would be spiritually inclined; of that wish I was born. But our marriage has not been consummated.

"After some time my attachment for my husband turned into non-attachment. Yet, I could not abandon him; a woman can abandon everything in this world but not her husband. However, I have only one desire now: and that is to be instructed by you. He too wishes to attain self-knowledge."

At her request I went over to her world-within-the-rock; but could not see the world, though I saw the rock! She continued: "I now see that what I previously saw in the rock is only in me. By repeatedly affirming the world within the rock, I began to experience it. **Ah, this is the only path to salvation: one should be totally devoted to the one desirable cause, one should be instructed in the right effort for its attainment and one should again and again engage oneself in such right action.**"

When I heard this, I entered into samādhi again. What appeared to be rock before shone as pure consciousness (cid-ākāśa). On account of the mysterious power of illusion, a notion arises for no reason whatsoever; paradoxically, the obvious is unreal and the unreal becomes obvious.

The subtle body is the first among these 'obvious' truths. The gross physical body exists in the ātivāhika or the subtle body, even as water exists in a mirage. When you realise that what seems to be obvious is unreal, what else is worth our consideration? How can we accept as real that which is established as real by the unreal? Thus what was seen by us as the world within the rock was unreal; it was pure consciousness only. Such a world is seen only by the ignorant who cling to the notion 'I am not enlightened'.

The celestial lady entered the world within the rock. I went in, too. She went to the Creator of that world. He was her husband. She asked me to enlighten both of them. He was in deep meditation. She brought him back to normal consciousness. He became aware of his limbs. These limbs were in fact different 'created' beings who arose in that awareness. He welcomed me. I questioned him concerning the lady and himself.

evaṁ sampadyate brahmā tathā sampadyate hariḥ
evaṁ sampadyate rudra evaṁ sampadyate kṛmiḥ (73/37)

VASIṢṬHA continued:

The 'Creator in the Rock' replied: "I am but a vibration in the one cosmic consciousness. I have not been created. I do not see anything else. What is seen here as you and I are mere vibrations or notions. Even so is this lady. She was not created as my wife! Now I wish to merge in the plane of infinite consciousness. Hence dispassion has arisen in me, signalling the onset of cosmic dissolution. Therefore dispassion has arisen in this lady who is also a notion! All notions cease. Just as a notion arises, it ceases; the yearning for the unconditioned inheres in conditioning.

"Time, space, matter, motion and so on are parts of consciousness, it is consciousness alone that exists as this rock. Countless worlds exist in that consciousness.

Having said this, the Creator entered into deep meditation. So did the lady. I, too, followed suit. When the cosmic person withdrew his consciousness from the notion called 'earth', it began to disintegrate. Great unrighteousness precedes natural and artificial catastrophies. When the earth had been destroyed, the water element deluged everything that existed. Unquenchable flames arose destroying everything. When the Creator withdrew his prāṇa or life-force, air abandoned its natural motion in space. What could live without life-force? Even stars and heaven, with its ruler Indra, began to disintegrate; for they were all only notions entertained by the Creator.

What survives is the eternal. It is beyond description. In relation to a mountain a subatomic particle is small; in relation to the infinite the entire universe is a subatomic particle. Creation is like a dream. As a particle of consciousness moves in space, it does 'there' what it did 'here' earlier; thus the sequence of time arises, as well as spatial distinctions like 'above', 'below' and so on. Though it is of the nature of pure space or void, it seems to become time, space, action, matter and awareness of the meaning of words. **Even so, this consciousness becomes Brahmā the creator; even so, it becomes Hari or Viṣṇu; even so does it become Rudra; and even so does it become a worm.** The entire universe is contained in a subatomic particle and the three worlds exist within one strand of hair.

The cosmic person has two bodies: the superior body is pure consciousness and the other is the world. He is able to view the world (like an egg) from outside it (as a hen does). He divided the egg into two: the upper part he called the sky or the heaven, and the lower part he called the earth. Heaven is his head, as it were, and the earth his feet. The other elements of the universe are his other limbs and parts of the body. However, since he is pure consciousness, all these are only notions. All actions that take place in this world originate in him. On account of him the world is seen to be real. He exists in that cosmic body as you exist in your heart when you are in meditation.

kākutstharudranāmāsāvahaṅkāratayotthitaḥ
viṣamaikābhimānātmā mūrtirasyāmalaṁ nabhaḥ (80/19)

VASIṢṬHA continued:

While the Creator continued to meditate, I looked around. I saw a sun arising in every direction — ten of them. Another arose from the bowels of the earth, the eleventh. Three more looked like the three eyes of Rudra; and together they formed the twelfth. The universe was reduced to ashes by the eyes of Rudra. Only two 'objects' remained unaffected: space, because it was all-pervading, and gold because it was pure. Nothing else was left. Future generations could only wonder, "Perhaps there was a world, a universe, a creation before".

Then terrible winds dried everything. This was followed by dreadful clouds which showered adamant and thunderbolt. There was total darkness. Only the vital air or prāṇa which presides over the disintegration of matter sustained the disintegrating objects. The entire space was filled with flying cities, demons, fire, serpents and suns, which looked like so many flies and mosquitoes. The three elements (water, fire and wind) were completely out of control. There was total darkness.

Devoid of the veil of creation, that which remains after the total destruction of what is known as creation alone existed. Once again there was fullness, the fullness that becomes apparent when the diverse creatures are destroyed, the fullness that was there all the time. There was no space. There were no directions. There were neither elements nor a creation. There was but one limitless ocean of consciousness. I saw the Creator seated in meditation surrounded by the first principles; the twelve suns also arrived there and entered into meditation. I saw them as one sees dream-objects or manifestations of mental conditioning, not as the materialisation of dream-objects. I then realised that all of them were pure void. That very instant they vanished from sight. Even the 'world of the Creator' had been destroyed.

I saw a fearsome form. He was like embodied dissolution of the universe. He shone by his own radiance. I thought "**This is Rudra**" and bowed to him. **O Rāma, he is the ego-sense. He is devoted to the disturbance of the equilibrium. His form is pure space or void.** Therefore, his colour is like that of space. The five senses are his faces. The five organs of action and their fields are his ten arms. This form of Rudra is but a small particle of the infinite consciousness. He exists as movement in cidākāśa (infinite consciousness) and as air in both the physical space and in living beings (as their life-breath). In course of time, when all his movements come to an end, he attains supreme equilibrium.

Since he is attained by goodness and his very existence is for the good of all, he is known as Śiva. He then attains to the state of supreme peace and is therefore known as Kṛṣṇa. He himself creates the whole universe, and he drinks the one ocean of cosmic being and attains to that supreme peace.

cetanatvāttathābhutasvabhāvavibhavādṛte
sthātuṁ na yujyate tasya yathā hemnā nirākṛti (82/6)

VASIṢṬHA continued:

Rudra began to dance in space. I saw a shadow behind him. How could shadow exist without the sun? As I was reflecting over this phenomenon, that shadow (female) stepped in front of Rudra and she was dancing, too. She was thin and huge. Her mouth emitted fire. She was Kālarātri (the Night of Death). Holy men call her Kālī. She playfully strung the mountains into a garland for herself. The three worlds became mirrors in the three parts of her body. The entire universe was in constant motion because she was dancing: from another point of view, of course, they were firmly established in her. Even as I was looking, they appeared, disappeared and reappeared. The revolving firmament looked like her flowing garment. But nothing really happened. By her dance she created and dissolved the universe moment after moment.

There was neither a male nor a female, nor did they dance. The cidākāśa itself is Śiva (Rudra). His own dynamic energy is non-different from him and inseparable. Only the eternal, infinite consciousness existed. The Lord himself took on the appearance of Rudra, but in fact he was formless. **It is not appropriate even to assume that the infinite consciousness, which had become manifest in all its glory on account of its inherent nature, would suddenly be without it: just as gold cannot be without any form whatsoever.** Consciousness is never without some movement within itself. Birth, death, māyā, delusion, wisdom, bondage, liberation, good and evil, you and I and all the rest of it, the deities and the natural forces are nothing but the infinite consciousness to the enlightened; he does not see diversity. I saw only that space which was supreme peace; and I experienced it in the form which I have described. No-one else saw it that way. That movement was experienced by me as the dance of the Lord, on account of my own psychological conditioning. The notion of motion in consciousness (which has no qualities) is ignorance.

Whatever there is and functions here is real to the self and not to another who does not perceive it and is unaware of it. An imaginary city is imagination, not city. Kālarātri is to the Lord what movement is to air. While she continues to dance in this fashion in space, by accidental coincidence she comes into contact with the Lord. She is instantly weakened and made thin and transparent. She becomes of the form of the Lord himself, like the river entering the ocean. The Lord shines one without a second. The energy of consciousness dances until it beholds the glory of nirvāṇa. When it beholds consciousness, it becomes pure consciousness.

Shortly after that, Rudra became as light as cloud and smaller than an atom. He became invisible. He had become one with the absolute Brahman or pure consciousness. All this I saw in that rock by the divine eye (awakened intelligence). Of course, if one sees the rock with the physical eye as if it lies at a distance, only the rock is seen. In every part of the rock I saw this creation, sustenance and dissolution take place. I saw the universe in the past, present and future.

evamrūpamahaṁ jālaṁ bhāvayan yattadāsthitaḥ
tadahaṅkāra ityadya kathyate tvādṛśairjanaiḥ (87/35)

VASIṢṬHA continued:

After thus contemplating the infinite consciousness for sometime, I suddenly realised that all this creation was within myself, just as the tree is in the seed. As I was thus observing creation, I had become atomic. I realised myself as a ray of light. Soon I had become gross. In this grossness there were the potentialities of sense experiences. When the consciousness 'opened its eyes', as it were, or became aware of its own inherent potentialities, the pure elements (tanmātrā) arose and then all the senses, which are in fact pure void, came into being. With the five elements and the five senses, their corresponding knowledge and experience arose in me irresistibly. All these were without substantiality, and illusory. Yet, **that state of my being is known by people like you as I-ness or ego-sense.** Though I am pure consciousness, I seem to have acquired a subtle body and an antaḥkaraṇa (mind and so on).

When I experienced space, I knew what earth was. I became earth. In that earth I experienced the existence of countless universes, without ever abandoning the awareness that I am the infinite consciousness. While I remained in the earth-consciousness I experienced the experiences of the earth. Truly, this was mental and I had myself become the earth; equally truly, this was not mental nor did I actually become the earth. Apart from the mind there is no earth. The notion that arises in consciousness is pure consciousness and nothing else. Hence, there is no notion as such, neither a self nor a world. When it is thus seen, the world does not exist; when it is not observed carefully, it seems to come into being.

It is pure consciousness alone that appears as this earth. It is the false notion entertained by countless beings in the three worlds that has attained relative or existential reality known as the earth. 'I am all this and all that is within all this.' With this realisation I saw everything.

Then I also experienced the water-plane by water-dhāraṇā. By contemplating water, I became water. Then I became the fire-element through the contemplation of that element (teja-dhāraṇā). I became the good colour (suvarṇa) in gold and so on. I became vitality and valour in men, in jewels I sparkled as their fire, in rainclouds I became the light of the lightning. Whatever I experienced in the states of earth, water and fire, I experienced only as Brahman. When one enters another state with this intelligence, out of his own wish, obviously one does not experience unhappiness or sorrow. When one touches a river of sparks which he fancies in his own mind, he does not experience pain. Such was the case with my elemental experiences.

Then I became the air-element by vāyu-dhāraṇā (contemplation of oneself as wind). I taught the grass, leaves, creepers and straw the art of dancing. Though the nether worlds were my feet, the earth my abdomen and the heavens my head, while I was wind, I did not abandon my subatomic nature.

svapnasaṅkalpasaṁśāntau svapnasaṅkalpapattanaṁ
yadā sā sukuṭī naṣṭā matsaṅkalpopaśāntitaḥ (93/15)

VASIṢṬHA continued:

After all this I re-entered my cottage or hermitage in outer space. I looked for my physical body. It was not there. But I found an aged sage sitting in that hermitage. He was in deep meditation. I thought he must also have been an aged sage who wanted to meditate in seclusion, who had found that cottage empty and therefore occupied it after throwing out my body. I wanted to let him have it. **When my desire to stay in the cottage ceased, the cottage disappeared. When a dream or a notion comes to an end the objects that arose in it vanish.** The hermitage fell. The sage fell. I too descended along with him onto the earth plane. The sage landed in the same state and posture in which he was in that hermitage. This was because, through the union of prāṇa and apāna, he had overcome the force of gravity. He did not even wake up from his meditation. His body was as strong as a rock and as light as cotton.

In order to rouse him, I assumed the form of a cloud and rained and thundered. He regained body consciousness and greeted me and told me his story. "I have wandered in the realms of the gods for a considerable time. I am tired of this saṁsāra. When all this is pure consciousness, what is it that we call pleasure? Pleasure is dreadful pain, prosperity is adversity, sensual enjoyment is the worst disease and pursuit of pleasure is disgusting. With the advancing of age the hairs turn grey and the teeth decay and the faculties diminish; only craving does not diminish. After a long time I have attained egolessness. I am not interested in heavenly pleasures. Like you, O sage, I too longed to resort to a secluded place. Hence I saw that hermitage in space." I requested him to continue to dwell in it. Both of us rose in space. He went where he thought fit and I went my own way.

I was roaming the heaven like a ghost. No one could see me, till one day I thought "May I be seen henceforth by these gods". They began to see me. In due course of time I came to have a physical or material body. To me there was no difference between the subtle and physical bodies: they were both pure consciousness in reality. Even here I appear to function in and through this body because of this discourse. There is no notion in me other than of Brahman. Hence even when I am engaged in diverse activities this realisation of Brahman does not cease. Because of the recurrent feeling of the ethereal Vasiṣṭha that arises in the minds of all of you and also in me, I appear to be seated here. In truth, however, all this is pure void and all these are only notions that arise in the mind of the Creator. When the truth is realised all these scenes of so-called creations vanish, even as a mirage ceases to be seen as water when its true nature is understood.

Liberation confers inner coolness (peace) on the mind; bondage promotes psychological distress. Even after realising this, one does not strive for liberation. How foolish are the people!

sarvāḥ śaṅkāḥ parityajya dhairyamālambya śāśvatam
mahābokttā mahākartā mahātyāgī bhavā 'nagha (9)

VASIṢṬHA continued:

Give up all your doubts. Resort to moral courage. Be a supreme doer of actions, supreme enjoyer of delight and supreme renouncer of all! Such triple discipline was taught in days of yore by lord Śiva to Bhṛṅgīśa by which the latter attained total freedom. Bhṛṅgīśa was a man of ordinary or traditional self-knowledge. He approached lord Śiva and asked: "Lord, I am deluded by this world-appearance. Pray, tell me the attitude, equipped with which I shall be freed from this delusion."

LORD ŚIVA replied:

Give up all your doubts. Resort to moral courage. Be a mahābhokttā (great enjoyer of delight), mahākartā (great doer of actions) and mahātyāgī (perfect renouncer).

He is a mahākartā (great doer of actions) who is freed of doubts and performs appropriate actions in natural situations (whether they be regarded as dharma [right] or adharma [wrong]) without being swayed by likes and dislikes or success and failure, without ego-sense or jealousy, remaining with his mind in a state of silence and purity. He is unattached to anything but remains as a witness of everything, without selfish desires or motives, without sorrow or grief, indifferent to action and inaction, without excitement or exultation but with a mind at peace. His very nature is peace and equilibrium or equanimity, which is sustained in all situations (in the birth, existence or annihilation of all things).

He is a mahābhokttā (great enjoyer) who does not hate anything nor long for anything, but enjoys all natural experiences; who does not cling to nor renounce anything even while engaged in actions; who does not experience though experiencing; who witnesses the world-play, unaffected by it. His heart is not affected by pleasure and pain that arise in the course of life and the changes that cause confusion, and he regards with delight old age and death, sovereignty and poverty and even great calamities and fortunes. His very nature is non-violent and virtuous and he enjoys what is sweet and what is bitter with equal relish, without making any arbitrary distinction 'This is enjoyable' and 'This is not'.

He is a mahātyāgī (great renouncer) who has banished from his mind concepts like dharma and adharma, pain and pleasure, birth and death, all desires, all doubts, all convictions, who sees the falsity in the experience of pain by his body, mind, etc., who has realised 'I have no body, no birth, no right, no wrong' and who has completely abandoned from his heart the notion of world-appearance.

VASIṢṬHA continued:

Thus did lord Śiva instruct Bhṛṅgīśa, who then became enlightened. Adopt this attitude, O Rāma, and transcend sorrow.

bhāvābhāvaviruddho 'pi vicitro 'pi mahānapi
nā·''nandāya na khedāya satāṁ saṁsṛtivibhramaḥ (116/10)

RĀMA asked:

Lord, you know all the truths. When the ego-sense is dissolved in the mind, by what signs does one recognise the nature of satva?

VASIṢṬHA said:

Such a mind, O Rāma, is untouched by sins like greed and delusion, even under the worst provocation. Virtues like delight (in the prosperity of others) do not leave the person whose ego-sense has been dissolved. The knots of mental conditioning and tendencies are cut asunder. Anger is greatly attenuated and the delusion becomes ineffective. Desire becomes powerless. Greed flees. The senses function on an even keel, neither getting excited nor depressed. Even if pleasure and pain are reflected on his face they do not agitate the mind, which regards them all as insignificant. The heart rests in equanimity.

The enlightened man who is endowed with all these virtues, effortlessly and naturally wears the body. **Being and non-being (like prosperity and adversity) when they follow each other creating diverse and even great contradictions, do not generate joy and sorrow in the holy ones.**

Woe unto him who does not tread this path to self-knowledge, which is within reach if he directs his intelligence properly. The means for crossing this ocean of saṁsāra (world-appearance or the cycle of birth and death) and for the attainment of supreme peace, are enquiry into the nature of the self (Who am I?) and of the world (What is this world?) and of the truth (What is truth?).

Your own ancestor, Ikṣvāku, even while he was ruling his kingdom, reflected within himself one day: "What may be the origin of this world which is full of diverse sufferings — old age, death, pain, pleasure and delusion?" He could not arrive at an answer. So, after having duly worshipped his father Manu, the son of Brahmā, he asked him: "Lord, your own will prompts me to place a problem before you. What is the origin of this world? How can I be free from this saṁsāra?"

Manu replied: "What you see here does not exist, my son, none of it! Nor is there anything which is unseen and which is beyond the mind and the senses. There is but the self which is eternal and infinite. What is seen as the universe is but a reflection in that self. On account of the energy inherent in the cosmic consciousness, that reflection is seen here as the cosmos and elsewhere as living beings. That is what you call the world. There is neither bondage nor liberation. The one infinite consciousness alone exists, neither one nor many! Abandon all thought of bondage and liberation and rest in peace."

etāvadeva khalu liṅgamaliṅgamūrteḥ
saṁśāntasaṁsṛticirabhramanirvṛtasya
tajjñasya yanmadanakopaviṣādamoha
lobhāpadāmanudinaṁ nipuṇaṁ tanutvaṁ (123/6)

VASIṢṬHA continued:

Manu concluded: "The actions of one who has attained self-knowledge are not motivated and are non-volitional; hence he is not tainted by their merit. He is beyond praise and censure. He is not agitated by others; he does not agitate others. He alone is fit to be worshipped. Not by rites and rituals but by the worship of such sages alone does one attain wisdom." Thus instructed by Manu, Ikṣvāku attained enlightenment. Adopt such an attitude, O Rāma.

RĀMA asked:

If such be the nature of the enlightened person, what is so extraordinary and wonderful in it?

VASIṢṬHA continued:

On the other hand, what is so extraordinary and wonderful about the attainment of psychic powers like the ability to fly in the air? The nature of the ignorant is the absence of equanimity. The characteristic of the enlightened one is purity of mind and absence of craving. **The enlightened one is not characterised by characteristics. He is devoid of confusion and delusion. Saṁsāra has come to an end. And lust, anger, grief, delusion, greed and such disastrous qualities are greatly weakened in him.**

The Lord assumes individuality (jīva). The elements arise in the cosmos without any reason whatsoever. The individual which emanated from the Lord experiences the elements (objects) as if they were created by him. Thus do all jīvā arise and function for no obvious reason. But from then on, their own individual actions become the causes for their subsequent experience of pleasure and pain. The limitation of one's own understanding is the cause for the individual's actions.

One's limited understanding and one's own notions are the cause of bondage, and liberation is their absence. Hence abandon all notions (saṅkalpa). If you are attracted by anything here, you are bound; if you are not attracted at all you are free. Whatever you do and whatever you enjoy, you do not really do, nor do you enjoy. Know this and be free.

All these notions exist in the mind. Subdue the mind by the mind. Purify the mind by the mind. Destroy the mind by the mind. Expert washermen wash dirt with dirt. A thorn is removed by another thorn. Poison antidotes poison. The jīva has three forms: the dense, the subtle and the supreme. The physical body is the dense form. The mind with its notions and limitations is the subtle body. Abandon these two and resort to the supreme which is the reality — pure, unmodified consciousness. This is the cosmic being. Remain established in it, having firmly rejected the former two.

nirvāṇavānnirmananaḥ kṣiṇacittaḥ praśāntadhīḥ
ātmanyevā ''ssva śāntātmā mūkāndhavadhiropamaḥ (125/4)

RĀMA asked:

Pray, describe the state of turīya which runs through the waking, dream and deep sleep states without being recognised.

VASIṢṬHA continued:

That pure and equanimous state which is devoid of ego-sense and non-ego-sense, of the real and the unreal, and which is free, is known as turīya (the fourth state). It is the state of the liberated sage. It is the unbroken witness consciousness. It is different from the waking and the dreaming states which are characterised by movement of thought: it is different from the deep sleep state which is characterised by inertia and ignorance. When the ego-sense is abandoned, there arises the state of perfect equilibrium in which the turīya manifests itself.

I shall narrate a parable, hearing which you will become enlightened, even if you are already enlightened! In a certain forest there was a great sage. Seeing this extraordinary sage, a hunter approached him and asked him: "O sage, a deer which had been wounded by my arrow came this way. Tell me which way it went." The sage replied: "We are holy men who dwell in the forest and our nature is peace. We are devoid of ego-sense. The ego-sense and the mind which make the activities of the senses possible have come to a rest. I do not know what are known as waking, dream and deep sleep. I remain established in the turīya. In it there is no object to be seen." The hunter could not grasp the meaning of the sage's words. He went his way.

Hence, I tell you, O Rāma, there is naught but the turīya. The turīya is unmodified consciousness and that alone exists. Waking, dream and sleep are states of the mind. When they cease, the mind dies. Satva alone remains — which the yogī aspire to reach.

This is the conclusion of all scriptures: there is no avidyā (ignorance) and no Māyā (illusion) in reality; Brahman alone exists. Some call it the void, others pure consciousness, others the Lord; and they argue among themselves. Abandon all these notions. **Rest in nirvāṇa without movement of thought, with the mind greatly 'weakened' and the intelligence at peace; rest in the self as if you are deaf, dumb and blind.** Inwardly abandon everything; externally engage yourself in the appropriate action. The existence of the mind alone is happiness, the existence of the mind alone is unhappiness. By remaining unaware of the mind let all these cease. Remain unaffected by what is attractive and what is unattractive; by just this much of self-effort, this saṁsāra is overcome! By remaining unaware of pleasure and pain and of even that which lies between the two, you rise above sorrow. Just by this little self-effort you attain the infinite.

yataḥ kutaścidānīya jñānaśāstrāṇyavekṣate
evaṁ vicāravānyaḥ syāt saṁsārottāraṇaṁ prati (13)

RĀMA asked:

How does one tread the seven states of yoga and what are the characteristics of these seven states?

VASIṢTHA continued:

Man is either world-accepting (pravṛtta) or world-negating (nivṛtta). The former questions: "What is all this liberation? For me this saṁsāra and life in it are better", and engages himself in the performance of his worldly duties. After very many births he gains wisdom. He realises that the activities of the world are a meaningless repetition and does not wish to waste his life in them. He thinks, "What is the meaning of all this? Let me retire from them." He is considered nivṛtta.

"How shall I cultivate dispassion and thus cross this ocean of saṁsāra?", thus he enquires constantly. Day by day this thought itself generates dispassion in him and there arise peace and joy in his heart. He is disinterested in the activities of the market place but engages himself in meritorious activities. He is afraid to sin. His speech is appropriate to the occasion, soft, truthful and sweet. He has set foot on the first yoga-bhūmikā (state of yoga). He is devoted to the service of holy ones. **He gathers scriptures whenever and wherever he finds them and studies them. His constant quest is the crossing of the ocean of saṁsāra.** He alone is a seeker. Others are selfish.

He then enters the second state of yoga known as vicāra, enquiry. He eagerly resorts to the company of holy ones who are well versed in the scriptures and in spiritual practices. He knows what is to be done and what is not to be done. He abandons evils like vanity, jealousy, delusion and greed. From the preceptors he learns all the secrets of yoga.

Easily thereafter he graduates to the third state of yoga known as asaṁsaṅga, non-attachment or freedom. He roams the forests in seclusion and strives to quieten the mind. Adherence to the scriptures and to virtuous conduct bestows upon him the faculty of seeing the truth. This non-attachment or freedom is of two types, the ordinary and the superior. One who practises the first type of freedom feels, "I am neither the doer, nor the enjoyer. I neither afflict others nor am I afflicted by others. All this happens on account of past karma, under the aegis of god. I do nothing whether there is pain or pleasure, good fortune or calamity. All these, as also meeting and parting, psychic distress and physical illness, are brought about by time alone." Thus thinking, he investigates the truth. He is practising ordinary non-attachment or freedom.

Note: Of course, vicāra means 'direct observation or looking into'.

saṁsārāṁbunidheḥ pāre sāre paramakāraṇe
ñāhaṁ karteśvaraḥ kartā karma vā prākkṛtaṁ mama (32)

VASIṢṬHA continued:

By the diligent practice of this yoga method, by resorting to the company of the holy ones and the avoidance of evil company, the truth is clearly revealed. **When thus one realises the supreme which is the only essence or truth beyond this ocean of saṁsāra, he realises 'I am not the doer but god alone is the doer; not even in the past did I do anything.'** He abandons vain and meaningless words and remains inwardly and mentally silent. This is superior non-attachment or freedom. He has abandoned all dependency, above and below, within and without, tangible and intangible, sentient and insentient. He shines like supportless and limitless space itself. This is superior freedom. In it he enjoys peace and contentment, virtue and purity, wisdom and self-enquiry.

The first stage of yoga presents itself to one by accidental coincidence, as it were, after one has led a pure life full of virtuous deeds. One who sets his foot on it should cherish it and protect it with great zeal, diligence and effort. Thus he should proceed to the next state, enquiry. By diligently practising enquiry he should ascend to the third state, freedom.

RĀMA asked:

How is it possible for an ignorant person born in a wicked family and who does not enjoy the company of holy ones, to cross this ocean of saṁsāra? Also, if one dies while yet in the first or second or the third state of yoga, what happens to him?

VASIṢṬHA said:

After very many lives, the ignorant man is awakened by accident coincidence. Till then he experiences this saṁsāra. When dispassion arises in his heart, then saṁsāra recedes. Even an imperfect practice of this yoga destroys the effects of past sins. If one leaves the body during the practice, he ascends to heaven and is then born in circumstances favourable to the pursuit of his practice. Very soon he ascends the ladder of yoga again.

These three states are known as 'waking state' because in them there is division in consciousness. However, the practitioner becomes an adorable person (ārya). Seeing him, the ignorant are inspired. He who engages himself in righteous actions and avoids evil is adorable (ārya). This adorable holiness is in a seed state in the first state of yoga, it sprouts in the second and attains fruition in the third. One who dies after thus having gained the status of an adorable one and who has obviously cultivated noble thoughts, enjoys the delights of heaven for a long time and then he is born as a yogi. By the diligent practice of the first three states of yoga, ignorance is destroyed and the light of wisdom arises in one's heart.

etāvāneva saṁsāra idamastvīti yanmanaḥ
asya tūpaśamo mokṣa ityevaṁ jñānasaṅgrahaḥ (85)

VASIṢṬHA continued:

In the fourth state of yoga, the yogī behold the one in all with a mind that is free from division. Division has ceased and unity is steady, and therefore they behold the world as if it were a dream.

In the fifth state, only the undivided reality remains. Hence it is likened to deep sleep. He who has reached this state, though he is engaged in diverse external activities, rests in himself.

After thus proceeding from one state to another, he reaches the sixth which is the turīya. In this he realises, "I am neither real nor unreal, nor even egoless. I am beyond duality and unity. All doubts are at rest." He remains like a painting of a lamp (hence, though he has not reached nirvāṇa — lamp without fuel — he is like a lamp without fuel, as the lamp is only a painted figure). He is void within, void without, void like an empty vessel; at the same time he is full within and full without, like a full vessel immersed in the sea.

They who reach the seventh state are known as 'the disembodied liberated beings'. Their state is not for words to describe. Yet, they have been described variously.

They who practise these seven states do not come to grief. But there is a terrible elephant roaming in a forest wreaking havoc. If that elephant is killed, then man attains success in all these seven states, not otherwise. Desire is that elephant. It roams in the forest known as the body. It is maddened by sensuousness. It is restless with conditioning and tendencies (vāsanā). This elephant destroys everybody in this world. It is known by different names: desire, vāsanā (tendency or mental conditioning), mind, thought, feeling, attachment, etc. It should be slain by the weapon known as courage or determination born of the realisation of oneness.

Only as long as one believes in objective existence does desire arise! **This alone is saṁsāra: the feeling 'This is'. Its cessation is liberation (mokṣa). This is the essence of jñāna or wisdom.** Recognition of 'objects' gives rise to desire. Non-recognition of objects ends desire. When desire ends, the jīva drops its self-limitation. The great man therefore abandons all thoughts concerning what has been experienced and what has not been experienced. I declare with uplifted arms that the thought-free, notionless state is the best. It is infinitely superior to the sovereignty of the world. Non-thinking is known as yoga. Remaining in that state, perform appropriate actions or do nothing! As long as thoughts of 'I' and 'mine' persist, sorrow does not cease. When such thoughts cease, sorrow ceases. Knowing this, do as you please.

Note: For the words 'thinking' and 'non-thinking' in the last paragraph above, the text uses the words 'samvedanam' and 'asamvedanam' which imply much more than mere thinking. Cognition, comprehension, feeling, experience and knowledge are also implied by 'samvedanam'.

bālānprati vivarto 'yaṁ brahmaṇaḥ sakalaṁ jagat
avivartitamānandamāsthitāḥ kṛtinaḥ sadā (28)

VĀLMĪKI said to Bharadvāja:

Having heard this quintessence of the highest wisdom and having been overwhelmed by śakti-pāta, Rāma remained immersed in the ocean of bliss for a while. He had ceased to ask questions, request answers and endeavour to understand them. He had become established in the highest state of self-knowledge.

BHARADVĀJA asked:

O preceptor! It is indeed a delight to hear that thus Rāma attained the supreme state. But how is it possible for us who are foolish and ignorant and who are of sinful disposition to attain that state which is difficult even for gods like Brahmā to reach?

VĀLMĪKI said:

I have narrated to you in full the dialogue between Rāma and Vasiṣṭha. Consider it well. For that is also my instruction to you.

There is no division in consciousness which can be called the world. Rid yourself of the notion of division by the practice of the secrets revealed to you. Both waking and sleep states are part of this creation. Enlightenment is characterised by the pure inner light. This creation emerges from nothing, it dissolves in nothing, its very nature is void, it does not exist. On account of beginningless and false self-limitation this creation appears to exist, creating countless confusions. You are deluded because you do not recollect repeatedly and frequently the truth concerning the infinite consciousness, but you partake of the poison of self-limitation and the consequent psychological conditioning.

This delusion continues till you reach the feet of the enlightened sages and gain the right knowledge from them. Dear one, that which did not exist in the beginning and will not exist in the end, does not exist even now. This world-appearance is like a dream. The sole reality in which it appears and disappears is the infinite consciousness. In the ocean of saṁsāra or ignorance there arises the notion of 'I', on account of the beginningless potential of self-limitation. Thereupon, the movement of thought generates other notions like 'mine-ness', 'attraction' and 'repulsion', etc. Once these notions strike root in one's consciousness, one inevitably falls a prey to endless calamities and sorrow.

Dive deep into the inner peace, not in the sea of diversity. Who lives, who is dead, who has come — why do you get lost in such false notions? When the one self alone is the reality, where is room for 'another'? **The theory that Brahman appears as the world (just as rope appears as snake) is meant only for the entertainment of the childish and ignorant. The enlightened ones rest forever in the truth which does not even appear to be different.**

yathā tṛṇādikaṁ kṣiptaṁ rumāyāṁ lavaṇaṁ bhavet
acetanaṁ jagannyastaṁ caitanye cetanībhavet (30)

BHARADVĀJA said:

Lord, I am now free from the subtle body and I am swimming in the ocean of bliss. I am the indivisible self which is the supreme self, and which itself possesses the two powers of consciousness and unconsciousness. Just as fire thrown into fire becomes indistinguishably fire, **just as straw etc., which are thrown into the sea become salt, this insentient world when it is offered into the infinite consciousness becomes one with it.** Just as a salt doll thrown into the sea abandons its name and form and becomes one with the ocean, just as water mixes with water and ghee mixes with ghee, even so have I entered into this infinite consciousness.

'I am that supreme Brahman which is eternal, omnipresent, pure, peaceful, indivisible and free from motion, which is devoid of gathering and scattering but whose thoughts materialise, which is free from merit and demerit, which is the source of this universe, and which is the supreme light, one without a second'. Thus should one contemplate. Thus does the mind cease to be agitated. When the movement of the mind has ceased the self shines by its own light. In that light all sorrow comes to an end and there is the bliss which the self experiences in itself. There is direct awareness of the truth, 'there is none but the self'.

VĀLMĪKI said:

Dear friend, if you wish that this delusion known as saṁsāra should come to an end, then give up all actions and become a lover of Brahman.

BHARADVĀJA said:

O guru, your enlightening discourse has completely awakened me, my intelligence is pure and the world-appearance does not stretch out in front of me. I wish to know what the men of self-knowledge do. Do they have any duties or none at all?

VĀLMĪKI said:

They who desire liberation should engage themselves only in such actions which are free from defects, and desist from selfish and sinful actions. When the qualities of the mind are abandoned, it takes on the qualities of the infinite. The jīva is liberated when one contemplates, 'I am that which is beyond the body, mind and senses'; when one is free from notions of 'I am the doer' and 'I am the enjoyer' as also from notions of pain and pleasure; when one realises that all beings are in the self and the self is in all beings and when one abandons the waking, dream and deep sleep states and remains in the transcendental consciousness. That is the state of bliss which is infinite consciousness. Immerse yourself in that ocean of nectar which is full of peace; do not drown in diversity.

Thus have I narrated to you the discourse of the sage Vasiṣṭha. Steady your mind by practice. Tread the path of wisdom and of yoga. You will realise everything.

dṛśanātsparśanācchabdātkṛpayā śiṣyadehake
janayedyaḥ samāveśaṁ śāmbhavaṁ sa hi deśikaḥ (61)

VĀLMĪKI continued:

Seeing that Rāma had become totally absorbed in the self, Viśvāmitra said to the sage Vasiṣṭha: "O son of the Creator, O holy one, you are indeed great. You have proved that you are the guru by this śakti-pāta (direct transmission of spiritual energy). **He is a guru who is able to give rise to god-consciousness in the disciple by a look, by a touch, by verbal communication or by grace.** However, the intelligence of the disciple is awakened when the disciple has rid himself of three-fold impurities and thereby acquired a keen intellect. But, O sage, please bring Rāma back to body-consciousness, for he has still many things to do for the welfare of the three worlds and for myself."

All the assembled sages and others bowed to Rāma. Then Vasiṣṭha said to Viśvāmitra: "Pray, tell them who Rāma is in truth." Viśvāmitra said to them: "Rāma is the supreme personality of godhead. He is the creator, protector and redeemer. He is the Lord and the friend of all. He is manifest variously, sometimes as a fully enlightened being, sometimes as if ignorant. In truth, he is the god of gods and all the gods are but his part-manifestations. Blessed is this king Daśaratha whose son is lord Rāma himself. Blessed is Rāvana whose head will fall at the hands of Rāma. O sage Vasiṣṭha, kindly bring him back to body-consciousness.

Vasiṣṭha said to Rāma: "O Rāma, this is not the time to rest! Get up and bring joy to the world. When people are still in bondage, it is not proper for the yogi to merge in the self." Rāma remained oblivious of these words. Vasiṣṭha thereupon entered the heart of Rāma through the latter's suṣumṇā-nāḍī. There was movement of prāṇa in Rāma and the mind began to function. The jīva which is of the form of inner light shed its lustre on all the nāḍī of the body. Rāma slightly opened his eyes and beheld Vasiṣṭha in front of him. Rāma said to Vasiṣṭha: "There is nothing I should do or should not do. However, your words should always be honoured." Saying so, Rāma placed his head at the sage's feet and then proclaimed: "Listen all of you! There is nothing superior to self-knowledge, nothing superior to the guru."

All the assembled sages and celestials showered flowers on Rāma and blessed him. They departed from the assembly.

Thus have I told you the story of Rāma, O Bharadvāja. By practice of this yoga, attain supreme bliss. He who constantly listens to this dialogue between Rāma and Vasiṣṭha is liberated, whatever be the circumstances of his life, and he attains knowledge of Brahman.

THUS SPAKE VASIṢTHA

A few great declarations from sections omitted in this edition
(The section number and chapter number are indicated e.g. Section II Chapter 2.)

III-2

There is a holy man named Ākāśaja (lit. born of space) who is in constant meditation and has the welfare of all at heart. He had lived for a long time, when death desired to devour him. When death approached him it had to struggle with a fierce fire that protected the holy man, and even after fending this off, it was unable to touch him! Bewildered by this extraordinary and unprecedented event, death went to Lord Yama who presides over the destinies of mortals, and questioned him: "Pray, Lord, tell me why it is that I am unable to grasp him."

Yama answered: "In fact, O death, you do not really kill anyone! Death is really caused by one's own karma (the fruits of one's own action). Hence, discover this man's fatal karma." But death could not discover the holy man's karma anywhere in the world. He reported this to Yama.

Yama said: "O death, this holy man Ākāśaja was truly born of space and is as pure as space, hence he has incurred no karma which can help you grasp him or devour him. Even as a barren woman's son, this holy man is not born. As he had no 'previous birth' karma, he has no mind and hence has not committed even a mental action which could bring him within your reach. He is nothing but a mass of intelligence.

> **prāṇaspando 'sya yatkarma lakṣyate cā 'smadādibhiḥ**
> **dṛśyate 'smābhir evai 'tan na tv asyā 'sty atra karmadhiḥ (25)**

He appears to be a living being only in our eyes; in him there does not exist any notion that could give rise to karma. Consciousness is reflected in consciousness; and the reflection assumes independence! It is the false assumption, not a real existence; and this holy man knows this truth.

IV-35

> **vicāraṇāsamadhigatātma dīpako manasyalaṁ parigalite 'vadhīradhīḥ**
> **vilokayan kṣayabhavanīrasā gatīr gatajvaro vilasati dehapattane (69)**

He who has an intelligence that has been rendered pure by the destruction of all inner impurities, has his heart illumined by the light of the self obtained through enquiry into the self; seeing the worthlessness of birth and death, he dwells without fear or anxiety in the city which is the body.

IV-36

> **cic cinoti citaṁ cetyaṁ tenedaṁ sthitam ātmani**
> **ajñe jñe tv anyadāyātam anyad astīti kalpanā (11)**

Consciousness reflecting in consciousness, shines as consciousness and exists as consciousness; yet, to one who is ignorant, though considering oneself as wise and rational, there arises the notion that there has come into being and there exists something other than this consciousness.

IV-59

What else is there in this world, O Rāma, except eating, drinking and sex? Hence, what is there in this world that a wise man would find worthy of seeking? This world of five elements, and the body composed of flesh, blood, hair and all the rest of it, are considered real by the ignorant, and they exist for his entertainment. The wise see in all this an impermanent and unreal but terrible poison.

V-56

He who has attained inner tranquillity and peace, finds peace and tranquillity everywhere in the world. He whose mind is agitated and restless finds the world full of restlessness.

> **dyauḥ kṣamā vāyurākāśaṁ parvatāḥ sarito diśaḥ**
> **antaḥkaraṇatattvasya bhāgā bahiriva sthitāḥ (35)**

The sky, the earth, the air and the space, the mountains and the rivers are all parts of the inner instrument (mind); they only appear to be outside.

VI.1-31

Just as one who is not dead wails aloud, "Alas, I am dead", and when she is not lost she weeps, "Alas, I am lost", on account of perverse understanding, even so the consciousness falsely imagines it is miserable or limited. Such imagination is irrational and unfounded.

***

If the prāṇa does not move, the mind attains a quiescent state.

> **yatra prāṇo marudyāti manas tatraiva tiṣṭhati**
> **yatra yatrā 'nusarati rathas tatraiva sārathiḥ (47)**

Where the prāṇa goes the mind follows, even as the rider goes where the vehicle goes.

VI.1-32

If only pure vāsanā or tendencies fill one's heart, all conflicts cease, and there is harmony, liberation and longevity.

VI.1-35

The infinite consciousness alone is fit to be adored and worshipped. However there is no use inviting it for the worship, no mantrā are of any use in its worship; for it is immediate (closest, one's own self) and hence does not need to be invited. It is the omnipresent self of all. The realisation of this infinite consciousness (which is totally effortless) is alone the best form of worship.

VI.1-37

The natural order is free from excitement but not purified of its limitation: that (the natural order) is what dances a dance-drama known as the world appearance.

VI.1-53

> **api kutsitam apyanyadapyadharmamayakramaṁ**
> **śreṣṭhaṁ te svaṁ yathā karma tathehā 'mṛtavān bhava** (14)

The performance of action appropriate to you — even if it is despicable and unrighteous — is the best. By its due performance become immortal here.

VI.1-56

The mind makes a moment appear like an epoch, it makes a little look like very much, it makes the unreal appear real instantly: thus has this delusion arisen.

VI.2-1

> **gaṁyadeśaikaniṣṭhasya yathā pānthasyr pādayoḥ**
> **spando vigatasaṅkalpastathā spandasva karmasu** (15)

When one has made up his mind to go to a certain place, his feet function without any mental activity. Function like those feet, and perform action here.

VI.2-2

The mind continues to exist as long as the body continues to live, whether the embodied person is enlightened or ignorant.

VI.2-11

He in whom the contact of sharp weapons and the contact of a naked woman produce the same experience — he is established in the supreme state. One should diligently engage oneself in spiritual practice until one reaches the state in which one's contact with the objects provokes the same reaction that it would if one were asleep.

VI.2-12

This world appearance is like an empire painted on canvas. Just as the canvas is made attractive by the use of different colours, this world appearance seems to be attractive with diverse sense-experiences.

***

The very moment a holy one is found, half the ignorance ceases in his company. Another one-fourth is dispelled by the study of scripture and the last part by self-effort.

VI.2-15

The world exists in the very meaning of 'ego-sense'; and the ego-sense exists in the very meaning of the word 'world'. They are thus interdependent.

VI.2-18

The air in the entire space is filled with the prāṇā of the departed ones. Mind exists in those prāṇā. And the world exists within the mind like oil in seeds.

VI.2-18

A sentient ball of iron may visualise within itself the potential existence of a knife and a needle, and so on. Even so, the jīva sees or experiences within itself the existence of the three worlds, though this is no more than a delusion or false perception.

VI.2-19

The personality arises of its own accord, grows, decays, expands and contracts, then ceases to be.

VI.2-21

One should strive to be a jñānī (man of wisdom or direct experience) and not a jñānabandhu, a pseudo-jñānī. Who is a pseudo-jñānī? He who studies the scripture for pleasure or profit like a sculptor studying art, and who does not live up to the teaching. His scriptural knowledge is not reflected in his daily life. He is more interested in applying scriptural knowledge to promote his physical welfare and sensual happiness. Hence, I regard an ignorant man as superior to a pseudo-jñānī.

***

Jñāna or wisdom is self-knowledge; other forms of knowledge are but its pale reflections.

> **atrā ''hārārthaṁ karma kuryādanindyaṁ**
> **kuryādāhāraṁ prāṇasaṁdhāraṇārthaṁ**
> **prāṇāḥ saṁdhāryāstattvajijñāsanārthaṁ**
> **tattvaṁ jijñāsyaṁ yena bhūyo na duḥkhaṁ (10)**

One should work in this world as much as is needed to earn an honest living. One should live (eat) in order to sustain the life-force. One should sustain one's life-force only for the sake of acquiring knowledge. One should enquire into and know that which frees him from sorrow.

VI.2-22

They who try to find the reason for the appearance of optical illusions are trying to ride on the shoulders of the grandson of the barren woman's son.

****

The ignorant fool who is bound to psychological conditioning extols scripturally-enjoined action because he is not spiritually awakened.

****

In every body the jīva exists like a snowflake, apparently heavy and large in heavy and large beings, and light and subtle in small beings.

****

There is really no difference between the ignorant and the wise (the knower of truth) except that the latter is free from the conditioned mind.

VI.2-24

Craving for pleasure never attains fulfilment, never finds satisfaction and, though all its aspirations end in failure, it (the craving) itself does not come to an end. In autumn the leaves dry up and fall away, but the desire for pleasure does not.

VI.2-25

It is consciousness alone which somehow thinks it is inert, and then the limitation bounces down into the conception of materiality, like a rock from a hill-top.

VI.2-26

There is no difference between the sage and the moon: both of them radiate joy. They are peaceful, cool and tranquil, full of immortalising nectar, and they enable one to see.

****

No one, from the Creator down to the smallest insect, can attain supreme peace unless he acquires perfect control of the mind.

****

The notion 'I am happy' experiences happiness and the notion 'I am unhappy' experiences unhappiness. All these notions are but pure consciousness.

VI.2-29

> **yathākramaṁ yathādeśaṁ kuru duḥkhamaduḥkhitaḥ**
> **bāṣpakrandādiparyantaṁ dvandvayukttasukhāni ca (4)**

Remain free from sorrow within yourself, but behave as if in sorrow in accordance with propriety and in accordance with local etiquette, even shedding tears and wailing and seemingly experiencing pleasure and pain. While enjoying the com-

pany of your wife and participating in festivals etc., manifest delight as if you were subject to mental conditioning . . . With your gaze turned inward, swimming in the bliss of the self and with your heart and mind at peace, what you do you do not do.

***

If such be the truth concerning the ego-sense, O sage, how do you appear here being called Vasiṣṭha?
Vasiṣṭha became totally silent. Rāma asked again: Why are you silent, O sage? There is nothing in the whole world which a holy sage is unable to answer.
Vasiṣṭha replied: I was silent, not because I could not answer, but because silence is the only answer to your question.

***

There are two types of questioners: the enlightened and the ignorant. One should answer the ignorant from the point of view of the ignorant, and the wise from the point of view of wisdom.

***

All verbal statements (whether they are verbose or brief, whether their purport is subtle or transcendental) are limited by logic, duality and division.

***

The purest truth is expressed only by complete silence.

VI.2-30

There is no fear of destruction in the battle painted on a canvas: even so, when the knower of truth is established in inner equanimity, activity does not affect him.

VI.2-32

Resort to the knowers of truth in privacy, not in public. For when different people express different points of view, your understanding may be stunted or perverted.

VI.2-33

Notions and ideas gradually cease to arise and expand in one who resolutely refrains from associating words with meanings in his own mind — whether these words are uttered by others or they arise in one's own mind.

VI.2-34

Just as the dream-experiences of two people sleeping side by side are not the same, and one does not know what the other is dreaming about, one's understanding and inner experience are personal and unique.

VI.2-42

Worship the self which is the supreme Lord with all your natural actions and experiences, including your wisdom. Worshipped with these articles, the self instantly bestows upon you the boon of spiritual unfoldment; in comparison, the worship of gods like Rudra and Viṣṇu is worthless.

> **vicāraśamasatsaṅgabalipuṣpaikapūjitaḥ**
> **sadyo mokṣaphalaḥ sādho svātmaiva parameśvaraḥ (30)**

The self which is the Lord immediately confers mokṣa or final liberation when worshipped with enquiry into the nature of the self, with self-control and satsaṅga (company of the wise).

VI.2-45

The ignorant person cannot meditate: nor is it desirable for him to do so . . . in the case of the wise, meditation becomes natural and effortless.

VI.2-46

If there is craving for pleasure, what is the use of something called meditation? If such craving does not exist, what is the use of something called meditation?

VI.2-47

Even the love and affection that the gods and the angels possess are nothing compared to the limitless love that flows from the holy ones.

VI.2-52

The notion of the existence of the world arises in the ignorant just as the awareness of its various limbs may arise in the 'mind' of a tree!

VI.2-69

What is seen here as you and I and what is seen as this dialogue between us are like two waves colliding in the ocean and making a sound.

VI.2-102

To one who has realised the supreme truth, even the rocks become friends and the trees in the forest are relatives; even when he lives in the middle of a forest the very animals become his kith and kin.

***

Powers like levitation and so on are gained by mantrā, drugs and so on, even by the ignorant people. He who is prepared to make the necessary effort can gain these, whether he is enlightened or not. It is the ego that makes the effort and gains the powers. These powers intensify the vāsanā or mental conditioning.

VI.2-124

Yogi can perform actions everywhere and experience all things in all the three periods of time, though apparently remaining in one place.

VI.2-125

The powers gained through contemplation and so on, can be seen by others; but the state of liberation that one attains cannot be seen by others.

VI.2-157

Yesterday's evil action is transformed into good action by today's noble deeds. Therefore, strive to be good and do good now.

VI.2-163

> cittamindriyasenāyā nāyakaṁ tajjayājjayaḥ
> upānādgūḍhapādasya nanu carmāvṛtaiva bhūḥ (6)

The mind (citta) is the commander-in-chief and the senses the armed forces. Hence, control of the mind is control (or victory) over the senses. If one's feet are covered with leather shoes, the entire world is covered with leather!

***

The knowledge that is gained by the study of this scripture is not gained by the study of any other scripture. This scripture bestows on you both efficiency in action and perfection in wisdom.

VI.2-167

'This is the self' and 'This is knowledge' — these are surely false notions that arise within, but they are not real. Abandon the words but remain established in the experience of the truth they indicate.

VI.2-170

The wise man's friend is his own action which arises spontaneously in him and in which there is no division or conflict.

VI.2-171

Just as ice is ever cool, the sage lives a natural life, doing what is natural to him, without aspiring for or abandoning anything. The characteristic of the ignorant man is that he strives to be other than what he is.

VI.2-172

I am not expounding the means of liberation for the benefit of ignorant people. It is only meant for those who have been awakened but who have some doubts concerning it.

VI.2-174

The practice of contemplation in which the mind is restrained from undergoing any modification is as good as supreme inertia; on the other hand, when such modifications exist in the mind, it is the seat of diversity or saṁsāra. By such contemplation a state of equanimity is not attained. If it is claimed that liberation is attained when the mind is forcibly restrained from all modifications, then why is it not attained in sleep?

VI.2-175

By a mere study of this scripture, ignorance is dispelled. The beauty of this scripture is that its student is not abandoned to his despair; if something is not clear in the first instance, a further study of the scripture makes it clear.

VI.2-187

Within the infinite space is the root-element of sound hidden, like a sprout in a seed. From this foolish people have spun theories concerning a material creation, for the entertainment of other fools.

VI.2-194

All cravings and desires come to an end in the awakened person; therefore nirvāṇa arises in him without his desiring it . . . Like a lamp in whose light all actions take place and in which the lamp is not interested, he lives and acts but is free from volition.

VI.2-197

Among those who study scriptures some attain pleasure, others wealth and yet others guidance in right conduct. Only these three are expounded in the scriptures; the attainment of the realisation of Brahman is beyond description and, therefore, it is not found in the teachings of the scriptures.

VI.2-203

O Rāma, you have heard all that is worth hearing and you know all that is worth knowing. What I have said to you and what you have studied in the scripture, now bring into harmony with your own direct experience.

VI.2-199

When somehow something has to be done at all times, why not do what is right? Whatever one does with a pure and clear mind which rests in equanimity, is right and appropriate, never defective. Amongst us, O Rāma, there are many who are involved in defective action but they are wise and clear-sighted.

There are some liberated ones who live the householder's life but without attachment. There are some who are royal sages like you who perform their royal duties without attachment and without agitation. There are some who perform the scriptural duties and rites. There are some who are devoted to god and meditation and to their own duties. There are some who have abandoned everything inwardly, but who live as if they were ignorant, engaged in all kinds of activities. There are some who dwell in dense forests totally immersed in meditation. There are some who dwell in holy places. There are some who roam in distant foreign lands in order to overcome all likes and dislikes. Some are constantly wandering from place to place.

***

Some have abandoned their natural duties and others are devoted to them. Some behave like wise men and others behave like mad men. Some are human, some are gods and others are demons.

In this world there are the fully enlightened ones, unenlightened ones and semi-enlightened who abandon right actions, too, and are thus neither here nor there. The forest-life is not essential for liberation, nor is living in one's own country nor an ascetic life, nor the abandonment of activity. Liberation is attained by one whose very nature is totally free and unattached. He whose mind is free and unattached does not get involved once again in this saṁsāra. O Rāma, you are the supreme state. Remain what you are, free from likes and dislikes, established in the supreme truth. In that Brahman there are no impurities, changes, veils, cravings or aversions. There is nothing more to say.

INDEX

INDEX

INDEX

INDEX